Art and the Critical Medical Humanities

CRITICAL INTERVENTIONS IN THE MEDICAL AND HEALTH HUMANITIES

Series Editors

Stuart Murray, Corinne Saunders, Sowon Park and Angela Woods

Critical Interventions in the Medical and Health Humanities promotes a broad range of scholarly work across the Medical and Health Humanities, including both larger-scale intellectual projects and argument-led provocations, to present new field-defining, interdisciplinary research into health and human experience.

Titles in the series

Abortion Ecologies in Southern African Fiction, Caitlin E. Stobie
COVID-19 and Shame, Fred Cooper, Luna Dolezal and Arthur Rose
Cocaine, Literature, and Culture, 1876–1930, Douglas R. J. Small
Medicalizing Difference, Stephanie M. Hilger
Medical Humanities and Disability Studies, Stuart Murray
Relating Suicide, Anne Whitehead

Forthcoming titles

Autism and the Empathy Epidemic, Janet Harbord
A Cultural History of Vertigo, Anindya Raychaudhuri
Disability in Contemporary American Poetry, Declan Gould
Reproductive Health, Literature, and Print Culture, 1650–1800, Ashleigh Blackwood

Art and the Critical Medical Humanities

EDITED BY FIONA JOHNSTONE, ALLISON MOREHEAD AND IMOGEN WILTSHIRE

BLOOMSBURY ACADEMIC
LONDON • NEW YORK • OXFORD • NEW DELHI • SYDNEY

BLOOMSBURY ACADEMIC
Bloomsbury Publishing Plc, 50 Bedford Square, London, WC1B 3DP, UK
Bloomsbury Publishing Inc, 1359 Broadway, New York, NY 10018, USA
Bloomsbury Publishing Ireland, 29 Earlsfort Terrace, Dublin 2, D02 AY28, Ireland

First published in Great Britain 2026

Cover image: Ruth Cuthand, Surviving: COVID-19, 2020. Glass beads, backing and thread, vinyl lettering on glass. Collection of the MacKenzie Art Gallery

A catalogue record for this book is available from the British Library.

A catalog record for this book is available from the Library of Congress.

ISBN: HB: 978-1-3505-0633-6
ePDF: 978-1-3505-0634-3
eBook: 978-1-3505-0635-0

Series: Critical Interventions in the Medical and Health Humanities

Typeset by Integra Software Services Pvt. Ltd.
Printed and bound in Great Britain

For product safety related questions contact productsafety@bloomsbury.com.

To find out more about our authors and books visit www.bloomsbury.com and sign up for our newsletters.

CONTENTS

PART II Visualizing knowledge and power

PART III Making and remaking medicalized bodies

PART IV Reproducing reproduction

FIGURES

CONTRIBUTORS

Angela Alves is a crip performance artist and artistic collaborator in the project team of Claire Cunningham's professorship at the University of Arts Berlin.

Monika Ankele is director of the Berlin Museum of Medical History at the Charité, professor for Medical History and Medical Museology at the Charité – Universitätsmedizin Berlin and co-director of the Institute for Medical & Health Humanities and Artistic Research.

Anna Arabindan-Kesson is Associate Professor of Black Diaspora Art at Princeton University, and directs *Art Hx: Visual and Material Legacies of British Colonialism.*

Vanessa Bartlett is an independent curator and Research Fellow at the University of Melbourne.

Suzannah Biernoff is a Reader in Visual Culture in the School of Historical Studies at Birkbeck, University of London.

Gemma Blackshaw is Professor of Art History at the Royal College of Art, and Inaugural Academic Associate of the Freud Museum, London.

Anna Burel is a visual artist and the illustrator of *Conceiving Histories*. Anna Burel and Isabel Davis have collaborated since 2015, holding an exhibition of their work in 2017.

Alice Butler is an interdisciplinary writer-scholar and Research Tutor at the Royal College of Art, where she initiated the MFA 'Poetics of Care' programme in 2023.

Kaira M. Cabañas is Associate Dean for Academic Programs and Publications at the Center for Advanced Study in the Visual Arts at the National Gallery of Art, Washington, DC.

Amanda Cachia is Professor of Practice in Museum Studies in the School of Art, Herberger Institute for Design and the Arts, Arizona State University.

Silvia Casini is a Reader in Film and Visual Culture at the University of Aberdeen.

Tania Cleaves (née Woloshyn) is an alternative academic (alt-ac) and Research Development Manager at the University of Nottingham.

Laura Cowley is an artist-researcher and a Wellcome-funded PhD student in History of Art at Birkbeck, University of London.

Jessica M. Dandona is Professor of Art History in the Liberal Arts Department at the Minneapolis College of Art and Design.

Isabel Davis is research leader in Collections and Culture at the Natural History Museum, London. She is the author of *Conceiving Histories: Trying for Pregnancy, Past and Present* (MIT Press, 2025).

Lorenzo Galgó is an artist based in Madrid. With Maria Morata, they work as the two-person collective cripxcess.

Leah Gipson is Associate Professor in the Department of Art Therapy and Counselling at the School of the Art Institute of Chicago.

Skye Haggerty is a Métis MA Graduate Student in Art & Design at the University of Alberta in amiskwaciwâskahikan (Edmonton).

Keren Hammerschlag is a Senior Lecturer in Art History and Curatorship at the Australian National University in Canberra.

Nora Heidorn is an interdisciplinary researcher, curator, and writer with a background in contemporary art.

Katharine Houpt is a psychotherapist practising counselling and art therapy in Chicago.

Suzanne Hudson is Professor of Art History and Fine Arts at the University of California in Los Angeles.

Anna Jamieson is a cultural historian and a British Academy Postdoctoral Fellow at the University of Birmingham.

Fiona Johnstone is Assistant Professor in Visual Medical Humanities at Durham University.

Céline Kaiser is professor of Media Cultural Studies and Scenic Research at the Hochschule für Künste im Sozialen, Ottersberg, and co-director of the Institute for Medical & Health Humanities and Artistic Research.

Ashley Lazevnick is a Faculty Research Support Officer at the University of New Mexico.

Chris Millard is Lecturer in the History of Medicine and Medical Humanities at the University of Sheffield.

Maria Morata is a curator, researcher and lecturer, born in Madrid and currently living in Berlin. With Lorenzo Galgó, they work as the two-person collective cripxcess.

Allison Morehead is Professor of Art History and in the Graduate Program in Cultural Studies at Queen's University, Canada.

Gabriella Nelson is Associate Director of Policy at Maternity Care Coalition, Philadelphia, USA.

Liz Orton is a visual artist living and working in London.

Kathleen Pierce is Assistant Professor of Art History at Smith College in Northampton, Massachusetts, USA.

Daniel Regan is a photographic artist and Founder and Executive Director of the Arts & Health Hub.

Camilla Mørk Røstvik is Associate Professor in History at the University of Agder, Honorary Research Fellow in Art History at the University of St Andrews, and Honorary Lecturer in the School of Medicine at the University of Aberdeen.

Natasha Ruiz-Gómez is a Senior Lecturer in Art History at the University of Essex.

Ilona Sagar is an artist and academic currently in residence at Somerset House Studios. She is a lecturer in the Department of Fine Art, Goldsmiths University London.

Tanya Sheehan is Ellerton M. and Edith K. Jetté Professor of Art at Colby College, USA. She chairs the Department of Science, Technology, and Society, and serves as Director of Academic and Scholarly Engagement at the Colby College Museum of Art's Lunder Institute for American Art.

Christine Slobogin is Assistant Professor of Health Humanities and Bioethics at the University of Rochester Medical Center.

Cera Smith is an Assistant Professor in the Indigenous, Race, and Ethnic Studies department at the University of Oregon.

Katie Snow is a Wellcome-funded Postdoctoral Researcher at University College Dublin.

Alison Syme is Associate Professor of Modern Art at the University of Toronto.

Arya Thampuran is an Assistant Professor at the Institute for Medical Humanities (Durham University).

Rebecca Whiteley is a British Academy Postdoctoral Fellow at the University of Birmingham.

Imogen Wiltshire is Senior Lecturer in Art History and Visual Culture at the University of Lincoln (UK).

Jessica Womack is an art historian and independent scholar based in Durham, North Carolina, USA.

Angela Woods is Professor of Medical Humanities and Director of the Institute for Medical Humanities and the Discovery Research Platform for Medical Humanities at Durham University.

FOREWORD

The role of art and of artists in engaging the public in matters medical and in educating clinicians has long been widely recognized. The role of art and of artists in generating new knowledge about health and illness much less so. *Art and the Critical Medical Humanities* envisages and enacts an intervention in the critical medical humanities that will reconfigure our collective understanding of what it is art and artists *do*. Editors Fiona Johnstone, Allison Morehead and Imogen Wiltshire have curated a work of global significance animated by lively writing, sumptuous and intriguing images, and novel scholarly formats. They waste no time dwelling on illustrative or instrumental accounts of art as being in service to medicine. Instead, *Art and the Critical Medical Humanities* is resolutely committed to entanglement and polyvalence, dialogue and dialogicity, allowing new voices to be heard and fresh questions posed. In conversations between humanities researchers and artists, for example, we start to glimpse the artist working in health, clinical and scientific settings as one who 'might bridge the gap between the abstract and the tangible' (Ilona Sagar), 'brokers dialogues around taboo topics' (Daniel Regan) and who can exercise 'certain privileges, to see things as an outsider, to ask difficult questions, and to be curious without having to necessarily solve anything' (Liz Orton).

The individual chapters in this volume will compel engagement from medical humanities and other scholars working across a wide range of areas, sites and scales: from eighteenth-century anatomical drawing to the contemporary radiography suite, from the singularity of Kenyan American artist Wangechi Mutu's *Cervical Hypertrophy* (2004–5) to the visual indices used across US dermatology. With authors unwavering in their attentiveness to the operations of power in and across these spaces, many of the chapters are exemplary of the intersectional, feminist, anti-racist and decolonial approaches that are increasingly driving research in the field.

What has resonated most powerfully for me about the volume as a whole, however, is its portrayal of intimacy. Its contributors portray intimacy by showing us how art can capture fleeting, inchoate, embodied aspects of experience, render them anew, and offer them for inspection, reflection and analysis. But *Art and the Critical Medical Humanities* also performs intimacy through acts of disclosure and care, through methods that centre tenderness and vulnerability, and by cultivating a kind of awe towards human existence. Intimacy, then, is both a thematic focus and a mode of enquiry, something the volume explores as well as something it enacts, something contributors and their subjects and interlocutors insist is indispensable to our understanding of health and illness.

Art and the Critical Medical Humanities will, I am certain, stimulate further conversations and new ways of thinking and working across art practice, art history and the critical medical humanities. My hope is that readers following the threads of intimacy woven through the volume will be as moved and as exhilarated as I am by their consequences for work in our field.

Angela Woods, Durham, January 2025

ACKNOWLEDGEMENTS

We are deeply grateful to everyone whose work appears within the pages of this book. Our appreciation extends to those who had hoped to contribute but whose work did not, for a variety of reasons, make it into the final manuscript. Thank you also to everyone who participated in the *Confabulations* event series, which allowed us to explore existing work in this area whilst generating new connections and lines of enquiry. The event series and the book have been generously funded by the Social Sciences and Humanities Research Council of Canada, the Institute for Medical Humanities at Durham University (via the Wellcome Trust), the Queen's University Scholarly Publication Fund, and the University of Leicester Wellcome Trust Institutional Strategic Support Fund.

A book workshop was delivered by the Creative Facilitation Unit, Institute for Medical Humanities, Durham University. Funding from the Institute for Medical Humanities at Durham University made it possible to offer travel bursaries for participants. The Health & Care Research Cluster at the Royal College of Art in London kindly offered space, inspiration, and hospitality, proving the ideal venue for animated discussion and debate.

We are grateful to our institutions for supporting our work on this project: Durham University, Queen's University, and the University of Lincoln. Thank you to colleagues who have read parts of the book manuscript and provided feedback at different stages: Harriet Cooper, Bentley Crudgington, Veronica Heney, Victoria Patton, Arya Thampuran, and Angela Woods. Comments from the book proposal's anonymous peer-reviewers helped shape the introduction to the volume. Hannah Darvin provided valuable assistance with obtaining image permissions. We are grateful to the series editors for Critical Interventions in the Medical and Health Humanities, and to our exemplary editor at Bloomsbury, Ben Doyle: thank you to Ben and the team!

* * *

Funding statement: This research was funded in part by the Wellcome Trust [Grant number 226798/Z/22/Z]. For the purpose of open access, the authors have applied a CC BY-NC-ND 4.0 public copyright licence to any Author Accepted Manuscript version arising from this submission. The e-book editions of this book are available open access under a CC BY-NC-ND 4.0 licence on bloomsburycollections.com. Open access was funded by the Social Sciences and Humanities Research Council of Canada and the Wellcome Trust [Grant number 226798/Z/22/Z].

Introduction

Confabulations: art practices, art histories, critical medical humanities

Fiona Johnstone, Allison Morehead and Imogen Wiltshire

This volume brings together three areas of critically engaged research: art practice, art history and critical medical humanities. Aimed at an interdisciplinary readership and aspiring to appeal to those who are 'art curious' or 'medical humanities curious', as well as those who already identify with those fields, it foregrounds ways in which art – its practices and its histories – can prompt new methods for asking and responding to pressing questions of human health. Many contemporary artists work on issues related to health and medicalized bodies without explicitly engaging the medical humanities or histories of art and medicine. Many art historians participate in conversations in the history of medicine but don't see themselves as contributing to or benefiting from contemporary art practices or the generative possibilities of critical medical humanities. And many scholars and practitioners working in the medical humanities remain unaware of the unique affordances of art as a critical methodology for interdisciplinary research. Our ambition is to bring these often-distinct 'worlds' – or, perhaps, methods for world-making – together.

Critical medical humanities emerged in the last decade, initially in the United Kingdom, to counter a service approach which had shaped medical humanities to that point. Especially when located in proximity to clinical training, medical humanities had valued the pedagogic, therapeutic and communicative qualities of humanistic research in the service of better healthcare, an admirable goal still central to many medical humanities programs. *Critical* medical humanities, as practised in the UK and now elsewhere, actively creates a different epistemological terrain that still aims at understanding and ameliorating human health experience, but – crucially – also probes the assumptions underpinning this objective: what is meant by 'better' health and healthcare, in what sense, under what conditions, and for whom? To answer these pressing questions, critical medical humanities emphasizes criticality, complexity, interdisciplinarity, intra-activity and entanglement. This book argues that art practice and art history can creatively and critically operate in this space. To this end, the artists, art historians, curators and others contributing to and represented in this volume offer distinctive approaches to addressing contemporary and historical structures of health- and medical-related experiences, knowledge, care, research and education. Collectively making a compelling case for the ways in which art deepens and diversifies interdisciplinary understandings of human health and its contexts, the texts assembled here pay urgent attention to constructions of gender, race, class, sexuality and disability as well as to how health, illness and medicine are unevenly and complexly distributed across different histories, geographies, communities and corporealities.

Confabulations

We sought contributions to this volume over a period of more than two years, starting with an international, online public programme of monthly events: *Confabulations: art practice, art history, critical medical humanities* (2021–2023). Working with both targeted invitations and open calls, sometimes brokering connections across disciplines, national borders and career stages, and sometimes ceding control over topic and format to guest curators, we strove to create an experimental online space where risks could be taken, access could be creatively negotiated, frictions and failures might be understood as often necessary and potentially generative, and different kinds of communities could be strengthened or emerge. We came to see our work as curatorial in the sense described by art historian Maria Lind: 'a way of linking objects, images, processes, people, locations, histories and discourses [...] an active catalyst, generating twists, turns, and tensions [...] a vital presence that strives to create friction and push new ideas' (2009: 103).

The series' title, *Confabulations*, aimed to foreground both conversation (*to confabulate*: from the Latin *con*, with or together, and *fabulari*, to talk, chat) and imaginative methods for making and re-making, knowing and unknowing, doing and undoing. In psychiatry, confabulation denotes the process by which the imagination fills in memory gaps with fabrications that are experienced as if they were real. For John Berger (2016), 'confabulation' describes the activity of writing as translation, implying the subtle shifts between different voices needed to convey the complexities of human bodily experience. 'Confabulation' thus draws attention to the problems of translating bodily experience into language, as well as to the breaches and omissions not only in individual memory, but also in the collective memories constructed in and through archives, disciplines, or fields of practice.

'Confabulation' also echoes Saidiya Hartman's 'critical fabulation' (2008), a method of research and writing that plays with the basic elements of a historical narrative in order to displace the dominant or authorized point of view. Art institutions – including art history – have long been dominated by strongly authorized perspectives, and in particular period- and geography-specific approaches that have constructed and reinforced hierarchical binaries, teleological and evolutionary narratives. 'Confabulation' therefore can insist on the necessity of decolonial, intersectional, trans-historical, transnational, trans-geographical, as well as radically local thinking about health, medicine and medicalized bodies. The richness of this term has shaped the content, form and purpose of this book: foregrounding knowledge as co-created whilst acknowledging the complexities of working between, across and through different disciplinary norms and practices, the texts assembled here critically engage with the institutional structures that delimit what can be known and what forms of knowledge are valued.

As organizers, based in the United Kingdom and Canada, who largely identify as white and as women, including one who is a settler, and as academics with full-time employment at the time of writing, albeit each with very different experiences of job (in)security over the last decade, we recognize the perversities and possibilities of editing and speaking from our current positions of relative stability and privilege. Especially given the precarity of working in (and making a living from) the arts and humanities, it will surprise few readers that art practice, art history, and medical humanities are spaces in which, like the academy in general but more acutely, white superiority is actively upheld. To connect our project with Hartman's 'critical fabulation', for instance, risks maintaining white superiority by extracting and tokenizing Black feminist labour to our ends. It's a risk we take advisedly and willingly, cognizant of the alternative of *not* citing the work of Black women such as Hartman and aware that contributors and readers will decide – should decide – whether *our* ends are theirs as well.

As part of the politics of *Confabulations*, we attempted to prioritize compensation for contributors who identified as independent, on short-term contracts, and/or precariously employed, using the fee schedule of Canadian Artists' Representation/Le Front des artistes Canadiens (CARFAC). This was explicit in our original calls for contributors to the series, and, as we pursued different sources of funding, including federal Canadian funding derived from the resources of Indigenous lands, we tried to pursue this ethic. We doubt that everyone who participated in *Confabulations* aligned with our policy or felt appropriately compensated for their labour. But we chose to risk the conversation as a way to increase transparency, mindful of the scarcity and the rapidly increasing consolidation of funding for research in art and the humanities. A project in keeping with the critical medical humanities' emphasis on radical interdependency, a project on art, health, illness, vulnerable bodies and caring could only proceed, we felt, in this way.

Key terms

Critical medical humanities

Over the last ten years, critical medical humanities has activated a range of methodologically innovative and theoretically engaged approaches that challenge a service-led framing of the relationship between the arts and humanities and clinical practice and biomedicine. The service model implicitly positions the creative practitioner or humanities scholar in an auxiliary role tasked with 'humanizing' healthcare, colourfully invoked in Des Fitzgerald and Felicity Callard's tongue-in-cheek caricature of the literary scholar 'lurking hopefully, poetry books in hand, at the edge of the clinical encounter's primal scene' (2016: 35). Aspiring to think through how the arts and humanities might intervene more *consequentially* in clinical practice and biomedicine, a series of influential publications propose that the arts, humanities and social sciences might be most impactful when viewed not as 'in service' to the clinical or life sciences, but rather as 'productively entangled' with biomedical cultures (Viney et al. 2015: 2).

The concept of entanglement, foundational to the new critical medical humanities, aimed to re-orient the debate away from fears about disciplinary hierarchies and hand-wringing over instrumentalization, instead emphasizing complexity, ambiguity, mutual dependence and intra-activity. Borrowed from Karen Barad's work on agential realism (2007), 'entanglement' describes the co-constitution of apparently discrete entities; considered in relation to (inter)disciplinary activity, entanglement draws attention to the practices of boundary making through which things – including differences – come to matter (Fitzgerald and Callard 2016: 38–41). Showing how practices of making, breaking and shifting boundaries actively constitute illness and healing, Fitzgerald and Callard proposed a radical rethinking of phenomena (including the figure of 'the human') taken for granted by earlier iterations of medical humanities scholarship.

No one definition of 'critique' or 'criticality' dominates critical medical humanities approaches. Posing the rhetorical question, 'What, then, is the "critical" work that is being enacted in and through the critical medical humanities?', Anne Whitehead and Angela Woods indicate that the answer is 'neither simple nor singular' (2016: 8), pointing to a diverse range of theoretical and practical legacies that include feminist theory and social and political activism. We are particularly struck by Bruno Latour's definition of the critic as 'not the one who debunks, but the one who assembles [...] the one who offers the participants arenas in which to gather' (2004: 30; cited Viney et al. 2015: 5); this seems to us apt for our own process of assembling – curating – a critical community and holding space for conflicting perspectives and constructive debate. We were similarly intrigued by the ways in which the language used in these influential calls for a newly critical medical humanities resembles the language of art practice, with recurrent metaphors of making and remaking as well as embracing mess, ambiguity, risk, experimentation and failure. To us, this suggests a shared (indeed, entangled) critical and theoretical heritage, a common (if not always precisely aligned) set of values, and rich possibilities for joint future endeavours.

Art practices

This volume engages with a particular set of practices that are for the most part designated as 'art' and exist (predominantly, but not exclusively) in traditional systems and spaces of art production and display such as museums and galleries – in other words, within 'art worlds'. Some readers may find this definition of art frustratingly narrow, even elitist; indeed, within much scholarship in the medical humanities, 'art' is often deployed in its broadest sense as a synonym for 'the arts', inclusive of literature, music, performance, television, cinema and online media. As scholars trained in the discipline of art history, we believe that there is a value in foregrounding writings and artworks that circulate within the institutions and networks of art; indeed, part of the argument of this book is that these kinds of art practices constitute particular *methods* of critical thinking. This is not to imply that more popular visual culture cannot be engaged with critically or constitute a critical tool in its own right – it clearly can, but this volume is explicitly concerned with addressing how the methods of criticality mobilized by art practices which operate in art worlds offer a distinctive and valuable approach to addressing vital questions of human health and flourishing.

In health contexts, the term 'art' often signifies not a method of critical thinking but instead a broad set of creative activities applied with practical outcomes in mind, including the generation of research data (in the case of arts-based research methods) or improvements in individual and public health (in the case of arts-in-health). These are quite distinct from the practices explored in this book. Without wishing to over-generalize, 'arts-based research' typically describes a process where methods from the arts, generally understood, are used to gather data as part of a research process; in such practices, the 'arts' element is typically (although not in every instance) regarded as a means to an end, with the 'aesthetic' output considered as subordinate to the 'research' output (see Leavy 2019). Whilst several of the contributors to this volume work in alignment with the aims and objectives of arts-in-health (also known as arts-and-health or creative health), we do not see the volume as explicitly in dialogue with this field, which we understand as primarily concerned with the ways in which the arts (again, broadly defined) contribute to health, wellbeing, social inclusion and healthcare practices. Our volume sits more comfortably with the concept of 'art as research'; that is, where art (as both process and output) is regarded not primarily as a tool for producing measurable health outcomes or research data, but as having a critical and aesthetic value in its own right.

Through the selection process, we sought to prioritize contributions that activate art-critical approaches to exploring – and often complicating – contemporary and historical perspectives on health and medicine. During the conversations about what to include and exclude there were many border instances where we were undecided on whether a particular object or image fitted within the contours of the definition of art delineated above: we have included some liminal cases (e.g., art therapy practices; medical illustrations; a Japanese tea bowl) precisely to point to the challenges of any hard and fast definitions. In many ways this issue also signals the porous boundaries of the (inter)discipline of art history, a field which, at its best, probes its own disciplinary margins, norms and limitations.

We have resisted solidifying an already-existing canon of health-related artworks. For example, the work of the British artist and activist Jo Spence – who visually documented her own experience of cancer treatment during the 1980s and early 1990s – is frequently used in clinical teaching as well as research and exhibition contexts, often shaping expectations of what art might do in relation to medicine. Yet, as curator Vanessa Bartlett points out in the opening chapter in this volume, Spence's ongoing valorization can distract attention from a wider variety of illness and other, less eloquent and coherent representations of those experiences, whilst also privileging certain forms of personhood such as white womanhood. This volume sets its sights beyond the more familiar and privileged case studies, aiming to think more richly and expansively about the work that art might do in responding to the making and remaking of health and illness. Accordingly, contributions explore artworks by self-identified crip artists (Alves, Ankele and Kaiser; Galgó and Morata) as well as by artists who resist identity labels

(Cachia on Jesse Darling); art as a critical research practice that addresses the health experiences of particular communities (Casini and Sagar); art as institutional critique of healthcare organizations and practices (Johnstone and Orton; Røstvik); and contemporary artworks as texts that can be read from different perspectives to generate a variety of meanings (Haggerty, Thampuran, Womack, Smith).

Art histories

This book also centres the criticality of art historical work, that is, the contextualization and analysis of both historical and contemporary art. In line with Saunders' assertion that a 'properly critical medical humanities is also a historically grounded medical humanities' (2016: 411) and other renewed calls for history (Bellis et al. 2024) and art history (Johnstone 2018; Biernoff and Johnstone 2024; Morehead 2024) to be more frequently incorporated into critical medical humanities research, this volume foregrounds different methods for 'doing' art historical work within critical medical humanities. These art historical methods include interpretive and evaluative practices which engage with and activate historical and contemporary art – for example, to demonstrate how historically and culturally specific ideas about health and illness emerge, come to be solidified and exert power (Lazevnick; Jamieson; Dandona); to show the ontological instability of concepts related to medicine (Pierce; Ruiz-Gómez, Cleaves and Hammerschlag); and, to surface the potential role of art in reinforcing and destabilizing categories and norms (Snow, Slobogin and Cowley; Arabindan-Kesson and Nelson; Syme). This art-historical work is less about instrumentalizing or revealing the past and more about highlighting the 'situatedness of medicine' through the worlds of art.

Many contemporary artists represented in the volume conduct historical work as part of an art critical research practice – for example, working with archives in ways that ask pressing questions of historical materials, narratives and legacies (Casini and Sagar; Davis and Burel; Blackshaw and Butler). Like more conventional forms of 'academic' (art) history, this creative-critical work opens up questions about the positionality and subjectivity of the researcher (addressed explicitly by several texts in this volume) and about the possibilities of refusal, relocation, subversion and reparation. Moreover, many art historians work in creative dialogue with contemporary art and artists. Therein lies one of the radical aspects of the work of Anna Arabindan-Kesson, an art historian of Black Diaspora art focusing on the long nineteenth century who regularly engages contemporary art as a way of thinking with and through histories of race, medicine and colonial visuality (2022). Focusing on gender and sickness, Gemma Blackshaw and Alice Butler also take historical 'flights' in their work, implicitly arguing that doing history can be a contemporary mode of creative practice, and that contemporary being and feeling via art can be a way of doing history. In line with these scholars' experimental work, we have insisted on art's practices *and* its histories sitting together in this volume.

This volume

Echoing the multiplicity of formats in the *Confabulations* series, this volume contains three different types of texts arranged in six thematic sections. 'Essays' are relatively conventional academic texts of around 6,000 words. Dialogic texts of approximately 2,500 words allow two or more authors to discuss a particular thematic, critical concept, or artwork; this multi-vocal format allows us to bring together different disciplinary, national or historical perspectives, and challenges the normative humanities model of individual scholarship to emphasize knowledge as collectively constituted. Shorter texts of under 1,500 words focus on a single artwork; these are intended to provide an accessible entry point for readers who do not normally work with art or visual methods, and will be particularly well suited as teaching resources (indeed, we see the production of such resources as an important part of facilitating interdisciplinary exchange).

From the outset of this project, we sought to foreground decolonial, intersectional, crip, queer and feminist methodologies; these appear throughout the volume, and are especially marked in contributions that explicitly challenge or redress the dominance of white, colonial and Eurocentric discourse in art and in medical humanities. However, while aspects of this volume may succeed in 'embracing' non-western perspectives and 'diversifying' an existing canon of scholarship, we recognize that the value of this supplementary approach is limited, and that a more radical restructuring of these fields with decoloniality and intersectionality at the centre is urgently required. Similarly, we recognize this volume's shortcomings in failing to adequately address, for example, experiences beyond gender binaries, despite significant work by artists and art historians in this area. We hope that these limitations will be taken up as a challenge in future projects and publications that will more boldly diversify and decolonize the field.

The contributions are grouped conceptually rather than organized around specific categories of illness experience, to avoid essentializing experience or reifying particular pathologies or clinical conditions, and to think expansively about health and illness. Many of the contributions exceed their thematic sections and the necessarily limited space afforded here. Many have a fluid quality, spilling outwards from this volume and running towards other projects, including edited collections and monographs currently in the making; where this is in the case, further readings are clearly signalled.

The first section of the volume focuses on **Lived Experience**, a key concept in critical medical humanities (Millard 2020) and often foundational to art practices that investigate and make visible aspects of health. The autobiographical artwork is frequently presumed to offer unmediated access to experiences of illness or disability. The texts included here complicate that formula, showing how the art-making process actively (re)makes experience. Recognizing the increasing importance of lived experience to social justice movements (both within academia and without), contributors resist the tendency to individualize and commodify lived experience, and instead think deeply and complexly about its embodied and connected nature, as well as its intrinsic entanglements with pressing social, political and environmental questions. This section opens with an essay by Vanessa Bartlett, who, as part of her curatorial research, has held extensive conversations with people living with chronic, yet medically undiagnosed, gut issues. For many of Bartlett's interlocutors, self-experimentation (e.g., gut bio-hacking) offers a practical strategy for agency when clinical medicine falls short. Bartlett argues that these 'creative collaborations with guts' are a form of imaginative health work that troubles binaries between amateur and expert knowledge and patient/artist identities. The second essay focuses on Ilona Sagar's film *The Body Blow* (2022), which explores the lives of retired labourers with long-term health conditions caused by exposure to asbestos, weaving the testimonies of patients, social workers, end-of-life carers and medical and legal professionals into a dense tapestry of interconnected experiences. In conversation with visual culture scholar Silvia Casini, Sagar discusses what it means to carry out artistic research using lived experience as method, the language of risk and care, and how certain kinds of bodies come to matter. Building on an ongoing conversation, artist Daniel Regan and historian Chris Millard explore how the concept of 'lived experience' resonates across their own spheres of practice. Regan's photographic works articulate his own experiences as a mental health service survivor, using the camera as a tool for documentation, communication and recovery; Millard researches the rise of 'personal' or 'lived' experience as a framework for academic writing. Together they explore the conventions, assumptions and experiences that variously underpin art practice and academic history, raising important points around disclosure, authority and hierarchies of knowledge. The section concludes with short texts addressing lived experience in relation to art making and art writing: Amanda Cachia on Jesse Darling's *Epistemologies (shamed cabinet)*, and Skye Haggerty on Ruth Cuthand's *Surviving: COVID-19*.

The second section, **Visualizing Knowledge and Power**, addresses the role of visuality in the production and mobilization of information, authority, and influence. Kathleen Pierce's essay uses nineteenth-century dermatology textbooks as a case study to advocate for a critical and capacious thinking about visuality modelled by art history at the core of efforts to address racism, sexism and other forms of inequality within healthcare systems and clinical training. A dialogic text authored by Katie Snow, Christine Slobogin and Laura Cowley considers humour in the context of medicine and health, looking at a range of visual sources including eighteenth-century caricature, cartoons of mid-twentieth-century operating theatres, and works by twenty-first-century self-identified disabled artists. Natasha Ruiz-Gómez, Tania Cleaves and Keren Rosa Hammerschlag ask how studying representations of the human body on a global scale might expand, complicate and enrich existing scholarship at the intersections of art history and histories of science and medicine. Finally, Anna Jamieson explores Thomas Lawrence's pastel *Mad Girl* (1787) in the context of the cultural feminization of madness in the late eighteenth century.

From precisely-detailed, hand-drawn anatomical illustrations to the software-generated data visualizations that are now an integral part of the contemporary clinical encounter, image-making has long been crucial to practices of modern medicine (as Michel Foucault recognized in *The Birth of the Clinic*, 1963; 1989). The texts in the third section of the volume, **Making and Remaking Medicalized Bodies**, probe the significance to clinical practice and patient experience of images in a variety of media and from different historical periods. Across these different texts, images are explored as sources of empirical evidence and as active players in processes of knowledge-creation; as spaces for articulating anxieties around professional medical identities; and as sites for questioning and strategically subverting norms and dominant clinical values. Ashley Lazevnick's essay considers the rise of professional medical illustration in the early twentieth century, focusing on the perceived tensions between (manual) drawing and mechanical (photographic) image-making, investigating the shared aspirations in surgical technique, artistic training, and photo-reproduction technologies of creating knowledge through embodied experience. In conversation with Fiona Johnstone, Liz Orton discusses her artist's book *Every Body is An Archive* (2020), which was created as part of a long-term collaboration with medical imaging practitioners and patients at University College London Hospital. Shorter texts by Rebecca Whiteley and Arya Thampuran address, respectively, a single printed illustration from William Smellie's 1754 midwifery atlas, and contemporary Kenyan American artist Wangechi Mutu's re-appropriation of a nineteenth-century medical diagram of uterine cancer.

The fourth section of the book, **Reproducing Reproduction**, considers a range of reproductive issues, addressing the histories and present-day realities of obstetrics and maternity care, infertility and abortion, paying attention to the uneven visibilities of different types of procreative experience, the pressing urgency to address reproductive healthcare inequities and the affordances of visual and material cultures for enhancing training for midwives, clinicians and other obstetric practitioners. Jessica Dandona's essay details the visual and material culture of obstetrical training in the late-nineteenth-century North Atlantic world, with careful consideration paid to how these highly affective objects and images resonate with obstetric practices and birthing experiences today. With a focus on contemporary reproductive justice, art historian Anna Arabindan-Kesson and Gabriella Nelson of the Philadelphia-based charity Maternity Care Coalition discuss the possibilities of an art-led response to the challenges of maternal healthcare and race. Jessica Womack studies Charmaine Watkiss's painting *Return of the Seed Keeper* (2021) to explore the reproductive agency of enslaved people. Researcher Isabel Davis and artist Anna Burel draw attention to the deep histories of infertility and un-reproductivity via Burel's collage illustration *Madonna della Misericordia* (2022), a work emerging from their long-running collaboration on invisible experiences of trying for pregnancy. With a focus on the intersections of private experiences and professional healthcare practices, Camilla Mørk Røstvik addresses Lyndsay Mann's video work *As You Were* (2023), which explores how the birthing experience of midwives and obstetricians is valued (or not) in institutional settings.

Histories of art and critical discussions in medical humanities have long marginalized therapeutic art practice. The thematic section **Rethinking Art and Therapy** takes an expansive approach to constellations of art and therapy; this includes critically examining 'art therapy' as a formalized mental health discipline developed in the context of Euro-American modernity, and exploring specific ways in which art-making – and art objects – might operate within therapeutic care, both inside and outside clinical settings (see Hudson and Sheehan 2024). Together these texts historicize and analyze the underpinnings and assumptions of therapeutic art practices, unsettle dominant power relations, and refigure relationships between art and psychiatry, opening up ways of rethinking and disrupting dominant ways of delimiting 'art'. In her essay art historian Suzanne Hudson uses her experience of 'retraining' in art therapy in a graduate MFT programme to discuss the role of diagnosis within art therapy's first decades in the United States, and to analyze art history's diagnostic tendencies and shared epistemic ground with medicine. Leah Gipson and Katharine Houpt take the image of the art therapist in Bong Joon-ho's film *Parasite* (2019) – and an essay about the film on the blog of the American Art Therapy Association (AATA) – as a starting point to analyze the politicized educational landscape of the art therapy profession. Arguing that the role of US-centrism and nationalist discourse in the field needs to be more closely examined, they suggest that critical studies in art and culture can oppose neoliberal modes of knowledge production and open up possibilities for establishing decolonial values in the profession. With a focus on therapeutic practices in Brazil, Kaira M. Cabañas shows how artist Lygia Clark's *estruturas vivas* (late 1960s) – simple objects made from interlaced rubber bands to form a flexible geometrical net – were later activated by artist and psychiatrist Lula Wanderley not only in a public mental health context, but also as part of a dance festival, affirming his patients' work as a form cultural citizenship.

Care is often summoned in fine art contexts (e.g. Jagoe and Kivland 2020; Blackshaw and Kivland 2021), conversations in the medical humanities (e.g. Mol 2008; Kristeva et al. 2018), and in activist public humanities spaces (*Care Syllabus* 2020–2022), with a shared set of theoretical references (e.g. Tronto 1993; Puig de la Bellacasa 2017). The term is necessarily fraught and activated in different ways in relation to healthcare. The texts in the expanded final section, **Caring, Collaborating, Curating,** take 'care' to signify not simply individual interpersonal relationships but a complex set of negotiations for time, space, power and resources. The section opens with an essay by Alison Syme which explores the entangled, creative, therapeutic and collaborative relationship between the British artist Vanessa Bell and the 'lady doctor' Dr Marie Moralt. Gemma Blackshaw and Alice Butler stage an epistolary exchange with and between two historical 'sick women', facilitating a reflection on embodied and auto-theoretical practices of feminist art history as praxis and care that also explores the challenges of creatively reconstructing historical health experiences. Artist and curator duo cripxcess (Lorenzo Galgó and Maria Morata) investigate the intersections between crip theory and ecological thinking, using the access rider – a document used for communicating the needs of artists with disabilities to arts institutions – as a framework for considering the relationship between diseased landscapes and sick bodies. Taking crip performance artist Angela Alves' installation *REST* (2019) as a starting point, Alves, Monika Ankele and Céline Kaiser explore the highly complex social, moral, political and physical implications of resting, from the late nineteenth century to the present day. Cera Smith reads Simone Leigh's installation *The Waiting Room* (2016) as an African American, female vision of healthcare rooted in holistic care and social justice movements. Suzannah Biernoff uses a fifteenth-century Japanese tea bowl repaired with the *kintsugi* technique as a surprising starting point for a discussion of reparative practices and neoliberal concepts of wellness and self-care. Inspired by the philosopher Adriana Cavarero (2016), who theorizes inclination as a model of the subject that is mutually dependent upon others, contrasting it with the modern, masculinist standard of the singular, upright able-bodied man, Nora Heidorn's visual essay brings together images of reclined and inclined bodies – common tropes include the psychoanalytic patient, the birthing woman, the fallen soldier and the reclining nude so prevalent in Euro-American art – drawing unexpected connections between imagery from the history of medicine, contemporary art and clinical practice. Closing this section, a short text by Allison Morehead articulates the inter-connections between care and curatorial practice, and a vision for a 'curatorial medical humanities'.

We have written this summary of the texts contained within this volume with gratitude for the work, including the artwork, entrusted to us. And we have endeavoured to hold these texts and works together without oversimplifying their similarities and differences. Our challenge has been to grapple with the curatorial and editorial challenges of an academic volume while remaining alive to the complexities and ambiguities of recognizing, simultaneously, the universality of our vulnerable bodies and the particularity of experiences of health, illness and disability. In doing so, we've tried to 'stay with the trouble' (Haraway 2016) of boundary crossing while critically reflecting on how boundaries (between disciplines, between sites of knowledge production, between bodies) are co-constituted, and what their making and unmaking can reveal and conceal.

This volume demonstrates how art recognizes, reconceives and transforms a rich variety of human health experiences, often while critically interrogating the assumptions that continue to shape dominant definitions of 'the human', 'health' and 'experience'. In doing this vital work, art shares common aims, questions, provocations and practices with critical medical humanities. Keenly aware of the tensions that characterize interdisciplinarity, we propose that 'art' and 'critical medical humanities' are most constructively approached not as neatly bounded entities that might be set in dialogue with each other, but rather as messy hybridities that are already mutually entangled. Offering a range of entry points for readers of all disciplines interested in exploring those inter-relations, this volume is not intended to be a definitive account of the intersections between art and critical medical humanities, but rather an experiment in articulating a fluid and open-ended assemblage of possibilities. We see its purpose as generative, rather than conclusive.

References

Arabindan-Kesson, A. (2022), 'Transmission and Transfer: Plantation Imagery and Medical Management in the British Empire', *Art History*, 45 (3): 472–97.

Barad, K. (2007), *Meeting the Universe Halfway: Quantum Physics and the Entanglement of Matter and Meaning*. Durham, NC: Duke University Press.

Bellacasa, M. Puig de la. (2017), *Matters of Care: Speculative Ethics in More than Human Worlds*. Minneapolis: University of Minnesota Press.

Bellis, R.T., F. Cooper, R. Knoeff *et al.* (2024), 'History at the heart of medicine' [version 1; peer review: 3 approved]. Wellcome Open Research 9:249 [https://doi.org/10.12688/wellcomeopenres.21229.1]

Berger, J. (2016), *Confabulations*, London: Penguin.

Biernoff, S., and F. Johnstone (2024), 'What Can Art History Offer Medical Humanities?' *Medical Humanities* 50: 529–38.

Blackshaw, G., and S. Kivland, eds. (2021), *Care(Less): A Supplement of On Care*, London: MA Bibliothèque.

Care Syllabus (2020–2022). Co-directed by Victoria Papa, Levi Prombaum and Laura. Thompson. www.caresyllabus.org

Cavarero A. (2016), *Inclinations: A Critique of Rectitude*. Stanford: Stanford University Press.

Fitzgerald, D., and F. Callard (2016), 'Entangling the Medical Humanities', in A. Whitehead and A. Woods, eds. *The Edinburgh Companion to the Critical Medical Humanities*, 35–49, Edinburgh: Edinburgh University Press.

Foucault, M. (1963; 1989), *The Birth of the Clinic: An Archaeology of Medical Perception*, trans. A.M. Sheridan, London and New York: Routledge.

Haraway, D. (2016), *Staying with the Trouble: Making Kin in the Chthulucene*, Durham, NC: Duke University Press.

Hartman, S., (2008), 'Venus in Two Acts', *Small Axe* 26: 1–14.

Hudson, S., and T. Sheehan, eds (2024), *Modernism, Art, Therapy*. New Haven: Yale University Press.

Jagoe, R., and S. Kivland (2020), *On Care*, London: MA Bibliothèque.

Johnstone, F. (2018), 'Manifesto for a Visual Medical Humanities', *Medical Humanities* (blog), 31 July. https://blogs.bmj.com/medical-humanities/2018/07/31/manifesto-for-a-visual-medical-humanities/.

Kristeva, J., M. R. Moro, J. Ødemark, and E. Engebretsen (2018), 'Cultural crossings of care: An appeal to the medical humanities', *Medical Humanities* 44: 55–58.

Latour, B. (2004), 'Why has critique run out of steam? From matters of fact to matters of concern', *Critical Inquiry* 30: 225–48.

Leavy, P. ed. (2019), *Handbook of Arts-Based Research*, New York: Guilford Press.

Lind, M. (2009), 'The Curatorial', *Artforum* 48 (2): 103.

Millard, C.J. (2020), 'Using personal experience in the academic medical humanities: a genealogy', *Social Theory and Health* 18: 184–98.

Mol, A. (2008), *The Logic of Care: Health and the Problem of Patient Choice*, Abingdon and New York: Routledge.

Morehead, A. (2024), 'Edvard Munch and the Medicalization of Modern Life: Towards a Curatorial Medical Humanities', *Journal of Medical Humanities*. https://doi.org/10.1007/s10912-024-09893-7.

Saunders, C. (2016), 'Voices and Visions: Mind, Body and Affect in Medieval Writing', in A. Whitehead and A. Woods, eds., *The Edinburgh Companion to the Critical Medical Humanities*, 411–27, Edinburgh: Edinburgh University Press.

Tronto, J. (1993), *Moral Boundaries: A Political Argument for an Ethics of Care*, London: Routledge.

Viney, W., F. Callard, and A. Woods (2015), 'Critical Medical Humanities: Embracing Entanglements, Taking Risks', *Medical Humanities* 41: 2–7.

Whitehead, A., and A. Woods (2016), 'Introduction', in A. Whitehead and A. Woods, eds. *The Edinburgh Companion to the Critical Medical Humanities*, 1–31, Edinburgh: Edinburgh University Press.

PART I

Lived experience

CHAPTER ONE

Curating beyond science communication towards embodied expertise: *creative collaborations with guts*

Vanessa Bartlett

Curators have responded with fascination to the emerging science of the gut-brain-microbiome axis. Over the past eight years, the Eden Project, UK, Medical Museion, Copenhagen, Melbourne Museum, Bloomfield Science Museum, and Science and Industry Museum, Manchester[1] have all staged major exhibitions exploring how microbes in the human gut could influence everything from human immunity to behaviour. This intense focus has prompted influential curator Jens Hauser to herald a 'bacterial turn' (2022) in art, design and architecture, where creatives are using microbes to create new visions of humans as complex ecosystems filled with organisms which collaborate and compete. In 2019, promotional material for the exhibition *Gut Feelings* at the Melbourne Museum called gut microbes 'magic creatures' which may 'cure peanut allergies, decrease anxiety, and even form future autoimmune therapies' (Mannix 2019; Museums Victoria

[1]Eden Project, *Invisible You*, 2015; Medical Museion Copenhagen, *Mind the Gut*, 2018; Melbourne Museum, *Gut Feelings: Your Mind, Your Microbes*, 2019; Bloomfield Science Museum, *Gut Feelings*, 2023; Science and Industry Museum Manchester, *Operation Ouch! Food, Poo and You*, 2024.

2019), demonstrating the scientific optimism that sometimes characterizes projects engaging with the gut microbiome.

Yet epidemiological research suggests that digestive dysregulation – interruption in the biological and cultural processes that turn food into energy in the human body – is rising exponentially across the globe, with profound implications for people's quality of life. Forty per cent of people globally report experiences in keeping with a functional gastrointestinal disorder, where digestive disruptions have no discernible organic cause (Sperber et al. 2021). People with functional conditions experience symptoms despite returning 'normal' results from blood tests and endoscopy/gastroscopy, and irritable bowel syndrome is the most recognized and publicly discussed. Meanwhile inflammatory bowel disease, an autoimmune condition that causes chronic inflammation in the bowel, more than tripled in Northern Europe between the 1950s and 1990s (Farrokhyar, Swarbrink and Irvine 2001). A significant proportion of patients either fail to respond to treatment, or lose their responsiveness over time. According to gastroenterologist Chamara Basnayake, 'gastrointestinal complaints that defy diagnosis are widespread', but current medical systems fail patients by adopting a siloed approach. He describes people being sent on a 'do it yourself' journey of joining the dots between psychologists, dietitians and other medical experts (Trounson 2020).

Acknowledging the failed connection between future-oriented promissory narratives of the 'microbiome revolution' (El-Omar 2023: 2) and people's lived experiences of poor digestion in the here-and-now gives a different kind of cultural urgency to the more traditional curatorial task of increasing people's scientific literacy via artworks and cultural artefacts. Gastroenterologists admit that the field of microbiome research is still 'short on mechanistic answers, but long on speculation' (Fasano and Flaherty 2021: 239), posing a complex ethical question about how such speculative science can contribute to a supportive cultural discourse for people living with unruly, chronically ill guts (Medvecky and Leach 2019).

Curators working with science and medicine are often driven by a desire to communicate new knowledge based on the premise that increasing the audience's scientific literacy is a form of public good. In *The Ethics of Science Communication*, Medvecky and Leach outline three ways that the communication of scientific information can contribute to an individual or collective's quality of life. The first is 'health communication' resulting in physical health improvements, an outcome that is often claimed for exhibitions exploring wellbeing (Chatterjee and Noble 2016). However, less directly utilitarian outcomes such as 'satisfying curiosity' and 'providing enjoyment' are also part of science communication's enrichment value (Medvecky and Leach 2019: 56). The exhibition *Mind the Gut* (2018) at Medical Museion (Figure 1.1) focused on communicating the 'complex, unsettled science' of the microbiome from a 'philosophical' perspective

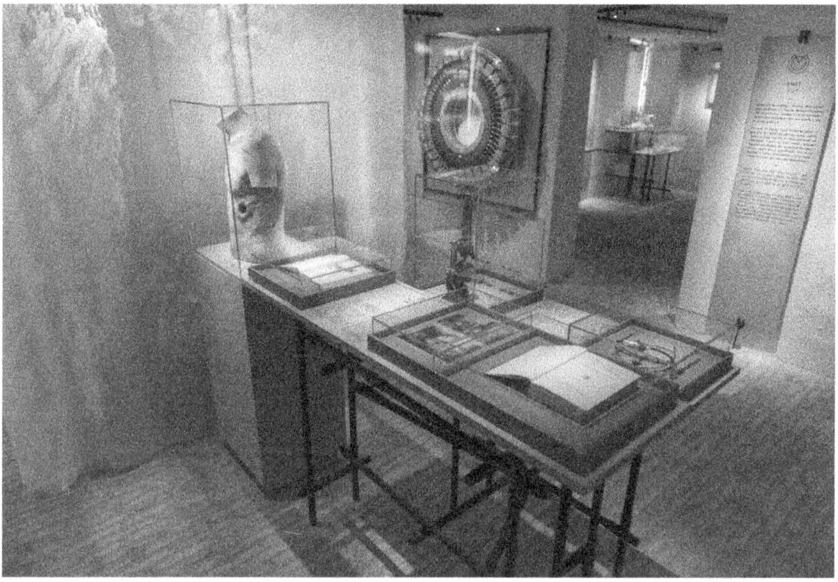

FIGURE 1.1 Exhibition view from *Mind the Gut* at Medical Museion, University of Copenhagen. Photograph by Morten Skovgaard.

(Bencard, Whiteley and Thon 2019: 136). All three types of engagement outlined by Medvecky and Leach appear to be guiding principles for Medical Museion, who describe their remit as 'adventurous public inquiries relating to the interests of the University of Copenhagen's medical faculty' (Arnold et al. 2021: 55). Yet, embedded within a university system and medical faculty, it is science communication rather than the complexities of lived experience, that appear to drive Medical Museion (Lillemose and Bencard 2022). Similar remits toward science communication have dominated most of the major museum exhibitions on the gut.

Beyond science communication: Toward lived experience as embodied expertise

In 2021, I began to consider what alternative forms of agency and expertise might be afforded to audiences of exhibitions about the gut and microbiome, beyond the invitation to enhance their understanding of science. My inquiry was spurred by an escalation in my own experiences of chronic, unruly digestion, which went largely unexplained by my doctor. As I worked to live with my symptoms in the absence of clinical guidance, I developed new insight into the different forms of agency and adaptation required to live with chronic, unexplained symptoms. This experience spurred me to invite individuals with undiagnosed gut issues to attend a series of conversations with me, and this chapter documents how these conversations have informed my curatorial thinking and practice. This move was driven by the major commitment of all of my scholarship on curating: that audiences, publics, and health communities are active collaborators in the production of meaning at the site of exhibitions (Bartlett 2020). It adds to a growing consciousness in complex interdisciplinary fields such as the medical humanities, that creative and curatorial thinking and practice can be recognized as a mode of research beyond illustrative or educational paradigms (Johnstone 2023). It offers the following provocation: that contemporary art might be made and read complexly in tandem with other everyday expressions of creative agency that thread the lived experience of illness under capitalism. It aligns with ideas being tested by other practitioners in this volume. Discussing her film *The Body Blow* (2022), visual artist Ilona Sagar proposes a revised conceptual frame for collaboration with people impacted by the devastating health legacies of asbestos. Pushing against the impulse to use bodies to 'represent' illness, she invites her collaborators to 'skew the hierarchical importance' of her artistic eye. According to one of Sagar's collaborators on a previous project, this approach nurtures networked knowledges that hold 'a collective gut reaction' (Casini and Sagar this volume).

Stone and Hooker argue that people with medically unexplained symptoms are subject to the same demands of self-regulation and performance as most bodies under capitalism. They are expected to work toward recovery and rejoin productive society, and for the chronically ill this can become a lifetime employment (2021: 50). In the area of gastrointestinal health, functional conditions operate as a catch-all term for symptoms with no 'organic' explanation, with many physicians deciding people simply need psychiatric treatment. Many patients fear their doctor thinks they are 'crazy' and avoid formal medical intervention (Black et al. 2020: 5). For many this initiates lifelong, self-imposed regimes of dietary modification, complementary medicines, independent research and changed social behaviours that supplement or simply replace formal medical care (Bartlett 2023). The availability of over-the-counter products like probiotics – which promise to adapt and change the microbial composition of the gut to achieve improved health (Yong 2017: 222) – supports a growing perception of personal agency and responsibility in relation to the gut, particularly in a neoliberal culture that regards an individual's health as their own responsibility. While people with medically unexplained symptoms are often dismissed by their doctor, they remain subject to the same social and economic pressures that demand their recovery. Without formal treatment pathways in place, this need to recover forms a complex burden.

Informed by my ongoing research, I formulated the following curatorial questions: *how can I curate an exhibition about the gut and microbiome from a lived experience perspective, one that accounts for the complex forms of expertise and agency required to live with dysfunction in parts of the body/mind that are poorly understood by science and medicine? Beyond communicating the emerging science, how can curating account for the forms of corporal, embodied knowing that digesting bodies bring to this visceral process, particularly the kinds of expertise and agency that people develop as they live with unruly guts that escape medical classification?*

These questions are well supported by theoretical frameworks from the critical medical humanities, particularly recent shifts in the field that understand art and creative practice as a site of knowledge production (Johnstone 2023). First wave medical humanities often promoted individual professional artists (who were often white and well educated) as revealing authentic, empathy inducing perspectives on illness. The artist Jo Spence, who documented her treatment for cancer in a set of compelling photographs and writings, repeatedly attracts attention from the most respected curators and scholars (Vasey 2020: Muñoz 2020). Spence's resourcefulness and intelligence radiates from her images and writing. In her 1988 text *The Picture of Heath*, she quips 'I found myself a delightfully bolshy socialist feminist naturopath', and remarks that she took 'several books on theories of representation' along for her most recent hospital visit (Spence [1988] 2020: 99–100). While Spence's work undoubtedly deserves attention, how much does her ongoing valorization distract from other people less equipped with the erudition and narrative skill that Spence displays? As Claire Hooker remarks, to privilege specific 'high culture works' illuminates 'particular forms of personhood' marked by 'disciplined' and 'self-improving' ways of being, and can exclude the perspective of people who are less resilient in the face of illness (Hooker 2014: 218).

Curatorial constellations: researching lived experience

The meeting point between art and the critical medical humanities invites practitioners to move beyond 'merely disseminating specialised medical knowledge to a non-expert public' and instead raises 'difficult ethical and philosophical questions about aspects of clinical knowledge' (Johnstone 2023: 2). But to raise complex ethical questions that push past limited definitions of medical subjectivity, I wanted to frame my approach to lived experience by looking beyond *my* experiences as a white, middle-class woman with undiagnosed gut issues *and* specific forms of educational and social privilege. I felt that I needed to listen to a range of voices. To fail to do so would risk undertaking a curatorial process that would simply reproduce my own lived experience. My conversations with people with lived experience were advertised via online forums and social media sites targeted at people with gut health issues. They took place via Zoom, were between forty-five minutes and 1 hour in duration, and were subject to research ethics clearance from the University of Melbourne Human Research Ethics panel. The aim was to explore how people were taking an active role in reimagining their own gut health outside of, or as a supplement to, clinical medicine. I conceived of these conversations as a way of developing relationships with an audience group who should be essential to any meaningful exhibition project on the gut. But I also considered them to be a form of curatorial research which could inform the key concepts of the exhibition.

This approach emphasizes curating as 'a specific system of knowledge production' (Sheikh 2015: 35) beyond researching and selecting artists for exhibitions. Curator Simon Sheikh invokes the form of the 'constellation' as a valuable metaphor for curatorial research in an 'expanded field' which includes undertaking art historical research into past exhibitions *and* collecting 'materials, data, sources' that investigate 'something other than art' and lead to the formation of a curatorial 'thesis' (2015: 36–37). Hosting conversations with people with lived experience allowed me to enact such a curatorial 'constellation' trained on developing a new stance on how curators might frame the gut and microbiome though lived experience. It also drew on the notion of curating as a 'practice of relations' that can activate 'new conversations and dialogue' between people (Hermon 2022: 63). My approach was influenced by 'Inclusive Curating', a practice-led curatorial methodology devised by Jade French with a group of intellectually disabled curators. Inclusive Curating empowers participants with no previous curatorial experience to curate an exhibition. Arts-based methods such as collage are used to leverage different ways of knowing within the curatorial process, helping participants to draw on their lived experience as part of the design and development of an exhibition. French argues that arts-based methods enable 'different ways of interpreting and representing human experience' and can be an effective aid for communicating 'the experiences of individuals or groups who have been oppressed and marginalised by dominant discourses' (French 2020: 52–53).

During my conversations with people with lived experience, I asked questions that focused on the history of their digestive disruptions, their relationship to clinical medicine, and how they had lived with undiagnosed gut issues. My key interest was to explore forms of expertise and agency which people developed while living with unruly guts. But it was my final question to each participant that became the most significant for my curatorial research: *if you had to think of an object or an artefact that could describe your relationship to your symptoms, what might it be and why?* This focus on objects was designed to be distinct from other questions about diet, lifestyle and medical marginalization that generated accounts of lived experience with a primarily narrative structure. Often people's responses to these more traditional questions unfolded in ways which reflected the complex burden of the medically undiagnosed as described by

Stone and Hooker (2021), where people were driven by a desire to return to a more normative ideal of digestive function.

I was committed to exploring people's accounts of their relationship with their gut, and the forms of expertise and agency that they displayed. But I was also alive to the risk of privileging forms of lived experience that reflect 'particular forms of personhood' (Hooker 2014). In first wave medical humanities, narrative accounts of illness were often celebrated as providing 'privileged access to the subjective experience of illness' (Woods 2011). However, narrative has also been critiqued for celebrating 'hero' narratives that seek mastery over symptoms, and recovery of more normative body behaviours (Frank 1995; Woods 2011: 73). Asking people to imagine an object to reflect their dysfunctional guts was designed to shift our discussion past the trajectory *toward* recovery, into a more image-based, imaginative account of guts. It introduced elements of arts-based research by inviting people to represent their lived experience in ways that 'adumbrate rather than denote' (Barone and Eisner 2012: 2), focusing on affective experiences rather than measures of health. I conceived of this question as curatorial, given practices of representing ideas, stories and histories via the collection and organization of objects and images.

Lived experience as embodied expertise

My exploration of guts as a site of agency speaks to a growing body of social research that examines relationships between people with digestive dysfunction and their guts (Beck 2021; Kolářová et al. 2023; Benezra 2023). This work has been prompted by imaginaries of microbial-human interactions that create what Beck calls 'corporal communication' that attends to 'the long ignored symbiotic relationship between human and microbe' (Beck 2021: 358). In her study of people who have experienced faecal microbial transplants, Beck describes people's sense of relatedness with their microbiome in the aftermath of the procedure. Faecal transplants replace a person's microbial ecosystem by inserting faeces from a 'healthy' donor into their gut via colonoscopy. Faecal transplants are used clinically to treat *clostridium difficile*, a tenacious bacterium which infects the gut causing aggressive illness. Owing partially to the status of faecal matter as a 'drug' which can be produced 'at home', a culture of do-it-yourself transplants has emerged outside of clinical spaces, where people are using the procedure to treat conditions like Crohn's disease without medical supervision (Yong 2017). Beck argues that this 'microbiome manipulation' can be understood as a 'physical engagement with microbial life that can be observed and felt by the user' (2021: 362). For Beck's research, participants' gut symptoms including 'digestive sensations of gut pain, nausea, diarrhoea or bloating'

(368) are experienced as expressions of the host body's ingestion of the new microbial community and its effects on their health.

Attuning to the body and its intestinal fluctuations prioritizes being in relationship with the gut as symptoms intensify and recede, more than it documents stories of achieving lasting mastery over unruly guts. Corporal communications can illuminate people's agency in relation to their gut, without equating agency with achieving normalized digestive health. Such agential relationships between people and their gut also work against the abstraction of the microbiome from lived experience in ways that mirror my own curatorial aim of complicating science communication via the embodied knowledges that people already possess. In their study of inflammatory bowel disease, Kolářová, Stöckelová and Senft argue that research on the microbiome has often been 'abstracted out of the particular materiality of bodies, environments, alimentary habits and eating practices' of people with dysfunctional guts. They suggest that biomedicine has tended to overlook the 'embodied expertise' of people with lived experience, but that people living with gut issues do in fact mirror insights from microbiome science in their habits and practices (2023: 1244). This is a rich prospect for a curatorial thesis which engages exhibition audiences as embodied experts in their own digestion. It suggests that an exhibition about the gut and microbiome might find innovative ways to complicate Medvecky and Leach's three key aims of science communication (health improvement, satisfying curiosity and providing enjoyment) by recognizing an audience's intuitive reflection of the emerging science in their habits and behaviour.

Creative collaborations with guts

The final section of this essay explores two examples from my conversations with people with lived experience of digestive dysfunction which demonstrate their embodied and agential relationships with their gut and the influence of these conversations on the development of my curatorial thesis *Creative collaborations with guts*. *Creative collaborations with guts* pushes past science communication towards a more participatory approach that explores the embodied expertise in digestion that audiences already possess. The significance of this participatory approach is not simply formed through listening to people with lived experience as part of my curatorial research. Rather it arises through the potential for collapsing boundaries between people's everyday health practices – their sensory-affective attunements to their guts – and curatorial thinking and doing. I will summarize each person's relationship with their gut as they expressed it, and then describe the object that they chose to represent their symptoms. The objects are not intended to be translated literally into an exhibit. They are speculative 'things to think with' (Muller and Seck Langhill 2021: 2) which bring me closer to the affective, embodied and interpersonal potentials of *creative collaborations with guts*, and how these could find form in an exhibition space. I will describe in brief how the objects shaped my own process of thinking curatorially with participants and start bridging a gap between research and the more practical process of devising, developing and making an exhibition. Only two conversations are described due to limitations of space. I have chosen different of examples to illustrate range.

Across my conversations, food was the most common tool that people used to influence their gut health. People restricted foods based on their embodied perception of symptoms after consumption, often finding that mainstream dietary advice was ill suited to their unruly guts. Sophie described how she has learned to test, modify and sometimes dismiss both clinical and colloquial dietary advice. After reading recommendations online to increase her intake of nuts and seeds she suggests that 'if I ate lots of seeds and nuts, I would probably end up in ED [emergency department] again'. Instead she has to 'bite the bullet' and engage in 'trial and error' experimentation with different foods. At the time of our conversation, Sophie had reached a place of equilibrium with her gut which allowed her to live a restricted, but relatively functioning life. But this has been hard won. In my research, she was one of two people with a diagnosis of Crohn's disease who had spent many years receiving ineffective medical care. She therefore identified with my project's invitation to people with undiagnosed gut issues. She worked with 'eight or nine different doctors' who all failed to diagnose her condition, resulting in multiple trips to hospital emergency departments with crippling, unexplained pain.

Kolářová, Stöckelová and Senft argue that clinical treatments for digestive dysfunction often involve dietary regimes that rest on ableist assumptions about healthy food (2022: 1245). Far from this digestive ideal, they suggest that people living with digestive dysfunction are forced to deepen their sensitivity to their interior life, and to experiment with different foods and their 'digestive aftermath' to identify what good food means for them. This generally involves 'a several-year process of searching, experimenting, and tracing' (1248) in which 'food becomes "good" based on how it moves (through) the body', and 'what "feelings in the belly" it produces' (1249).

Attunement to 'feelings in the belly' were in evidence across most of my conversations with participants, both in relation to food, but also as a more general demand of living with unruly guts. When asked to select an object or an artefact to describe her relationship to her symptoms, Sophie selects three similar, highly relational 'things to think with' that illuminate her attunement to her gut: They are: 'a new kitten trying to learn the ways around the house'; 'a puppy' and a young child who frustrates and delights in equal measure; 'my sister she's got three boys like there's times where she's like "Oh my gosh, it's so frustrating ... but you just have to deal with it. But then the good times are really, really good"'. These images figure

Sophie's gut as an animal or infant to be cared for. They compare life with dysfunctional guts to the fluctuating, up-and-down, enduring labour of parenting (humans and animals), in ways that recall Beck's framing of corporal communication with microbes as an unstable 'agile' practice of care between humans and nonhumans (Beck 2021: 367). They illuminate the deep embodied knowledge and self-care that the chronically ill develop.

Sophie's images have offered me a point of entry into how people's intangible self-care practices could be translated into my curatorial process. Previously, while curating exhibitions exploring mental health, I have used maternal imagery to frame my approach to exhibition design and object selection as a way of enacting curatorial care for audiences (Bartlett 2020). This was intended to support visitors while they experience the complex embodied sensations that can arise in response to the subject of illness. Exploring the exhibition as a 'container' for overwhelming or 'difficult' feelings allows an exhibition to reflect the complex social and cultural dimensions of mental distress and present them back to the viewer in a more 'digestible' or accessible form (Bartlett 2020). This approach captures the crux of curating from the perspective of lived experience rather than science communication. It makes space for audiences to *feel into* the frustrations and fluctuations of living with a chronic health condition, rather than simply learning new scientific information. This approach is slowly gaining traction in the field, for example in the exhibition *Misbehaving Bodies: Jo Spence and Oreet Ashery* (2019), curators Bárbara Rodríguez Muñoz and George Vasey developed the exhibition design to help people feel they were 'being hugged' (Vasey 2020). This was intended to help people process the potentially traumatic subject of cancer in a very public venue with high footfall, particularly showing Ashery's work in 'cocooned' 'den-like' spaces (Vasey 2020) that held the viewer. Sophie's 'new kitten' or 'puppy' invites a curator to consider how performing a holding function could bring exhibition visitors closer to the transient, unpredictable experience of chronic digestive dysfunction, in ways that feel safe and supportive. They ask how an exhibition could be framed around self-care in its most radical form (Sharma, Sainte-Marie and Fournier 2020) as a way of complicating more paternalistic health education agendas trained on learning science.

For Sophie, *creative collaborations with guts* describes forms of attunement that support living in harmony with unruly guts. For a second participant, Ama, their relationship with their gut was equally entangled, but it was also fraught with distressing symptoms that she struggled to control. Born in Sri Lanka, Ama grew up in a family that placed great value on Ayurvedic medicine, a tradition from the Indian subcontinent that works to create union between body and mind. As an adult she has used Ayurveda to develop a more 'holistic' approach to her health. Her relation to her gut is defined by abrupt and violent symptoms stimulated by emotionally charged relational experiences. She describes receiving upsetting text messages and then 'rushing to the toilet'. Her gut appears to be attuned to her social world, which has led her to conclude that her symptoms are emotionally triggered: 'I know that for a fact ... I've noticed patterns'. When pressed to explain this, she says she has a deep personal sense that her digestive system is more sensitive than others: 'I've literally been to the toilet like seconds after seeing text messages which are like deeply hurtful and troubling'.

Ama has married into a family that includes multiple doctors trained in Western medicine, who have discouraged extensive medical testing because they believe the symptoms have psychological causes. Ama's complex interface with Ayurveda and Western medicine traces ways of knowing that often characterize the experience of living with unruly guts. Several research participants used so-called alternative knowledge systems like Ayurveda to address symptoms that were not seen as 'biological' or serious enough to warrant attention from their doctor. Such alternative practices often support the development of what Kolářová, Stöckelová and Senft name as 'an embodied language – a gut semiosis – that supports individuals to understand their "interior life"' (2022: 1250). As people live with unruly guts, they often find allies in traditional healing practices with greater tolerance for attuning to visceral sensory information that guts produce.

Ama chose a mobile phone as her object to reflect her relationship to her symptoms, based on her strong physical reactions to text messages, and her own sense of her gut's 'abnormal' behaviour. 'I always talk about the phone ... when I talk about gut health ... it's not normal to look at the phone and be in the toilet the next second'. Ama views her gut's responsiveness to the world as 'incomprehensible to a normal person', reflecting her perception that there is a 'normal' state of digestive health to be recovered. The corporeal communication between Ama and her gut is boisterous and immediate – the gut reacts emphatically to bad news.

For feminist theorist Elizabeth Wilson, the gut is nothing less than 'an organ of mind', linked through the complex networks of the nervous system. Capable of rumination and deliberation, anger and depression, the gut ingests the social and relational facets of lived experience, and sometimes responds violently (2015: 5, 65). *Creative collaboration with guts* acquires a different nuance here, where communicating with guts includes the generation of powerful sensory expression that interrupts the expected flow of living. For Beck, corporal communication demands agility, and allows for both partners to be painfully out of sync. She quotes Donna Haraway: 'An embodied communication is more like a dance than a word. The flow of entangled meaningful bodies in time – whether jerky and nervous or flaming and flowing.' (Haraway 2008: 26). Ama's gut finds forms of expression that are jerky, nervous and flaming.

A curatorial approach to the lived experience of digestive dysfunction must account for complex forms of agency that manifest beyond digestive normalcy, embracing the gut's capacities for chaos and rage. Feminist philosopher Jane Dryden has argued that the 'imperative of normalcy' which governs bodies under capitalism has been refigured via the microbiome, where microbiome therapies are being developed to 'cure' 'conditions' such as autism and obesity. She argues that 'the complexity of the gut microbiome ought to encourage us to rethink our conception of ourselves' rather than becoming 'one more tool for controlling unruly bodies' (2023: 131). There is a risk that positivist health outcomes dominate cultural discourse of the microbiome, and it is crucial that this is critically addressed in the curation of exhibitions.

In her essay *How to Be a Person in the Age of Autoimmunity*, visual artist Carolyn Lazard illuminates how living with Crohn's disease has forced her to embrace her guts' radical expression and how this works against the demands of capitalism. She cites *The Autoimmune Epidemic* (Nakazawa 2008) – the rapid rise of autoimmune conditions like Crohn's in industrialized nations – as part of the body's revolt against demands for hyper-productivity. Due to all this forced activity the body begins to attack itself. Critiquing the medicalized language of 'fighting back', Lazard reframes illness as cultural phenomena and argues for greater social acceptance of the physical symptoms of digestive unrest: 'I sacrificed entire days to incessant shitting. I was forced into more intimate relations with my body – relations that underscored my lack of control, thus my lack of civility, and ultimately my body's radical realness' (Lazard 2017).

Individuals like Ama prompt a desire in me to reframe shitting as a gutsy protest. The mobile phone – the object that Ama chose to reflect her symptoms – has become a popular cultural image of the demands placed on bodies to constantly work and socialize in the neoliberal era. It speaks to a sense of anticipation, the pressure of receiving bad news. It reflects a fear of symptoms manifesting suddenly, which was in evidence across many of my conversations. A curatorial response could include selecting an artwork such as Zhou Xiaohu's installation *Even in Fear* (2008). Xiaohu is a Shanghai-based artist who works across sculpture, installation and digital media, often critiquing the ways that technology and propaganda shape Chinese and global society. In this work, a giant weather balloon slowly inflates, its rubbery skin stretched thinner and thinner, growing more like a giant stomach or bladder. Watching the piece grow, the viewer knows that it must eventually burst as the pressure builds. Perhaps her body tenses – taut muscles, shallow breathing, clenched anus. For the artist, this speaks to 'the pressures experienced at every level of contemporary society'. For a curatorial project about unruly guts, the work could shape an exploration of the pressures that capitalism exerts, and the violent protests bodies can mount in response. Pushing past the desire to educate audiences about microbiome science, *creative collaborations with guts* asks audiences to feel into the body under pressure – its patterns of holding and release, surges of adrenaline and bile. In this way it collaborates curatorially with guts and their visceral sensations, rather than simply representing guts through abstract scientific forms.

Curating with guts: future directions

My intention in this essay has been to develop a curatorial thesis for the gut and microbiome grounded in the lived experiences of increasing proportions of the global population living with chronic and difficult to diagnose gut issues. *Creative collaborations with guts* has emerged as a way of accounting for the things people do with their gut where clinical medicine is unable to offer clear pathways towards treatment and recovery. It illuminates people's agency in relation to their health, while guarding against narratives that promote recovery of stabilized digestion.

Methodologically, *creative collaborations with guts* forges a path towards a more socially engaged way of curating that could support a polyphonic, less individualist way of representing lived experience at the meeting point between art and medical humanities. But this is not simply formed by introducing conversations with lived experience participants as part of my curatorial research. Rather it arises through a willingness to enact a form of 'creative boundary crossing' (Fitzgerald and Callard 2016) between people's everyday health practices – their sensory-affective attunements to their guts – and creative and curatorial work. This interdisciplinary move draws on James Thompson's recent book *Care Aesthetics*, which builds on histories of socially engaged art to collapse boundaries between artworks that emphasize care for participants, and everyday care-giving practices such as nursing. Socially engaged and participatory art practices have long promoted human interaction and agency as the primary material of the work of art. Thompson uses socially engaged artist Mierle Laderman Ukeles as an example of how bodily and domestic demands (washing, cooking, cleaning) have been integrated into art practice (Thompson 2022: 87). In her 1969 *Manifesto for Maintenance Art*, Ukeles highlights the everyday administrative and domestic duties required to manage the life of the family as a new mother, and her integration of these demands into her practice, leading her to the proclamation that 'everything I do is art' (Ukeles 1969: 2). Using literature from the field of social care, Thompson then frames the sensory affective dimensions of caring environments and interactions to frame 'nursing as an art' (2022: 108). This move rests on an expanded definition of aesthetic experience as sensory immersion in the world at large, which includes, but is not limited to, engagement with the arts. If, as Ukeles claims, domestic work is an art, can the forms of bodily attunement demanded by dysfunctional guts become curatorial?

Fundraising is underway for the next phase of this project, which will push *creative collaborations with guts* more firmly towards acts of

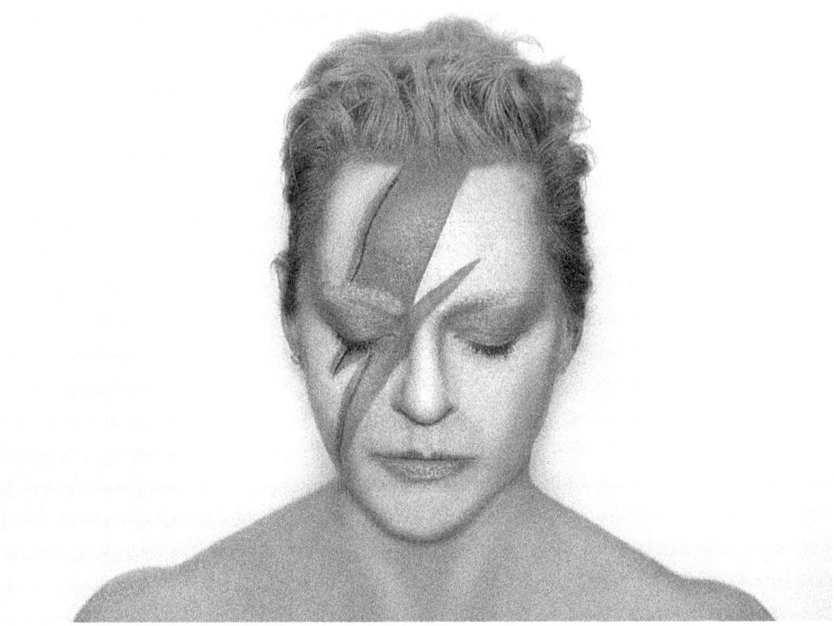

Figure 1.2 Kathy High, *Kathy As Bowie*, 2015. Photographer Eleanor Goldsmith.

collaborative exhibition making. This work is supported by a wider turn toward gut microbes as collaborators in contemporary art, which offers a rich field of practice to draw on curatorially with participants. In *After Eating: Metabolising the Arts*, artist and scholar Lindsay Kelley documents an emerging wave of 'poop art' that appreciates 'metabolic waste ... as communication from the microbiota at work in the digestive tract' (2023: 114). Contemporary art's past uses of poo to represent disgust or humour – for example tin cans filled with the artist Piero Manzoni's shit (1961) – are being joined by a metabolic art practice in which 'reactions must become dialogues' (Kelley 2023: 115). Kelley uses American interdisciplinary artist Kathy High's work as an example of poo's 'value, vitality and communicative capabilities' (2023: 128). In 'Kathy As Bowie' (2015, Figure 1.2), High solicited poop from pop-star David Bowie for use in a transplantation (the request was never fulfilled due to Bowie's death). A friend asked High who would be her ideal poo donor, and High was curious about the potential to 'become a bit of Bowie' via this microbial exchange (High 2019: 66). High is both an artist and a person living with Crohn's disease, but her interest in faecal transplants is more conceptual than medical – she has never actually done a transplant because she believes the health benefits may be temporary (Interview with the artist 2022). Yet High's work makes tangible the complex forms of knowing *beyond representation* that take shape when people enter microbial dialogues, both as art practice and everyday health practice. As such, it offers a rich starting point for curating with guts. The field of medical humanities offers a supportive ground for future development of this curatorial project, allowing for a sometimes awkward, but often productive entanglement between different fields and practices.

Note: The author would like to thank collaborator and project co-lead Dr Rachel Marsden, and all of the interview participants.

References

Arnold, K., et al. (2021), 'Museum as Academy: Research Practices at Copenhagen's Medical Museion', *The Garage Journal* (3): 52–81.

Barone, T., and E. W. Eisner (2012) *Arts Based Research*. LA: Sage.

Bartlett, V. (2020), 'Psychosocial curating: A theory and practice of exhibition-making at the intersection between health and aesthetics', *Medical Humanities*, 46 (4): 417–30.

Bartlett, V. (2023), *Stomach Ache: An Arts-led Exploration of the Gastrointestinal System. Project Report*, Melbourne: University of Melbourne.

Beck, A. (2021), 'Microbiomes as companion species: An exploration of dis- and re-entanglements with the microbial self', *Social & Cultural Geography*, 22 (3): 357–75.

Bencard, A., L. Whiteley and C. H. Thon (2019), 'Curating experimental entanglements', in M. V. Hansen, A. F. Henningsen, and A. Gregersen (eds), *Curatorial Challenges*, 133–46, London: Routledge.

Benezra, A. (2023), *Gut Anthro: An Experiment in Thinking with Microbes*, Minneapolis: University of Minnesota Press.

Bishop, C. (2012), *Artificial Hells: Participatory Art and the Politics of Spectatorship*, London: Verso.

Black, C. J., D. A. Drossman, N. J. Talley, J. Ruddy and A. C. Ford (2020), 'Functional Gastrointestinal Disorders: Advances in Understanding and Management', Lancet (London, England), 396: 1664–74.

Chatterjee, H., and G. Noble (2016), *Museums and Wellbeing*, London: Routledge.

Dryden, J. (2023), 'The Gut Microbiome and the Imperative of Normalcy', *IJFAB: International Journal of Feminist Approaches to Bioethics*, 16 (1): 131–62.

El-Omar, E. M. (2023) 'Future directions in the microbiome field: An editor's perspective', *eGastroenterology*, 1(1). Available at: https://doi.org/10.1136/egastro-2023-100003.

Farrokhyar, F., E. T. Swarbrick and E. J. Irvine (2001), 'A critical review of epidemiological studies in inflammatory bowel disease', *Scandinavian Journal of Gastroenterology*, 36 (1): 2–15.

Fasano, A., and S. Flaherty (2021), *Gut Feelings: The Microbiome and Our Health*, Cambridge, MA: MIT Press.

Fitzgerald, D. and F. Callard (2016), 'Entangling the Medical Humanities', in A. Whitehead, A. Woods, S. Atkinson, J. Macnaughton and J. Richards (eds), *The Edinburgh Companion to the Critical Medical Humanities*, Edinburgh: Edinburgh University Press.

Frank, A. W. (1995), *The Wounded Storyteller: Body, Illness & Ethics*, Chicago: University of Chicago Press.
French, J. (2020), *Inclusive Curating in Contemporary Art: A Practical Guide*, new edn, Leeds: Arc Humanities Press.
Haraway, D. (2008), *When Species Meet*, Minneapolis: University of Minnesota Press.
Hauser, J. (2022), 'Toward a "Bacterial Turn", in Art, Architecture and Design', *CCCB LAB: Cultural Research and Innovation*, 28 September. Available at: https://lab.cccb.org/en/toward-a-bacterial-turn-in-art-architecture-and-design/
Hermon, R. (2022), 'I Care By … ', in G. Blackshaw, N. Heidorn, R. Hermon, S. Baluch and M. Fraser (eds), *I Care By …*, 63–65, London, UK: Royal College of Art.
High, K. (2019), 'Ways In? Processing Messages Received', *Public: Art, Culture, Ideas*, 59: 61–71.
High, Kathy (2015). *Kathy As Bowie*, photographic prints.
High, Kathy (2022). Interview with author.
Hooker, C. (2014), 'Ethics and the Arts in the Medical Humanities', in P. Macneill (ed.), *Ethics and the Arts*, 213–24, Dordrecht: Springer Netherlands.
Johnstone, F. (2023), 'Collaborations in art and medicine: Institutional critique, patient participation, and emerging entanglements', *Leonardo* [Preprint]. Available at: https://direct.mit.edu/leon (Accessed 12 May 2023).
Kelley, L. (2023), *After Eating: Metabolizing the Arts*, Cambridge, MA: MIT Press.
Kolářová, K., T. Stöckelová and L. Senft (2023), 'Disability and the (dysbiotic) gut: Sensing, tasting and knowing with food', *Sociology of Health & Illness*, 45 (6): 1242–58.
Lazard, C. (2017), *How to Be a Person in the Age of Autoimmunity*, Project Row Houses. Available at: https://projectrowhouses.org/howtobeapersonintheageofautoimmunity/ (Accessed 1 October 2024).
Lillemose, J., and A. Bencard (2022), 'Embracing the Complex and the Unfinished', in A. Bencard et al. (eds), *The World is in You*. Medical Museion and Department of Public Health, University of Copenhagen.
Mannix, L. (2019), *Be nice to your gut microbes, says new exhibit, so they'll be nice to you. The Age*. Available at: https://www.theage.com.au/national/victoria/be-nice-to-your-gut-microbes-says-new-exhibit-so-they-be-nice-to-you-20190318-p5156g.html (Accessed 16 October 2023).
Manzoni, P. (1961) *Artist's Shit*. Tin can, printed paper and excrement.
Medvecky, F., and J. Leach (2019), *An Ethics of Science Communication*, Cham: Springer.
Muller, L. and C. S. Langill (2021) *Curating Lively Objects: Exhibitions Beyond Disciplines*. 1st edn. London: Routledge.
Muñoz, B. R., ed. (2020), *Health*, Cambridge, MA: MIT Press.
Museums Victoria (2019), *Meet your microbes!, Museums Victoria*. Available at: https://museumsvictoria.com.au/media-releases/meet-your-microbes/ (Accessed 16 October 2023).
Nakazawa, D. J. (2008), *The Autoimmune Epidemic: Bodies Gone Haywire in a World Out of Balance – and the Cutting-Edge Science that Promises Hope*, New York: Simon and Schuster.
Sharma, S., L. Sainte-Marie and L. Fournier (2020), 'Antinomies of Self Care', in B. R. Muñoz (ed.), *Health*, 147–50, London: Cambridge, MA: MIT Press.

Sheikh, S. (2015), 'Toward the Exhibition as Research', in P. O'Neill and M. Wilson (eds), *Curating Research*, 32–46, Amsterdam: Open Editions.
Spence, J. ([1988] 2020), 'The Picture of Health', in B. R. Muñoz (ed.), *Health*, 98–103, Cambridge, MA: MIT Press.
Sperber, A. D., S. I. Bangdiwala, et al. (2021), 'Worldwide Prevalence and Burden of Functional Gastrointestinal Disorders, Results of Rome Foundation Global Study', *Gastroenterology*, 160 (1): 99–114.e3.
Stone, L., and C. Hooker (2021), 'Medically unexplained symptoms and the ethics of diagnosis: What does it mean when the doctor says there's nothing wrong?', in C.-A. Farkas (ed.), *Reading the Psychosomatic in Medical and Popular Culture*, London: Routledge.
Thompson, J. (2022), *Care Aesthetics: For Artful Care and Careful Art*, London: Routledge.
Trounson, A. (2020), 'How Treating Gut Disorders Needs to Be a Team Effort', *Pursuit*, 15 July. Available at: https://pursuit.unimelb.edu.au/articles/how-treating-gut-disorders-needs-to-be-a-team-effort.
Ukeles, M. L. (1969), 'MANIFESTO FOR MAINTENANCE ART, 1969! Proposal for an exhibition'. Available at: https://feldmangallery.com/exhibition/manifesto-for-maintenance-art-1969 (Accessed 30 May 2024).
Vasey, G. (2020), 'Misbehaving Bodies: exhibiting illness', *Science Museum Group Journal*, (14). Available at: https://dx.doi.org/10.15180/201402/001.
Wilson, E. A. (2015), *Gut Feminism*, Durham: Duke University Press. https://doi.org/10.1215/9780822375203.
Woods, A. (2011), 'The limits of narrative: Provocations for the medical humanities', *Medical Humanities*, 37 (2): 73–78.
Yong, E. (2017), *I Contain Multitudes: The Microbes Within Us and A Grander View of Life*, London: Penguin Random House.

CHAPTER TWO

After images: technologies of the body and the archive

Silvia Casini and Ilona Sagar

In this dialogue, researcher-curator Silvia Casini and researcher-artist Ilona Sagar explore the concept of the after image as a method for valuing research materials beyond their objective and operational functions. Whether in the trace left in an archive, the production of medical diagnostic images, or the realization of architectural plans, the after image represents the residual imprint left when a body is passed through an observational technology. Rather than offering a conventional chronological history of Sagar's practice, this conversation focuses on key works such as *The Body Blow* (2022), with further reference to *Deep Structure* (2019) and *Correspondence O* (2018). Engaging with the power of images, archives, and collaborative knowledge-making, Sagar's practice weaves together archival materials, expert and lived experiences, quantitative data, and techniques from both documentary and experimental filmmaking traditions. Drawing on the conceptual and material coordinates offered by literature in the medical humanities, science and technology studies, and critical theory, Casini and Sagar address the principles of co-enquiry, the role of lived experience in research and the language of risk, care and maintenance. At the core of their exchange is the question of whose bodies matter and for whom.

Silvia Casini (SC): Why keep making images in a world already saturated by them? Some encounters with images can re-open the entire field of our experience, making us question the modalities of our apprehension and ways of seeing, even prompting us to action. After all, an image can save the world and not merely diagnose it, as the great film theorist Nicole Brenez once stated.[1]

Images do not simply represent things, but they *happen*, they intervene between us and the world, they work on us, and they sometimes stay with us – as after images.

This dialogue is critical *and* personal; not a literal, chronological history of your work, Ilona, but a tapestry of lines and intensities. Our dialogue starts, for me, with a precise memory and an indefinite after image inextricably woven together. First, our encounter at the Wellcome Collection in London after I saw your two-channel moving-image installation *Correspondence O* (2018) and, then, the memory of a series of almost imperceptible gestures and movements occurring across the two screens: a hand scratching the back of the neck, the absorbed glance of a young woman looking through a transparent building, hands pulling on a rope. But this is not a series of still images that can serve as a hinge or as a fixed reference to a concept or to an object. They are images that come *after*.

Back then I was doing research for my book on biomedical imaging technologies and art practices. *Correspondence O*, which was part of the exhibition *Living with Buildings* (2018–19), anchors the exploration of the private body carried out by medical imaging to discourses and practices of public/private health that occurred in certain spaces such as the Pioneer Health Centre in Peckham in England. *Correspondence O* struck me for how it placed imaging technologies such as Magnetic Resonance Imaging (MRI) and Light Detection and Ranging (LiDAR) into a wider infrastructural network of exchanges between bodies, technologies, scientific procedures, and medical archives. It left me wondering to whose bodies I was given partial access: that of a building, that of a woman, that of an archive. Our conversation continues as does our commitment to collaborate further, especially since both our work trajectories, albeit in different ways, are informed by methods that foreground lived experience, processes of co-enquiry, and techniques of re-igniting life into archives.

Ilona Sagar (IS): I think what you're drawing on here is our shared interest in exploring the materiality of the body and its mediation within a wider sociological and technological context. Your book *Giving Bodies Back to Data* (2021a) is a significant contribution to the discourse surrounding the instrumentation of optical images and functional image-making, considering how such embodied and situated technologies render the invisible aspects of the body visible. Machinic eyes penetrate the world and see better than

[1]Brenez's words come from the documentary film *Experimental Conversations* (2006), written and directed by Fergus Daly. The film features well-known filmmakers and critics including Nicole Brenez, Philippe Grandrieux, F. J. Ossang, Maeve Connolly, Grace Weir, Clare Langan, Gerard Byrne, Vivienne Dick, and Maximilian Le Cain. *Experimental Conversations* highlights the fact that experimental cinema can be an aesthetic and philosophical international dialogue.

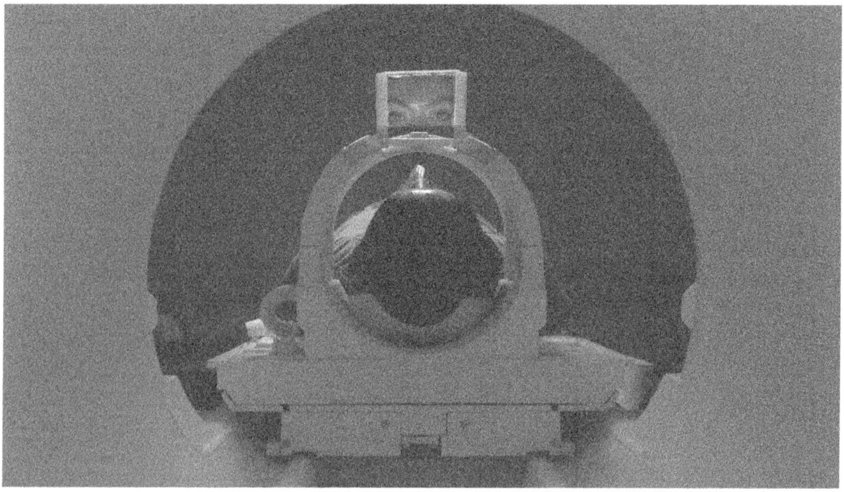

FIGURE 2.1 Ilona Sagar, *Correspondence O*, 2018. HD digital film, dual-screen, stereo sound (still, courtesy of author).

us and without us. This is not only a question of optical penetration, but of social materiality and agency. Who is being watched and what is the apparatus of the observer? Scientific vision and data aesthetics should not be understood as factums of truth but as practices that muddy the dichotomy between private and public space. That is to say, the actions of being counted and accounted for articulate a regime of publicness defined and re-defined by our systemic visibility within its social and scientific observational structures.

SC: I remember attending a talk you gave at S1 ArtSpace in Sheffield connected to another work of yours, *Deep Structure* (2019), a film and exhibition which explores connections between architecture, health and community wellbeing on Sheffield's Park Hill Estate. One of the most unusual aspects of Park Hill's design process was the emphasis placed on the residents themselves. The planners encouraged social interaction and uniquely involved tenants within a closely observed consultation throughout the design process and the building's initial use. The film uses scanning, spatial analysis techniques and psychosocial data sets from the Park Hill archives to unpick the ways in which buildings and bodies are surveilled, both through official bureaucratic structures and shared social experiences. The application of algorithms and data visualization becomes a mode of navigation within the film, and reflects how scientific reasoning is authored and inscribed into both the body and civic systems.

IS: I'm glad you mentioned the talk series at S1 ArtSpace, as it feels particularly pertinent here. 'What is it to count and to be counted?' is a provocation Professor Alex Taylor made to me during one of three open panel discussions I brought together around the exhibition of *Deep Structure* (2019). Taylor's question riffs on feminist geographer Joni Seager's 'What gets counted counts' (Seager 2016). Modes of collecting and counting are rendered into visual languages, charts, tables, maps, and other forms of representation that catalogue and order through technical means. Data, both digital and analogue, has a weight, it can be generated, classified and archived, but it always refers to something outside of itself: publics, places, events, figures silhouetted behind their statistical quantification. Data images become instruments, interfaces, a porous skin between the subject of monitored regulation and their quantifiable visualization, allowing the boundaries between image, representation and archives to blur.

SC: And, yet, you always manage to avoid fetishizing technologies. In your work technologies become tools for navigating through or folding in different histories and spaces, both public and private. This reminds me of the strategies of the artist Camille Henrot in her work *Grosse Fatigue* (2013), a video in which the artist's gesture of mining archives and their taxonomies builds a fictional but plausible origin story about the creation of the universe, blending scientific histories with narratives from different knowledge systems such as anthropology, the history of technology, and ethnography. You activate a wide range of sources (among others, material from archives, qualitative data coming from lived experience of people you collaborate with, statistics). Although your works cannot be labelled as 'films', you employ techniques proper to the expanded cinema tradition, for example by pushing the relationship between the audience and the multiple screens you often use in your installations. What are the challenges and the opportunities of combining such a wide range of sources and methods?

IS: It's interesting that you are reluctant to name my work 'film' as I also struggle to find a comfortable label for what I do. My practice, my writing, and the discursive space between the two activate film as a site of mediation, channelling different knowledges and situated relationships that allow for exchange and dialogue with different experiences and expertise. By involving co-participants, expert opinions, and a variety of perspectives, a dialogue results that isn't only a method of accumulating research material, but a mode of producing a pluralistic position and narrative. A former resident of Park Hill Estate who I worked with on *Deep Structure* (2019) suggested 'that this way of working isn't documentary, it's about a collective gut reaction, it's a feeling of a place, it's the stuff you can't say that's felt rather than spoken about'. What they described was a process, less about an emphatic certainty, than a shared navigation of a subject that was physically felt, an act of tapping on things and seeing what bounces back. This sentiment resonated powerfully with me as it perfectly describes how I approach these sites, their significance, their wholeness and complexity, negotiated in an embodied way, a felt way, an unfixed and unsettled experience of a place. My approach to moving-image transmits ideas not through the continuity of images, objectivity, and notions of impartiality, but among the interwoven gaps between image, voice, audience and material. I consider how these histories, knowledges and lived experiences might spatially intersect. A collective searching out of different ways to destabilize or entangle how a topic might be understood, complicates an official narrative that might exist around a place, its ideology and archival imprint. The gallery space and exhibition of the work takes on an active role. This splitting of the subject relies on viewer participation to make meaning from the assemblage, the viewer spatially engaged in the film. The films become part of an environment that invites the audience to extend and challenge ideas articulated within the exhibition space. The moment of display becomes constituent to knowledge creation through its activation rather than a summative instant of presentation. This is not a curatorial process, but engrained into how the works are formed and developed through my relationship with everyone who has contributed to these projects.

SC: As a scholar and a curator, I often question my own subject position in collaborations with scientists and artists. How can one avoid an extractive relationship to knowledge from the 'field' of enquiry and from collaborators' lived experiences? Reflecting on my own role in art-science projects (Casini 2021b), I embraced Donna Haraway's ironical concept of the 'modest witness' (Haraway 1997), which revisits Shapin and Schaffer's concept of witnessing (Shapin and Schaffer 1985). In their text the (male) witness was the guarantor of the experiment's objectivity, the neutral conduit of nature's alleged objective meanings without interfering with any of these meanings with his views or with his body. As Haraway highlights, however, the scientist's desire to give up all claims to power and authority as objective observers of the world is exactly what gives them this power. The question of who gets to speak and who is considered a reliable witness informs how you remediate the voices, experiences, and bodies foregrounded in your work.

IS: I am interested in the hybrid language that is developed by working outside my practice. What new knowledges are created in those intersections? A significant aspect of my practice is the broad cross-disciplinary dialogue generated through collaboration with a range of people with lived experience of a place or situation, architects, material scientists, neurologists, human-computer interaction designers, medical professionals, social workers. This mode of working creates a space for me to experimentally mediate multiple perspectives, applying their experience, techniques, technologies and discourse as tools to navigate the subject of focus. I attempt to understand positions of knowledge within a network of expertise. I do not work with specific groups or practitioners at the instruction of an institution or in a way that is conditional to funding requirements. I find the people I work with through a process of research and encounter that begins with the site, its conditions, its archives, its current usages, and then spirals out into a wider, more sprawling network of connections. It's a process of finding the gaps, wondering how someone else's perspective might collide with another's, testing or confronting the site in unexpected ways. It is a more intimate process than only seeking out people that 'represent' a type of knowledge – a neuroscientist, a resident, an architectural historian – but finding personal connections with people who are open to a process that is malleable and fluid. This is a move away from participatory modes of art making where invited participants are asked to respond to a fixed brief demarcated by the artist, its success driven by demonstrable outcomes. To dodge the extractive optics of collaboration, co-enquiry feels a more fitting way to describe the types of exchanges central to my methodology and practice. The methods I have developed are not grounded in the optics of collaboration or a visual expectation of how these situated knowledges should be presented, they hold a spatial and material physicality. As an artist, I am not placed to illustrate the work of the contributor and the contributor is not placed to serve my concepts. This practice of co-enquiry enables me to skew the hierarchical importance of my eye as an artist, forming relationships that allow for other means of thinking and becoming together. This mode of work is a slow process of finding the slippery languages and common desires in the space between disciplines and lived experience. For these forms of working together to take place there needs to be a shared openness to 'not knowing', a meaningful, common space of enquiry between the questions of the researcher and the questions posed by the artist. Assembling layers of professional and lived experience acts as a refusal of finite narrative, instead addressing the entwined resonances of a subject. I don't categorize these types of co-enquiry and exchange as holding separate values within the work, but they are given equal weight.

SC: Critical medical humanities scholarship interested in visuality has thought through some of these issues. Johnstone (2023), for example, has recently interrogated the genealogy and process of collaboration in sci-art and arts and health collaborative projects. She highlights how art making is a knowledge-production activity and discusses the challenges of involving patients as co-participants. The critical medical humanities have long foregrounded the value of 'experimentation, reflective practice, collaboration and modes of sceptically risky thinking' (Viney, Callard and Woods 2015: 4). Artists, though, can further ground in practice what, otherwise, risks remaining too abstract and not conducive to any visible change. Can you expand on how you co-design a collaborative methodology?

IS: It's fascinating to consider how artists might bridge the gap between the abstract and the tangible. Yet, in assessing the success of approaches, we run the risk of problematically conforming the measurement of outcomes to a scientific standard that prevents a richer, more complex value being placed on these hybrid knowledges. I would resist modes of collaboration that render art an application of theory, the artist merely a didactic illustrator of scientific knowledge or a tool for public outreach; rather, collaboration must recognize art as a method of knowledge-production that allows for a subversion of scientific reasoning.

To return to a phrase I introduced earlier in this discussion – it is in the 'not knowing' that artists and scientists find common ground. 'Not knowing' is descriptive of a gap, an undetermined and unnamed space that connects the site of knowledge to a shared vulnerability and willingness to not know, to work alongside, to search out and undo received knowledges. This approach can be found in the shared moments that happen with neuroscientist Professor Paul Fletcher and architectural surveyor, Tom Bell in *Correspondence O* (2018), or with Professor Laura Vaughan's Space Syntax investigations and my work with residents of Park Hill Estate and material scientist Professor John Provis in *Deep Structure* (2019). This is a way of working that doesn't seek to reproduce a known participatory power dynamic, one where the artist enforces a perspective on another, whether they are a community collaborator or a professional discipline. Instead, I set out to find a shared language that sits in between. These methods present an opportunity to understand co-enquiry as a shared space between approaches to a subject. My relationship with collaborators isn't about illustrating an idea or extracting from them but producing a shared navigation of the subject of the work.

SC: Your creative works often entail a morphological understanding of archives which implies considering archives as organisms. Goethe coined the term 'morphology' in 1797 to describe the science which illustrates and makes testable the processes of formation and transformation of organisms under certain conditions. When studying the metamorphic processes in plants, Goethe investigated the conditions under which the formation of leaves made possible the appearance of a specific plant. It is a process whereby a certain matter acquires a new form (Goethe 2000: 32–37). The task of morphology was to provide a depiction of life phenomena: it was more about presenting than explaining a phenomenon. One could say that archives should not be conceived of as repositories of dead objects waiting to be brought back to life, but as the secretions of living bodies.

IS: Your reference to Goethe's concept of morphology is a compelling entry point for rethinking the ontology of archives. By situating archival material not as static residues but as dynamic forms undergoing continual transformation, we begin to perceive archives less as containers of fixed memory and more as sites of living processes, subject to conditions, environments, and temporalities that shape their emergence and expression. Described by English historian Vivian Hunter Galbraith in 1948 as `the secretions of an organism' (1948), a form of embodied transmission whose peripheries are vague and malleable. Archives are not static: they are living, shifting, visceral and morphological spaces that operate as intersections. They have 'limits', 'impulses', and 'fevers', 'constituting' the boundaries of the archive as distinct, but volatile (Mbembe 2002; Foster 2004; Derrida 1995; Enwezor 2008). There has always been a temptation to hermetically protect historical material to guard against the fear of cross-contamination, solidifying its identity and defending a definitive narrative. My work isn't about reanimating the archive, nor is it a testimonial, an urge to physically resurrect a particular historical moment. Instead, I am attempting to acknowledge its liveness and to reopen the questions that it poses. This conception of the livingness of archives resonates closely with Stuart Hall, who considers the constituting of an archive away from the 'dead works' of museums, instead seeing them as 'on-going, never completed project[s]' (Hall 2001: 89). Within my own practice I explore the idea that a fragmentary approach to archives might not be a process of fictioning, a romantic longing for what is lost, but rather a transgressive platforming of present-day knowledges, situated within the debris of those materials, addressing questions that such archives ask outside the institutional frames of the museum and civic collection that otherwise could not be asked of them.

SC: You intertwine different layers of temporalities in your work, for example by engaging closely with both archival material and cutting-edge operational images such as medical diagnostic tools. For instance, in the multi-channel installation *The Body Blow* (2022),[2] you reactivate operational images from surgical and radiological procedures editing them with clips from mesothelioma research and archival sources to explore how the historical legacy of asbestos continues to have a devastating health impact. I am bringing the topic of operational images into our conversation for the medical humanities seem to struggle to engage 'hand-to-hand', so to speak, with images, particularly technical and operational ones, following the example set by scholars in image-science (Bredekamp et al. 2015), media archaeologists (Parikka 2023) and artists (Farocki 2001). Operational images do not represent an object; they are made neither to entertain nor to inform, but they serve specialized tasks and are made by and for machines. Operational images embody a nuanced relationship with temporality as they concern the present, the past (memory, the archive), and the future (operational images as forecasting systems). With these images,

[2]*The Body Blow* (2022) was commissioned by Serpentine Gallery for 'Radio Ballads', a project which explored labour and care, alongside other artwork by Sonia Boyce, Helen Cammock and Rory Pilgrim.

the human fields of perception and action become embedded with those of the nonhuman, alternating instances of human looking with all the nuances of the term (glimpse, glance, peek, gaze, stare) with automated, machinic processes of 'looking for', a goal-oriented type of vision. Operational images do not quite make the human eye anachronistic as Farocki implied, rather they encapsulate all the actions and structures that enable – or not – human and non-human bodies to operate, often in synergy.

IS: Are there other ways to comprehend the value of nonhuman ways of seeing that antagonize their social, historical and embodied application? This question seems to be at the forefront of both of our research. Something that has preoccupied me across a number of different projects is thinking about how we encounter different kinds of technical images as agents themselves. Jussi Parikka extends the notion of the operational image suggesting it 'ties to infrastructures, logistics, and all manner of actions that function to sustain, mobilize, analyze, and synthesize the thing we have grown to call "images"' (2022). By delving into the peripheries and limitations of human vision and technology, I find that new, transgressive, machinic possibilities develop outside their original purpose. I became very interested in the perceived objectivity of technical images when in fact they can be incredibly subjective. How we understand sight in the context of observation, objectivity and analysis highlights 'the complexity and complicity of vision, the differences for example, between looking, glancing, seeing and staring, and about the social and historical nature of sight' (Cosgrove 2008: 5). For me, the relationship between the camera eye and the embodied space of film has the potential to open up different encounters between visuality and corporeality, between time and tense, the felt and representational.

The collision between apparatus and subject are what constitutes the material of my practice, the result of the networked act of editing, making and discussion, opened out into the public forum of the exhibition. The spectator extends, complicates, and aggregates the meaning of these laden phrases and interactions. By employing the vision technologies enfolded into my practice beyond their intended application, such as LiDAR, MRI, microimaging and Space Syntax, I make them intelligible in specific ways – opening up different encounters with these ways of surveying or analysing societal, bodily space that doesn't render my use of data aesthetics as only poetic, but keeps them critically alive. The computative potential of such technical images not only extends the eye but generates spatial testimonies. In previous works, I explore the ideological implications of spatial conditions as an observational instrument. In *The Body Blow*, this understanding of observable bodies and archives is extended through the techniques of the survey as a diagnostic tool that drives a solutionist approach to complex social problems, considering the cumulative effect such methods of surveying have on the bodies they organize. Such encounters with technical images, then became a way to value them outside of their objective and operational function. The survey, the body and its attendant technologies become key tools to test and provoke the boundaries active within the archive, between observed and observer, body and building, modernity and obsolescence.

When we linger with material, analyze its directions and pull apart its structures, new figures appear. Data bodies, social bodies and individual bodies are entwined and interdependent, through a long history of civic analysis and attempts at quantification with both progressive and repressive potential. The social and spatial conditions of the body are not positioned in my work as a categorical object, separate 'to' the historical subject of research. The distinctions and relation between personal experience entwines with the archive and the historical subject: this exposes archives not as hypothetical abstractions confined to institutions, but something to be worked through the body.

I am interested in the schism, the sense of loss, those silent figures locked in table data and statistical charts, bodies hidden behind the data they generate. These figures don't haunt us, but become visible in the burning glow of their after image. An after image does not produce meaning in and of itself, but always refers to an image from elsewhere, the retinal intensity that is seared into the eye by staring at images for far too long. The after image becomes a way to think about the subjectivity found in our encounter with these research materials, a way to value them outside of their objective and operational function.

SC: In *The Body Blow* (2022) the bodies of workers, end-of-life carers, and medical and legal professionals are intertwined with words taken from fragments of conversations, legal texts, and archival materials. The film seems to emerge out of the coordinates represented by the concepts

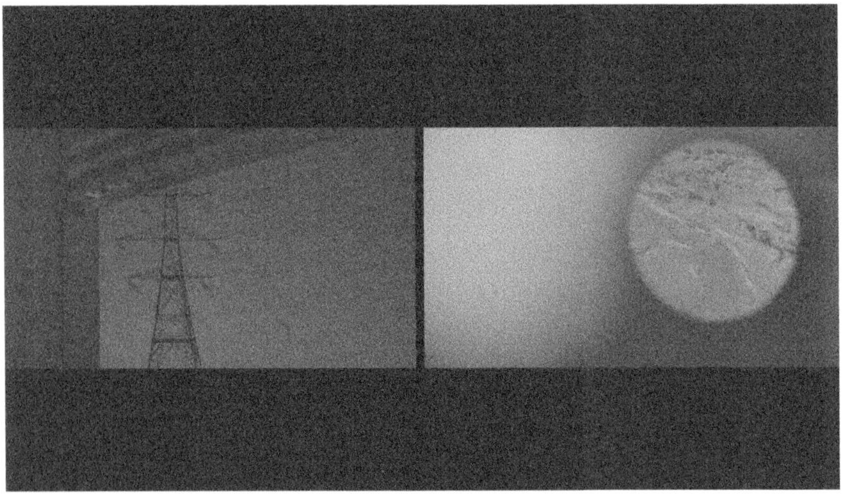

FIGURE 2.2 Ilona Sagar, *The Body Blow*, 2022. 4K digital film, dual-screen, stereo sound (still, courtesy of author).

of the body-as-archive (Sekula 1986) and the body-as-capital (Bourdieu 1978, 1986); that is, the body conceived as a place of investment whereby a wide variety of behaviours and health practices are understood as assets. This second concept is important to work that critically interrogates the relationship between bodies and media in the medical humanities. Bonah and Laukötter (2020), for example, have carried out historiographical research on health-related issues by treating moving images as a performative corpus of historical sources that can inform understandings of bodily perceptions and practices in a different, perhaps deeper way than written sources alone. *The Body Blow* (2022) is situated within a genealogy of works showing the performative power of visual media and its entanglement with the body-as-capital.

IS: *The Body Blow* (2022) was developed through long-term collaboration with those with lived experience of asbestos cancers, social workers, end-of-life carers, asbestos removal experts, campaigners, medical and legal professionals. Focused on ideas of 'acceptable bodily risk', the film considers what risk means in the context of care, work and our health, reflecting on how health inequalities are enmeshed within work and the built environment.

Sufferers of mesothelioma or asbestos exposure are stuck between different layers of legal and bureaucratic languages, from the benefits and welfare system and medical treatment through to the legislative frameworks of litigation and law. Many are navigating complex compensation claims, constantly confronting the various ways their bodies are framed within these contexts.

Throughout the project I worked closely with lawyers and solicitors who defend those who experience asbestos exposure. I came across the types of quantification and statistical analysis that they use in their work to fight on behalf of claimants, such as *Kemp & Kemp: Quantum of Damages* and the book of general damages which are annually updated with data from the Office for National Statistics. The actions of being counted and accounted for allows body parts to be financially evaluated: risk is measured depending on several factors including life expectancy, age, level of education, and type of employment. This becomes your body's dissected value. The way that we imagine data is as something objective and emotionless; a good data set is assumed to eliminate 'human error'. But I would argue this is anything but the case. This abstraction of bodies into simple categories of data captures the individual as a measurable, computable currency. This does not necessarily enable a deeper understanding of our world or result in greater freedoms; rather, it has the potential to become the apparatus of a different means of power, a form of embodied citizenship which makes the body an object of political and economic control.

Historically in the UK the people who were exposed to asbestos were in traditionally working-class jobs: factory workers, dock yard workers and

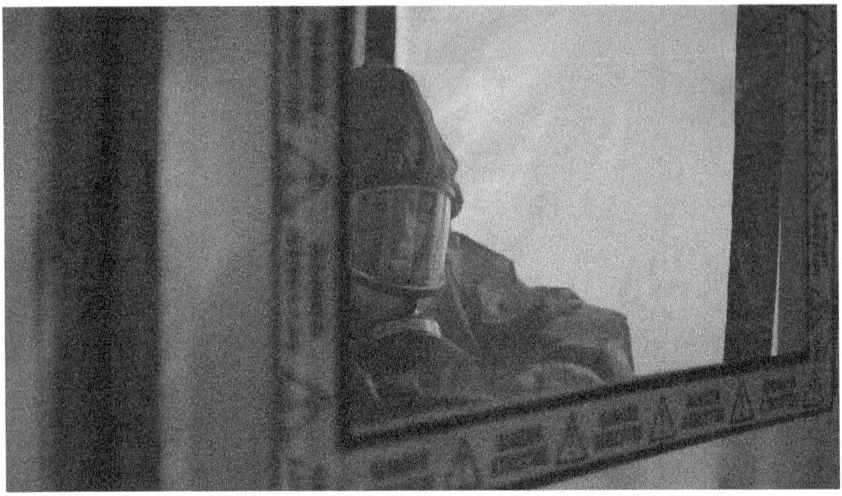

FIGURE 2.3 Ilona Sagar, *The Body Blow*, 2022. 4K digital film, dual-screen, stereo sound (still, courtesy of author).

laggers. Outside the UK it was miners and their families in countries such as South Africa where the asbestos mineral was extracted. Asbestos was banned in the UK in 1999, but it remains embedded in housing estates, post-war council properties, schools, hospitals and waste grounds. Now it's illegal, it's the people who remove it who are exposed: construction workers, site foremen, plumbers, electricians and asbestos removal workers. The ongoing crisis of asbestos is related to the invisibility of those voices. It's that idea that's really key to this project; who is allowed to be exposed to risk and how is risk quantified? Whose bodies matter and how do they matter?

SC: This is a matter of bodies and privilege, of whose bodies become visible and whose bodies fade into the background. In *The Body Blow* (2022) medical and legal professionals help workers with asbestos-related illnesses navigate the complex language of bureaucratic papers required to obtain economic compensation and/or care support. Viewers are exposed to images, gestures and words that have to do with care practices. Naive understandings of care as based exclusively on the individual or on affectivity have since long been challenged by scholars working across medical humanities and science and technology studies. Care and technology are not opposite terms: care is no other to technology but includes it, whether we understand technology as highly complex imaging-generating techniques or language itself as a form of technology (Mol, Moser and Pol 2010).

In the context of my work on biomedical imaging technologies, I foregrounded the importance of attending to the complex machineries built to diagnose patients. Ensuring the accurate functioning of a machine across time (maintenance) is a way of anticipating the patient's body and of expanding care work outside and beyond the clinical encounter (Casini 2023). It seems to me you are also interested in expanding beyond care, for example by paying attention to the protocols that ensure the proper functioning of a machine, or to the correct understanding and navigation of bureaucratic procedures that guarantee workers to have their rights respected.

IS: I worked very closely throughout the project with a group primarily of women, who work with people who have been exposed to asbestos, as well as directly with people with asbestos-related cancers. I think what I found most surprising about the project was the interdependent web of care that asbestos and its administration exposes through differing governing structures in ways that aren't immediately obvious: social workers, end-of-life carers, coroners, legal professionals, campaigners, the unnamed and limitless care of partners, families and kin. Care is material, a constellation of physically designed and planned decisions. It sits between the soft effects of an infrastructure of emotional and moral relationships to an economy of material and practical forces. Care becomes an ecosystem, an infrastructure. Social and personal care zoom in and out at different scales from one body, to communities, civic systems, infrastructural bodies and societies. That's why asbestos is so devastating as a way to antagonize systems of care because it slices through them in such violent ways.

Care is often talked about in very individualized terms: 'maintenance' describes an idea of care that is more networked and transgressive. Within my practice, I have found 'maintenance' helpful in articulating acts of care, attention, inspection, and acknowledging, that connects materiality with archives, on a collective rather than individual level. As time moves and agendas change, so too does what is being maintained. From the body, its clinical treatment and self-care to public infrastructure, 'maintenance' was a terminology that made these conditions and their historical underpinning live.

SC: I think the critical medical humanities ought to pay attention to the nuanced relationship between care and maintenance in the network of bodies and technologies. Bodies, language, and technology are attuned to one another, and they are part of the same infrastructure.

IS: Maintenance is done in dialogue with others, it's an activity that acknowledges our interdependency. Maintenance is the inverse of wilful neglect; it highlights a choice to uphold something. That might be a belief system or the physical structure of a building – do we ideologically invest in something or not? Whose life will be protected and maintained and whose will be collateral? I think these questions are painfully apparent in our present: we are revealed as infrastructural, networked and socially seen bodies. What I do is a different kind of care and attendance to these complex physical and bodily histories, that does not seek to restore, but asks questions of what is allowed to be maintained, what survives and is valued.

References

Bonah, C., and A. Laukötter, eds. (2020), *Body, Capital and Screens: Visual Media and the Healthy Self in the 20th Century*, Amsterdam: Amsterdam University Press.

Bourdieu, P. (1986), 'The Forms of Capital', in J. G. Richardson (ed.), *Handbook of Theory and Research for the Sociology of Education*, in 241–58, New York, NY: Greenwood Press.

Bourdieu, P. (1978), 'Sport and Social Class', *Social Science Information*, 17(6): 819–40.

Bredekamp, H., V. Dunkel and B. Schneider, eds. (2015), *The Technical Image: A History of Styles in Scientific Imagery*, Chicago: University of Chicago Press.

Casini, S. (2021a), *Giving Bodies back to Data. Image-makers, Bricolage, and Reinvention in Magnetic Resonance Technology*, Cambridge MA: MIT Press.

Casini, S. (2021b), 'What Counts as Data and for Whom? The Role of the Modest Witness in Art-Science Collaboration', in H. S. Rogers, M. K. Halpern, D. Hannah, and K. de Ridder-Vignone (eds), *Routledge Handbook of Art, Science, and Technology Studies*, 49–62, London and New York: Routledge.

Casini, S. (2023) 'Visibilizing the Patient's Body through Anticipation. A Matter of Care', *Reti, Saperi, Linguaggi. Italian Journal of Cognitive Sciences*, 24(2), 291–311.

Cosgrove, D. (2008), *Geography and Vision: Seeing, Imagining and Representing the World*. New York: Bloomsbury.

Derrida, J. (1995), 'Archive Fever: A Freudian Impression', *Diacritics*, 25(2): 9–63.

Enwezor, O. (2008), *Archive Fever: Photography Between History and the Monument*. Göttingen, Germany: Copublished by the International Center of Photography, New York, and Steidl Publishers.

Farocki, H. (2001), *Eye / Machine I* (original German title: *Auge / Maschine I*), two-channel video part of the thrilogy *Eye / Machine*. Germany, colour, sound, 25 min.

Foster, H. (2004), 'An Archival Impulse', *October*, 110: 3–22.

Galbraith, V. H. (1948), Studies in the Public Records. London: T. Nelson and Sons, p. 3.

Goethe, J. W. Von (2000), *Werke*, München, Hamburger Ausgabe: DTV.

Hall, S. (2001), 'Constituting an archive'. *Third Text*, 15(54): 89–92.

Haraway, D. (1997), *Modest_Witness@Second_Millennium. FemaleMan©_Meets_OncoMouse[a]: Feminism and Technoscience*, New York and London: Routledge.

Henrot, C. (2013), *Grosse Fatigue*, high-definition video, Paris, colour, sound, 13 min.

Johnstone, F. (2023), 'Collaborations in Art and Medicine: Institutional Critique, Patient Participation, and Emerging Entanglements', *Leonardo* 56(4): 424–29.

Mbembe, A. (2002), *The Power of the Archive and its Limits*. Cape Town: New Africa Books.
Mol, A., I. Moser and J. Pols, eds. (2010), *Care in Practice. On Tinkering in Clinics, Homes and Farms*, Bielefeld: Transcript Verlag.
Parikka, J. (2023), *Operational Images. From the Visual to the Invisual*, Michigan: University of Minnesota Press.
Parikka, J. (2022), *Operational Images – Preface in the forthcoming book*. [Online] Available at: https://jussiparikka.net/2022/02/16/operational-images-preface-in-the-forthcoming-book/ [Accessed 10 May 2022].
Seager, J. (2016), *Missing Women, Blank Maps, and Data Voids: What Gets Counted Counts, talk at the Boston Public Library*. [Online] Available at: https://civic.mit.edu/index.html%3Fp=1153.html [Accessed 20 June 2022].
Sekula, A. (1986), 'The Body and the Archive', *October*, 39: 3–64.
Shapin, S., and S. Schaffer (1985), *Leviathan and the Air-Pump: Hobbes, Boyle, and The Experimental Life*, Princeton: Princeton University Press.
Viney, W., F. Callard and A. Woods (2015), 'Critical medical humanities: Embracing entanglement, taking risks', *Medical Humanities*, 41: 2–7.

CHAPTER THREE

How close is too close? The practice and politics of lived experience in contemporary art, academic history and the medical humanities

Daniel Regan and Chris Millard

This text has emerged over some years of discussion between Chris Millard (CM) and Daniel Regan (DR). Chris is a historian of medicine and psychiatry who has written about the use of personal experiences in the medical humanities (Millard 2020), and is writing a forthcoming book about 'the personal' in history-writing. Daniel is a visual artist whose work explores the phenomenology of complex experiences, including his own struggles with mental health. His work brokers dialogues around taboo topics such as mental health, grief, self-injury, suicide and racism.

Talking and thinking across disciplines is exciting and challenging; it is difficult to render such work in the conventional, single-voiced output. We have kept our thoughts distinct but interacting because the politics of personal experience in producing artworks and producing written history are substantially different. But as the conversation goes on, commonalities are revealed. There is only limited value in presenting this similarity at the top, which risks forgetting the distance. The discussion is not resolved, and no firm conclusions are possible. However, there are suggestions for supporting (funding) those who wish to explore their experiences in their work, and a firm commitment not only to ask questions about experience and its relation to marginality and authenticity, but to be precise when thinking about what personal experience is, and how it relates to different people, and different kinds of artistic and scholarly work.

CM: One striking thing to emerge from our discussions is the distance between our starting points. The significance of 'personal experience' in academic history and the medical humanities is shrouded in ambiguity, ambivalence and defensiveness. Historians appear reluctant to disclose any personal experience that has relevance to their published research, in their published research. This is the case even when they might talk about it more or less publicly in other fora (blog posts, podcasts, interviews, at conferences).

DM: I think that because the origins of my creative practice are so bound up with the onset of my own mental health difficulties as a young person, exploring my personal experiences in relation to a subject matter is often the *only* starting point when I approach making new work. I have not always been as open about this as I am now, simply because of the shame or stigma associated with mental health difficulties. Now, in order for me to *make* something I need to *feel* something, and often it is in the excavation of my own past experiences that something is stirred up and piques my interest. I think often we give permission to artists to make from lived experiences because creating requires a source, a stimulus, a catalyst. It baffles me that in academia a similar passion for and connection to a research subject is not afforded the same permission to acknowledge the roots of why it might personally interest you.

CM: The term 'permission' is apt here because there are places, at the margins of academic texts (in prefaces, forewords, afterwords, epilogues and acknowledgements) that are more permissive regarding personal experiences. Often quite traumatic experiences seem 'dumped' in these places, between the hardback covers of expensive monographs. Sometimes these experiences are deemed to be of fundamental significance to the research. However, the 'main text' often contains no acknowledgement of the significance of this experience deposited at the margins. For example, the acknowledgements to Ellen Ross's *Love and Toil: Motherhood in Outcast London* begins: 'The catastrophe of my little son's ghastly three-month-long hospitalization with a brain tumor and his death in December 1989 transformed this project for me and for everyone who knew me'. For Ross, her book 'took on new layers of significance when I resumed work on it' and even though it was 'unfashionable intellectually' to relate emotionally to the historical actors one was studying, Ross 'took solace and sometimes inspiration from my historical subjects, mothers themselves, many of whom had also sat at their children's deathbeds, women who carried on with their own lives after doing all they could for the sick child'. This deep emotional investment in the sources and the work is kept at a distance (because, 'intellectually unfashionable'), and instead the book 'has retained the conventional scholarly form I imagined for it' when she commenced the research process in 1984 (Ross 1993: vii). Perhaps because history retains a methodological conservatism, an attachment to a very empirical, objective tradition around sources, and feels a duty to describe a past that really happened, this distrust of personal experience has only recently – with important exceptions (Steedman 1987; Friedlander 1993; Hartman 2006) – begun to soften.

DR: This makes me think about value and the currency of lived experience. Not all artists acknowledge in depth their personal connection to the stories in their work, or cite individual experiences as the inspiration. Yet culturally the value of having an experience close to the work that you have created is often acknowledged and appreciated. We favour novels about the lives of women written by women, or may question the plausibility of a white author's ability to accurately portray the life of a Black protagonist. The currency of lived experience here is that we gain trust and hopefully validity in the creator's work because of their lived experience and connection to the subject matter, not in spite of it. It is interesting that in academic research the presence of lived experience could somehow be seen to jeopardize that validity, that the presence of their humanity could somehow undo the work.

CM: This reminds me of a quotation from literary critic Michael Bérubé, who argues that 'as long as the scholarship in question concerns humans and is written by humans, readers should at least entertain the possibility that nothing human should be alien to it' (1996: 1065). In literary criticism, ideas of 'personal criticism' have been debated and developed since the 1980s; in anthropology the project of 'autoethnography' – explicitly foregrounding the identity of the author who observes their 'own group' – has been around just as long. However, for historians, the idea that one's experiences (or one's identity) might inform one's academic research is still thought dangerous. Women writing about the history of childbirth, motherhood or domesticity risk their work being reduced to their gender; something similar can happen with Black scholars writing about the history of racism, segregation and slavery. But there is also a powerful politics of authenticity – around the history of race, homosexuality or mental illness, for example – where the identity and experiences of the historian become relevant grounds for critical engagement. Jacqueline Jones, a white historian, ends her chapter in the collection *Historians and Race: Autobiography and the Writing of History* in a very defensive way: 'I have always considered the story of African Americans to be the story of America, and I reject the currently fashionable position that declares certain kinds of history off-limits to certain kinds of people ... I suggest that we focus not on an author's background but her footnotes, and avoid reading too much between the lines' (1996: 130). Similarly, in Paul Gilroy's preface to an edition of Peter Fryer's *Staying Power*, an influential history of Black people in Britain, Gilroy notes how: 'As a white, communist Englishman who had not only dared ... to take possession of this subaltern history but was also prepared to render himself accountable for his choices, Peter Fryer was often treated unfairly ... the destructive, hateful treatment which was dished out by resentful, lazy and hostile community spokespeople ... because this particular history of suffering was their own special property' (2010: xii). In both cases, 'the personal' and the 'lived experience' of the historian is acutely relevant but in a different way.

DR: In most arts contexts, we elevate a person's experience because it makes sense that they would make work about their lives and its events (regardless of whether you like the work). There are however difficult conversations in relation to socially engaged arts practices, particularly around working with marginalized communities. Questions arise about who should (or could) be working with participants, such as those from refugee backgrounds or within psychiatric hospitals. I am really interested in how the value of lived experience – in these examples connection to culture, experience of being an asylum seeker, or having been hospitalized – can be seen as assets in the work that artists do. Can having similar life experiences – whilst also having the professional skills and adequate recovery/support – create a greater experience for the beneficiaries of socially engaged creative practices? From my perspective it is not either/or – you may have a connection to a community's lived experience but lack the practical and creative skills needed to teach and facilitate. Similarly you may have excellent creative skills but lack the interpersonal skills to hold space, regardless of whether you identify with that community or not. Sometimes an artist's lived experience can be a hindrance in participatory practices – it can render too close to the surface and trigger trauma responses, even with time having passed. In my own participatory practice I avoid working on certain projects in specific places because it is *too close* to my lived experiences.

CM: These are exactly the difficult conversations that I think historians struggle to have. How close is too close? It's vital to have this space for considered discussion. There is another aspect too, when 'lived experience' shades (unremarked) into ideas of identity. Having certain experiences *can* certainly become the basis of an identity – an experience of severe mental ill-health, or of being sectioned, can mean that one becomes a 'psychiatric survivor'. In the same way, experiencing child abuse or cancer can mean that one has an identity as a 'survivor' of those things. But this is a different relation to the experience of racism, and the identity of being Black. In this case, the latter identity does not easily or simply depend on the experience of racism. Similarly, is it useful to talk of 'lived experience of being gay'? Is this different to 'identifying as gay'? And what about those who are not marginalized – can one have 'lived experience' of being heterosexual? I am not sure how useful it would be to claim that.

DR: The politics of labels and ownership is interesting to me given my intersecting identities as a queer person, with a disability, of mixed heritage. The terminology around lived – and even living – experiences is fascinating because it is so uniquely individual and informed by our experiences and can become a semantic minefield. Examples can include people's personal identification within mental health services (patient, client, service user etc.) and how difficult experiences in our lives inform what we want others to know about us (i.e some wear the label of survivor proudly, others less so).

We all have lived and living experiences, but it seems we identify or reclaim them when these experiences sit outside of the norm, or when that identity is marginalized and/or one that is minoritized. One can have a lived experience of being white and heterosexual, but within the cultural context of being within the majority, we assume (rightly or wrongly) that these identities pose less of a potential struggle given their afforded privilege. In the work that I do in mental health the term 'lived experience' is synonymous with having experienced ill mental health specifically. The understanding of the term 'lived experience' is as varied as the actual experiences people place under the term itself.

CM: How one learns how to be a historian – the years of graduate training and work towards a PhD – is crucial. Much PhD training and supervision has no sense of how one might include one's personal experiences (if they are relevant to the topic at hand). In fact the training process in history often encourages the active removal of anything personal, and the adoption of a 'scholarly tone' that is distanced and supposedly 'objective'.

DR: I cannot say that my experience in studying at art schools proposed anything different from what you have described. Whilst making my works – which were deeply personal about my mental health experiences – I felt like my tutors were unsure of how to support me. At times they simply suggested that I not make the work at all.

In my own teaching I have noticed a rise in students making personal works relating to their own mental health experiences. In the past two decades the stigma of some mental health difficulties (namely anxiety and depression) has undoubtedly reduced. The prevalence of mental health issues amongst students has also risen – from 2010/11 to 2020/21, conditions reported by students increased by nearly 7 per cent (Lewis and Bolton 2023).

Whilst it is encouraging that some students feel more comfortable to use the arts to unpick and navigate their challenges, it may also compound the pressure placed on staff to navigate difficult discussions, and the impact that sharing their work has on their peers. This can be another stressor on already overstretched and under-resourced staff who are now trying to sensitively facilitate sessions on often emotionally heavy content without additional support themselves, and often without an understanding of trauma-informed pedagogy.

Conclusions

Despite the different starting points, there is plenty of common ground here. The issue of training and teaching is one that would repay detailed further study. The question of different lived experiences, different identities and the problem of proximity (or 'how close is too close?') are also very interesting to explore further. This discussion has brought out how complicated 'lived experience' is when one looks closely at it. Ideas of authenticity, marginality, power and privilege swirl around it. It also raises urgent questions about providing (and funding) appropriate support in both history and art to help students and practitioners explore *how* lived experiences might interact with the artwork and scholarship being produced. Artworks and histories are produced by humans – how these objects relate to the conditions of their production is a broad and complicated question. But personal experience is always a part of the story.

References

Bérubé, M. (1996), 'Against subjectivity', *PMLA*, 111(5): 1063–68.

Friedlander, S. (1993), *Memory, History, and the Extermination of the Jews of Europe*. Bloomington; Indianapolis: Indiana University Press.

Gilroy, P. ([1984] 2010), 'Introduction', in P. Fryer (ed.), *Staying Power: The History of Black People in Britain*, x–xii, London; New York: Pluto Press,

Hartman, S (2006), *Lose Your Mother: A Journey Along the Atlantic Slave Route*, New York: Macmillan.

Jones, J. (1996), 'Autobiography and Scholarship', in P. Cimbala and R. Himmelberg (eds), *Historians and Race: Autobiography and the Writing of History*, 111–30, Bloomington; Indianapolis: Indianapolis University Press.

Lewis, J., and Bolton, P. (2023). 'Student mental health in England: Statistics, policy, and guidance'. London: House of Commons Library. Available online: https://researchbriefings.files.parliament.uk/documents/CBP-8593/CBP-8593.pdf (accessed 11 November 2024).

Millard, C. (2020), 'Using personal experience in the academic medical humanities: A genealogy', *Social Theory & Health*, 18(2): 184–98.
Ross, E. (1993), *Love and Toil: Motherhood in Outcast London, 1870–1918*, Oxford: Oxford University Press.
Steedman, C. (1987), *Landscape for a Good Woman: A story of Two Lives*, New Jersey: Rutgers University Press.

CHAPTER FOUR

Cripistemology of the cabinet: Jesse Darling's *Epistemologies (shamed cabinet)*

Amanda Cachia

Jesse Luke Darling (he/him/his) is a British-born, Berlin-based transmasculine disabled artist who uses sculpture, video, text, performances, sound and installation to explore both the formation and re-formation of sociopolitical bodily subjects. Lauded as one of the most brilliant artists of his generation (he was awarded the prestigious Turner Prize in 2023), Darling has long been interested in exploring somatic vulnerability and imperfection. In 2016, the artist experienced a neurological disease after giving birth to his child, resulting in partial paralysis and the loss of full use of his right arm. While this life-changing event precipitated a focus on the signifiers of disability, damage and the prosthetic body, the artist's commitment to exploring issues of malfunction and pain in his work long predate this. Darling modifies and adapts sculptural objects – including medical assistive and prosthetic devices – so that they become dilapidated, spindly, contorted and wonky. Considering the prosthetic impulse to cure and normalize (adapting to a prosthesis is very much a learning process, rather than automatic), Darling situates his praxis in the context of the larger frameworks of patriarchy, imperialism, white supremacy, ableist machismo culture and the medical/psychiatric/diagnostic industrial complex.

This chapter is an extract from the author's monograph, *Hospital Aesthetics: Disability, Medicine, Activism*, Manchester: Manchester University Press, 2025.

Darling resists being co-opted into the simplistic categorization of 'disability artist', an identity label which museums are eager to deploy to demonstrate more inclusive policies. Instead, aiming to undo the master narrative underpinning the medical model of disability, he prefers to embrace what Louise Hickman and David Serlin (2018) have called a 'cripistemological' approach. Cripistemology heeds a call by disability studies scholars for a crip-based approach to method, where crip experience animates research and/or practice questions from the ground up. Darling's praxis mobilizes cripistemology as methodology, through a concern for the prosthetic object and its function(s). I use this text to show how Darling engages this method in his work *Epistemologies (shamed cabinet)* (2018), part of a series that also includes *Epistemologies (limping cabinet)* (2018) and *Epistemologies (collapsed cabinet)* (2018). Bound up in Darling's use of cripistemology is a desire to resist the curative imperative and the cultural logic to repair, regularly deployed by the medical industrial complex, and to instead embrace the normativity of the wonky, the broken and the unstable. The prosthetic device in Darling's work therefore allows us to consider how centring these unsteady states provides a generative space for the production of new forms of knowledge.

Epistemologies (shamed cabinet) (2018) is a glass museum cabinet, animated by bent legs suggestive of walking and motion (see Figure 4.1). Yet, despite the cabinet's apparent desire for freedom, its damaged form renders it unable to move. Inside the glass case, a series of archival binders are piled up on top of each other. Upon closer inspection, one sees that the binders are filled with blocks of concrete: rather than indicating movement, the sharply angled legs of the cabinet are collapsing under the weight of its contents. These archival binders reference historical medical records of 'deviant' bodies measured, documented and scrutinized in the pursuit of clinical science: from a contemporary vantage point, these archives read not as a narrative of progress, but as evidence of the skews and prejudices in the construction of white Western medical knowledge. Indeed, this is an epistemology that must be shamed. By freighting the archival binders with concrete (an apt metaphor for the heaviness of the subject-matter), Darling rejects the white medical heteronormative imperative to collect and collate, cripping a museological archive of Western knowledge acquired through the extractive and violent methods of colonization. The legs of the cabinet literally buckle under the weight of this history and oppression.

The title of the work, and the title of this essay, reference Eve Kosofsky Sedgwick's *Epistemology of the Closet*, a defining book in queer theory which critiques a binary model of hetero- and homosexuality (Sedgwick 2008). Darling's cabinet shames the closeting of homosexuality, disability and debility within the museological space, referencing a long and problematic history of spectacularizing particular bodies while refusing to centre forms of knowledge generated by queer or crip experience. In the 1980s, the Native American artist James Luna put his own indigenous body on display

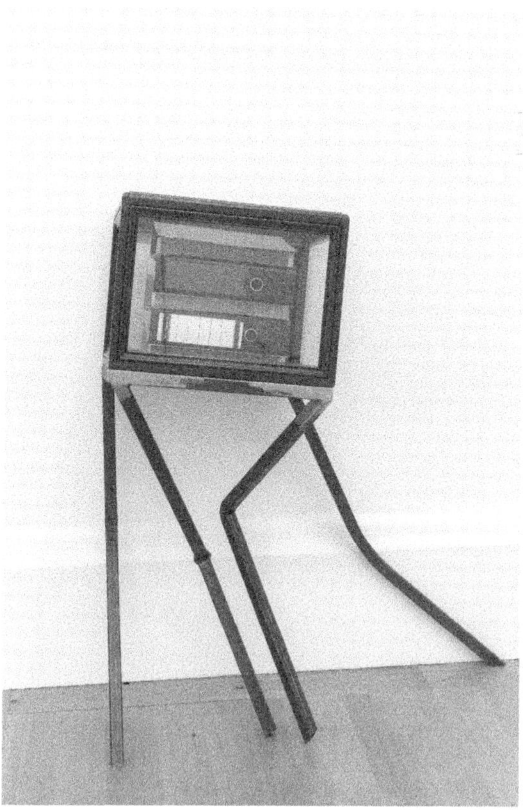

FIGURE 4.1 Jesse Luke Darling, *Epistemologies (shamed cabinet)*, 2018. Mahogany, glass, steel, linen, archival binders, concrete. Courtesy: the artist and Arcadia Missa, London, photograph: Matt Greenwood.

to imitate standard museum practices of the time, where wax figures of indigenous people were presented within idealized tableaux that elided the realities of those communities' experiences. Likewise, Darling shows how museological structures literally foreclose the possibility of making visible the knowledge and experiences of the communities to which he belongs. Luna's living and breathing body – which startled museum visitors initially believing themselves to be looking at a waxwork – challenged the idea that a cabinet must contain legible knowledge or be an artefact of an objective 'truth', offering instead a visual taxonomy no longer controlled by the museum. Darling's cabinet does similar work, using a cripistemological framework.

Although the cabinet is loaded with a weighty past and present, Darling empowers it with an agential discontent which invites a reading of its (lack of) mobility from a different point of view. As David T. Mitchell, Susan Antebi, and Sharon L. Snyder note, disability has an 'ongoing potentiality to reshape the world' (Mitchell et al. 2019: 1). A posthumanist approach to disability rejects the curative impulse typically associated with the medical model, providing instead 'an opportunity to encounter disability more viscerally as an active participant in the trans-historical, intraspecies, and cross-cultural interactions of materiality, sociality, structures, and environments' (Mitchell et al. 2019: 2). More than simply 'representing' disability in positive and affirming ways, a posthumanist approach recognizes disability as an active participant in meaning-making. Darling's epistemology of 'cripistemology' makes this manifest: in his literal re-assemblage of support structures, he is reassembling the meaning of support, rethinking how bodies can carry and be carried. Indeed, while metaphors of the prosthesis have been deployed ad-nauseum by scholars as a signifier within techno-culture or trauma-informed narratives, here, Darling fleshes his cabinetry with mobilizing form so that it becomes a vehicle for new and empowered knowledge production and epistemologies. The cabinet's unstable state offers an opportunity to consider what generative new knowledges may emerge.

References

Hickman, L., and D. Serlin (2018), 'Towards a Crip Methodology for Critical Disability Studies', in *Interdisciplinary Approaches to Disability: Looking Towards the Future, Volume 2*, edited by Katie Ellis, Rosemarie Garland-Thomson, Mike Kent and Rachel Robertson, London: Routledge.

Mitchell, David, T. S. Antebi and S. L. Snyder, eds. (2019), *The Matter of Disability: Materiality, Biopolitics, Crip Affect*, Michigan: The University of Michigan Press.

Sedgwick, E.K. (2008), *Epistemology of the Closet*, Berkeley, California: University of California Press.

CHAPTER FIVE

Beads, breath and memory: Ruth Cuthand's *Surviving: Covid-19*

Skye Haggerty

'I am trying very hard to be as true to the teller as I can possibly be. I do that by being not only aware of words but even more aware of breath'.

– Maria Campbell (in Gingell 2004)

I begin with the above quote by a Métis elder which transformed my understanding of the relationship between breath, the act of beading, and cultural memory. In 2019, at the Royal Alberta Museum, I encountered Ruth Cuthand's *Trading* series. The series, which debuted ten years prior, depicts eleven diseases brought to North America (with one taken back to Europe and rendered in quillwork). For the small selection of works at the RAM, in their tubular, Petri-dish-like display cases, they invite the viewer to step closer and study the medical image–inspired works. True to Cuthand's intentions, I was drawn in by the seductive beadwork only to be repelled by its subject. The negative connection between beads and disease for our people had not occurred to me before that moment. Still, I would continue to think about these, in Cuthand's own words, 'terrible but gorgeous' works long after leaving the museum (Cuthand 2021).

The *Surviving* series (2011–ongoing) addresses diseases after the signing of Little Pine Nation to Treaty 6 in 1879. Like the preceding works, the beaded discs are mounted on a black suede board and depict electron microscope images of each virus. Cuthand continues her work to expand and challenge perceptions of beading by seeking new subjects and images to bead. Appropriately, these beaded images tell stories in ways that differ from typical units of measurement. Ruth Cuthand's *Surviving* series breathes life into cultural memories through the practice of beading.

The chosen image here for COVID-19 is a complex representation. The disc is divided broadly into three colours – blue, purple and yellow – and mounted at the centre of a rectangular suede board. Overlapping the blue and purple hemispheres, shades of yellow and orange compose the uneven, coin-like bodies of the virus emerging from healthy cells. To the right of the centre, a light purple cell separated from the purple mass alludes to this transformative infection process. At the bottom, we see the word COVID-19 printed in grey vinyl lettering applied to the black mounting. The original image that Cuthand used as a model was colourized and coded by a lab's visual medical arts office (see Wamsley 2020). Human hands are behind the creation of these images, a thought narrowing the gap between artist and technician (Fung 2006).

For Ruth Cuthand, beads and disease go hand in hand (Robertson 2017). While Cuthand refers to disease transmission through human encounters along the trade of beads, there is an additional relationship between beads and disease. But first, we must address beads' history before discussing their effects. Seed beads were early trade objects that quickly became popular upon their introduction in the eighteenth and nineteenth centuries. Kate Duncan (1989) states that, on average, fifteen to twenty bead colours and types were available to a beadworker at the trading posts before the twentieth century. Some of the bead types available were greasy beads (named for their oily finish), steel cuts (ranging from steel to brass) and Charlotte beads – to name but a few. Venetian glass factories dominated the bead trade until their decline in the latter half of the nineteenth century, after which Czech beads became the standard for trade (Francis 2008). Pale blue, as seen in Cuthand's work, was a popular colour, and Indigenous beadworkers preferred Venetian beads for their vibrancy in colour despite inconsistency across batches. The varying shades of colour within the hemispheres of the work additionally allude to this inconsistency while creating the illusion of a teeming, textured and moving surface rather than a static state. Although the beads could not themselves carry disease, the exposure and proximity to European traders and the subsequent movement of beads from person to person carried the viruses far ahead of the colonial project.

Alongside this history, we can connect beading to disease through its healing potential. Beading and other forms of needlework continue to be a socially grounded practice that finds its roots in traditional artmaking for Plains women such as Cuthand. As Indigenous women travelled, they shared designs and ideas across communities through beading circles (Schneider 1983: 107; Berry 2011: 58; Robertson 2017: 15; Fey, 2017: 45). These spaces, often within a domestic setting, help forge communal ties and provide opportunities for sharing intergenerational knowledge. This community-building practice is present even in the cross-cultural spaces of institutions. From the 1940s to the 1960s, the Canadian government forcibly sent First Nations, Inuit, and Métis peoples for tuberculosis treatment at 'Indian Hospitals', and they were absent for years from their community (Komarnisky 2021). Further links to the medical treatment of Indigenous bodies in Cuthand's work emerge through her memory of using discarded paper for yearly X-rays (testing for tuberculosis) for art as a child. The occupational therapy programs of hospitals, such as the Charles Camsell in Edmonton, Alberta, were an important space where the displaced Indigenous patients could connect to songs, stories, and relationships with 'the human and beyond human' in a restrictive, colonial setting (Komarnisky 2021: 356–57). Beading was one of the varied practices available to individuals who could learn from other patients who already possessed beadworking skills.

In her 2019 residency at the University of Saskatchewan's Health Sciences, Ruth Cuthand brought the healing aspect of beading forward by leading a beading circle for medical staff and students. The participants were primarily, though not exclusively, women. As time passed, patients from the psychiatry ward were also permitted to join, recognizing that their participation was beneficial. The beading circle became a place of casual chit-chat and a place where the participants helped one another. Beading, while capable of being a deeply personal expression and practice, becomes a meditative act of healing through the rhythmic experience of sewing with others and sharing a common experience (Cuthand 2020a, 2021; Farrell Racette 2017: 119).

Breath, as Métis Elder Maria Campbell shares, is essential in storytelling because it connects us to rhythm (Gingell 2003). A storyteller chooses their words to fit a breath as carefully as a beadworker decides upon beads to fit a design. Each stitch is akin to punctuation, barely noticeable between the beads if registered at all. Beading is taxing work for the eyes and hands but also mindful work. In measuring, stringing, and stitching, the body settles into a breathing pattern, like in meditation, while the head and hand work together to bring a work into being. Storytelling requires a similar focus and pacing, one which our body comes to know intuitively through practice. In Cuthand's 2019 beading circle, some students treated beading as practice for learning to suture (2020a). The necessity for focus, even spacing and patience extends across these three spaces: storytelling, beadwork and healing. The individual parts may have changed, but the practice stays the same across generations, connected not necessarily by beading but by sharing knowledge.

For some, the repetitive motion which instills us with muscle memory also activates cultural memory. Black suede board evokes memories of the black silk velvet and cotton velveteen our Indigenous grandmothers used to make wall-pockets and other decorated textile belongings (Duncan 1989: 68; Phillips 1998: 159). The black, luxurious surface of the material was difficult to work upon and demonstrated the skill of the beadworker while highlighting the vibrancy of the beads' colours – seen here in this example of Cuthand's work (Figure 5.1). But encased additionally in each laid stitch are memories of each easy laugh, frustrated sigh, and quiet breath in creating the work. In the predecessor to the *Surviving* series, Cuthand sourced inspiration from a shipment of beads which dazzled her with their appearance (2020b). She wondered if her reaction was the same as the women who saw those glass beads for the first time, connecting herself (and us) to a cultural memory through a framework of storytelling. Standing before these monstrous images, they draw us in with their terrible beauty and the memories they hold (Smetzer 2021). *Surviving: COVID-19* compels us to think about our experience of the pandemic and imagine the suspended cells caught in a moment of memory just as we are.

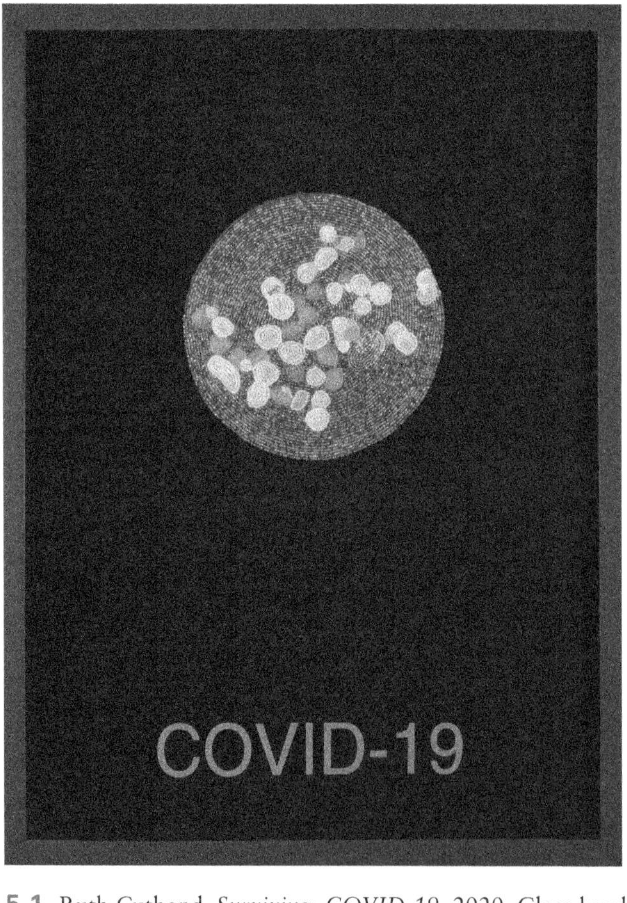

FIGURE 5.1 Ruth Cuthand, *Surviving: COVID-19*, 2020. Glass beads, backing and thread, vinyl lettering on glass. Collection of the MacKenzie Art Gallery.

Look at the image. Focus on the intricate work of the design, the seemingly effortless curves and the thumbprint-like surface of the cells. Extend your mind to the practised hands which string and tack each section of beads, working your way past the quiet rhythm of their hands to the voices in the room. Hear cups of *maskihkîwâpoy* (tea, lit: liquid medicine) and spoons clinking with the comfortable silences between conversations. Now, think of those lungs labouring to catch their breath and to talk without spasming and coughing. Does a change of breath not modify our speech patterns or disrupt the rhythm of our words? How do we share our stories if we cannot speak to them? Look at the image again.

Tuberculosis was once known as the thief because it stole people from their homes, loved ones, and communities (Meijer Drees 2013; Komarnisky 2021). It also took their breath in cases where it took the form of respiratory infections, like COVID-19. For many of them, it took their stories, as evinced by the profusion of anonymous works in museums and private collections. Cuthand's beadwork speaks not only to the survival of our traditions and practices but to the survival of our memories and the breaths, or beads, through which we share them.

References

Berry, S. (2011) 'Recovered Identities: Four Métis Artists in Nineteenth-Century Rupert's Land', in S. Carter and P. A. McCormack (eds), *Recollecting: Lives of Aboriginal Women of the Canadian Northwest and Borderlands*, 29–59, Edmonton: Athabasca University Press.

Cuthand, R. (2020a), 'Artist Spotlight: Right Cuthand's Don't Breathe, Don't Drink', Art Gallery of Ontario, July 10. Available online: https://youtu.be/i9Cre372UFI?si=sVlPmdjLgbbTGGYu (accessed 28 April 2024).

Cuthand, R. (2020b), 'Ruth Cuthand Interview – MacKenzie Art Gallery', MacKenzie Art Gallery, December 8. Available online: https://youtu.be/yupq1_nzbWA?si=w2AcsbWSds2JLa_ (accessed 28 April 2024).

Cuthand, R. (2021), 'Bluecoat Talk with Artist Ruth Cuthand', Science North, September 23. Available online: https://www.youtube.com/live/kKeohaaIEYI?si=ArCjH42n05W385G7 (accessed 28 April 2024).

Duncan, K. C. (1989), *Northern Athapaskan Art: A Beadwork Tradition*, Tokyo: University of Washington Press.

Farrell Racette, S. (2017) 'Tuft Life: Stitching Sovereignty in Contemporary Indigenous Art', *Art Journal*, 76 (2): 114–23.

Fey, A. (2017), 'From Women's Hands: An Object Biography of the McTavish Collection', MA diss., University of Manitoba, Winnipeg.

Francis, P. Jr. (2008), 'The Venetian Bead Story', *BEADS: Journal of the Society of Bead Researchers*, 20: 62–80.

Fung, K. (2006) 'Artwork Using 3D Computed Tomography: Extending Radiology into the Realm of Visual Art', *Leonardo*, 39 (3): 187–226.

Gingell, S. (2004) '"One Small Medicine": An Interview with Maria Campbell'. *Essays on Canadian Writing*, 83: 188–205.

Komarnisky, S. (2021), 'From the Sanatorium to the Museum and Beyond: The Circulation of Art and Craft Made by Indigenous Patients at Tuberculosis Hospitals', in B. Lemire, L. Peers and A. Whitelaw (eds), *Object Lives and Global Histories in Northern North America: Material Culture in Motion, c.1780–1980*, 346–76, Montreal: McGill-Queen's University Press.

Meijer Drees, L. (2013), *Healing Histories: Stories from Canada's Indian Hospitals*, Edmonton: University of Alberta Press.

Phillips, R B. (1998) *Trading Identities: The Souvenir in Native North American Art from the Northeast, 1700–1900*, Hong Kong: University of Washington Press.

Robertson, C. (2017), 'Land and Beaded Identity: Shaping Art Histories of Indigenous Women of the Flatland', *RACAR: revue d'art Canadienne / Canadian Art Review*, 42 (2): 13–29.

Schneider, M. J. (1983) 'Women's Work: An Examination of Women's Role in Plains Indian Arts and Crafts', in P. Albers and M. Medicine (eds), *The Hidden Half: Studies of Plains Indian Women*, 101–121, Washington: University Press of America.

Smetzer, M. A. (2021), *Painful Beauty: Tlingit Women, Beadwork, and the Art of Resilience*, Seattle: University of Washington Press.

Wamsley, Laurel. (2020), 'IMAGES: What New Coronavirus Looks Like Under the Microscope', NPR, February 13. Available online: https://www.npr.org/2020/02/13/805837103/images-what-new-coronavirus-looks-like-under-the-microscope&sa=D&ust=1584133843276000 (accessed 28 April 2024).

PART II

Visualizing knowledge and power

CHAPTER SIX

Looking well: art historical interventions for a more equitable medicine

Kathleen Pierce

In *Image Matters*, Tina Campt (2012) deftly calls attention to the tensions inhered in the act of scrutinizing imaged bodies for physical evidence. As she recounts her efforts to locate people of Afro-Caribbean descent within the Birmingham City Archive as part of her larger effort to surface social histories buried, in part, by systemic racism, we see Campt struggle with her own disciplining gaze. Even as she applies a visual acuity honed over years of careful study (124), she comes to find that that same visual acuity, untempered, risks replicating the very systems of power she writes against: 'As if standing beside myself, I watched myself scanning with effort each plate for visible clues of racial difference, in the process reinscribing all the essentialisms this good black feminist postructuralist disavows'.

Campt's nuanced attention to the entanglement of visual acuity and the equivocal power of looking have long resonated with me as an essential lesson for a more ethical and equitable medicine. From at least the nineteenth century onwards, European and North American trained physicians, too, have often aimed to cultivate an exacting visual acuity. Physicians and medical students frequently honed this visual acuity to more readily perceive the discernible symptoms of illness or health. It might equally be trained on rendering aspects of identity legible so as to more easily apply categories like gender or race in prophylactic or diagnostic thinking – an act, as we will see, sometimes itself framed as addressing structural oppression in healthcare.

In a medicalized refraction of Campt's description, socially constructed categories can become a visual heuristic, where facets of identity operate as powerful filters by which practitioners calculate the possibility for illness or particular health outcomes.[1] Under this rubric, a patient may or may not *look like* someone likely to experience a certain disease, a diagnostic fact that fundamentally shapes the kind, quality, speed, and duration of care a patient receives.

It was partly my own experiences navigating chronic illness that crystallized how Campt's insights might (re)shape medical systems. I frequently reflect on a 2016 doctor's appointment, midway through my graduate studies in art history. The clinician entered with my chart in hand and repeated a ritualized corporeal and perceptual act I had witnessed – and read about – hundreds of times before: she looked me up and down, applying the oft-discussed diagnostic or clinical gaze (Foucault [1963] 1973; Jordanova 1989; Callen 2018). When she finally made eye contact, she introduced herself and said: 'You don't look like the sort of person I expected to see!' Her tone was friendly; this statement was no doubt intended to put me at ease. The scene reified with exacting precision the stakes of a critical visual medical humanities. The trouble with the clinician's summative *you don't look as I expected* expands beyond questions about the power inhered in the clinician's gaze (most pointedly articulated by Foucault), or the question of empathy – worthy subjects in their own right. Rather, I want to emphasize how this scene points up a multivalent kind of looking within the context of the medical encounter. Here, beyond parsing divides among 'the normal and the pathological' (Foucault [1963] 1973: 35), looking simultaneously comprehends efforts to determine patients' identities (especially age, sex, gender, race, ethnicity, ability) via visual rubrics forged within and without medical education and practice, and, subsequently, efforts to gauge how and whether the information communicated before or during the visit – by way of the chart or patient narratives – may or may not map onto various clinical possibilities. Campt's warnings resound at high volume.

---

[1]The Society for Maternal-Fetal Medicine's Vaginal Birth After Cesarean Section (VBAC) calculator offers a powerful example of these strategies at play. The calculator ostensibly provided clinicians with a tool that might help guide discussions with patients considering a VBAC. The original calculator's algorithm was based on the experiences of 11,856 patients who gave birth in United States hospitals between 1999 and 2002. The calculator allowed for the input of six variables, one of which was 'Black or Hispanic race/ethnicity'. With all other variables remaining the same, selecting either a Black or Hispanic racial or ethnic identity (where, notably, *only one* race/ethnicity could be selected) caused the calculator to offer lower chances of a successful VBAC. As Darshali A. Vyas et al. have argued (2019: 201–3), this is especially alarming given the vast racial and ethnic disparities in maternal morbidity and mortality in the United States. Within the VBAC calculator, socially constructed categories (themselves shifting, contested, and more plural than the calculator allows) are presented as both biological and knowable by the clinician. In effect, the calculator captured the systemic racism that shaped racial and ethnic disparities in maternity care, and re-presented these disparities as biological truths.

Established critical histories of medicine, such as Foucault's *The Birth of the Clinic*, have located the gaze at their centre, and numerous important scholarly works have teased out the particular roles of representation, perception, or visuality in specific times, places, and medicalized experiences. Yet the crucial role of *looking* and *seeing* as core ways of knowing across diverse aspects of medical education and practice, past and present, as well as the larger stakes of bringing – or failing to bring – interdisciplinary thinking about visuality to the study of these ways of knowing, remains undertheorized. Even as medical schools increasingly partner with arts institutions in collaborative curricular programming, the central role that methodologies and ways of thinking from art history, media studies, and visual studies might play in a critical medical humanities remains underacknowledged, though scholars of visual culture (Johnstone 2023) have emphasized its significance – a project to which this very volume attests. Fiona Johnstone (2018) calls for just such a recognition in her 'Manifesto for a Visual Medical Humanities':

> A visual medical humanities is not limited to an investigation of images ... but is grounded in an expanded understanding of the visual as an embodied perceptual experience that also involves the other senses .... It is essential that a visually engaged medical humanities pay attention to the phenomenological and emotional dimensions of visual experience, as well as to the issues of representation, power and ideology that have dominated to date.

The present essay offers a provocation around this theoretical work. Capacious and critically attuned ways of thinking about the gaze, visuality, representation, and how they intersect must be at the core of efforts to address racism, sexism, homophobia, ableism and other forms of oppression within health-care systems. Visual studies, art history, and related fields offer crucial epistemological frameworks for doing this work. I anchor my attention to looking as it collides with representation and visuality in the field of dermatology. As one of the 'most visual of all medical subspecialties' (Ott 2010: 92), dermatology evinces what is just under the surface in other contexts. Visual histories of dermatology also comprise the primary area of my own research (Pierce 2020; Pierce 2025). But more than this, because of the ways racial formation projects distilled in western European and American scientific practice have emphasized skin colour within processes of racialization – what Frantz Fanon ([1952] 2008) named 'epidermalization' – dermatology has emerged as a poignant site for thinking about racial equity and its absence in medicine and healthcare. I focus my attention on twentieth- and twenty-first-century efforts to describe and categorize skin colouration in the name of improving health, especially as they relate to the Fitzpatrick scale: a tool developed for this purpose in 1975, and which remains omnipresent in medical research, practice, and education.

A note on terminology

Phrases like 'skin of colour' have become popular in medical literature as a way to describe *both* patient populations who identify as people of colour *and* patients with darker skin tones. I understand how such phrasing might be politically useful for healthcare practitioners who wish to signal efforts to increase equity in their practice, or align their care with social justice movements. Yet skin colour does not map easily onto race or ethnicity; likewise, it is possible for clinicians to discriminate against their patients based on each of these facets of identity – skin colour, race, and ethnicity – separately, or in combination. 'Skin of colour' collapses skin tone into the social categories of race and ethnicity. Throughout this essay, I aim to recognize, with specificity, the complex relationships among skin colour, race, and ethnicity, as well as racism and colourism. Within my own descriptions, I primarily use relative terms to describe skin colour, especially the adjectives 'lighter' and 'darker', and only use phrases such as 'race' or 'ethnicity' to signal these social categories.

* * *

The late twentieth century witnessed the emergence of a visual rubric for describing and classifying skin that has had and continues to have an outsized influence on medicalized thinking about the relationships among skin colour, race, ethnicity and health: the Fitzpatrick Skin Phototype Scale. In 1975, Thomas Fitzpatrick formally proposed (1975: 33) the classification of patients' skin into one of four categories depending on the skin's purported susceptibility to 'tanning' or 'burning'. These 'phototypes' ranged from 'type 1', 'an individual incapable or only very slightly able to tan', to 'type 4', 'an individual who does not get sunburns'. Fitzpatrick, then Chairman of the Department of Dermatology at Harvard Medical School and Chief of the Dermatology Service at Massachusetts General Hospital, had been researching the prevention, diagnosis, and treatment of melanoma throughout the 1960s and 70s. Thinking about skin cancer and its prevention thus fundamentally informed his development of the phototypes (Mihm et al. 2004: xxxii). His initial publication (Fitzpatrick 1975: 33–34) framed the phototypes' usefulness in relation to emergent professional discourse around sun protection, skin cancer prevention, and phototherapy. As Fitzpatrick noted in 1988 (869), he primarily developed the phototypes 'to classify persons *with white skin*' (emphasis in original). By 1988, a cluster of articles (Fitzpatrick 1988: 869) argued for the expansion of the scale to include six phototypes, where the addition of types V and VI were said to comprehend people with 'black and brown' skin. The six-part scale continues to comprise a standard both within and without dermatology (Ware et al. 2020: 77–9), not only for describing patients' potential response to sunlight and UV radiation, but also for documenting and communicating skin colouration within patients' charts, frequently as a proxy for the social category of race. Researchers (Ware et al. 2020: 77; Coleman et al. 2023: 726) ascribe the scale's prominence to its purported universality: its singularly wide adoption in medical education, research, and practice. As just one measure of its influence, Unicode used the Fitzpatrick scale (Robertson et al. 2021: 350:1–2) as the basis for the emoji skin-tone modification options released in 2015.

What might transform if we hold Campt's insights in mind as we consider the Fitzpatrick scale's prominence and, as we will see, its critics? Or if we think alongside the definition of 'visuality' Nicholas Mirzoeff articulates (2011: 3) in *The Right to Look*? For Mirzoeff, visuality comprehends: 'a set of relations combining information, imagination, and insight into a rendition of physical and psychic space' which 'classifies by naming, categorizing, and defining'; 'separates groups so classified as a means of social organization'; and 'makes this separated classification seem right and aesthetic'. As we will see, the scale comprises a visual and conceptual framework around which numerous actors make scopic, representational, hierarchical, categorical, political, technological, and bureaucratic choices, whose consequences bear on life, death and how it feels to live within a particular body on a day-to-day basis. What might become possible to know, question, or imagine when critical paradigms for understanding the visual, like Mirzoeff's, are meaningfully brought into reassessments of dermatological thinking and practice?

Although the earliest descriptions of Fitzpatrick's phototypes were textual, they quickly accrued visual language; eventually, authors began to communicate the phototypes through diverse kinds of representation. Initially, Fitzpatrick (1975: 33) advised practitioners to observe and consider patients' skin, hair, and eye colour only secondarily when classifying phototypes. He emphasized (Fitzpatrick 1988: 869) that practitioners should lend particular weight to patients' responses to questions like: 'how painful is your sunburn?' Very quickly, however, authors began to attach descriptive language to the scale and, subsequently, encourage clinicians to actively evaluate patients' appearances. In one of the first papers to argue for expanding the number of phototypes, in this case from four to five, Madhu A. Pathak et al. (1986: 227–31) describe types not only in terms of a propensity to 'burn' or 'tan', but also in relation to skin tone, race, and ethnicity. For example, Pathak (1986: 227–8) terms phototype I skin 'very fair', likely someone 'with Celtic background – Irish and Scottish', while skin linked to phototype III is 'medium' in its colouration. To phototype

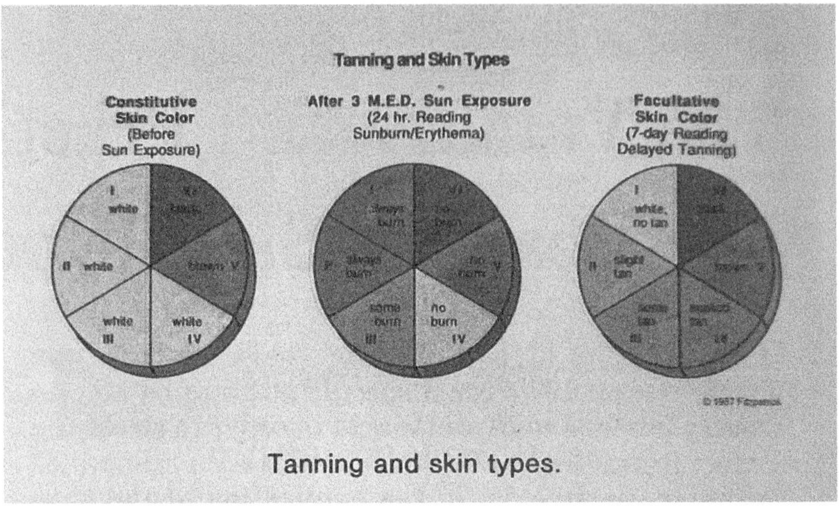

FIGURE 6.1 Thomas B. Fitzpatrick, 'Tanning and Skin Types', *c.* 1987, published in Fitzpatrick, 'The Validity and Practicality of Sun-Reactive Skin Types I Through VI', *Archives of Dermatology* 124, no. 6 (June 1988): 870.

V, Pathak (1986: 231) appends the labels 'markedly tan' and 'dark', as well as language used within eighteenth- and nineteenth-century efforts to demarcate racial typologies. These authors encourage practitioners to assign phototypes based on their close looking at and interpretation of patients' skin, eye, and hair colour, and/or how they perceive their race or ethnicity.

In 1988, Fitzpatrick (870) supplied a representational diagram to help clarify the scale (Figure 6.1). This same diagram later appeared in other publications, including his co-authored textbook (Fitzpatrick et al. 1993: 1693), *Dermatology in General Medicine*. The illustration presents readers with three pie charts tracking changes in skin colouration over time: pre-sun exposure, twenty-four hours after an hour of noon sun exposure, and seven days following the hour of noon sun exposure. Each chart has been divided into six wedges labelled with a phototype (I–VI) and filled with a solid colour. Within the pre-exposure chart, the wedges signifying types I–IV have all been labelled 'white' and filled in with the same light beige hue; the wedges representing types IV and V have been labelled 'brown' and 'black' and filled with sienna and umber pigments, respectively. Within the third chart (signifying the passage of one week), each wedge and, subsequently, each phototype, has been assigned a distinct colour ranging from the same light beige hue for type I, to light and medium ochre pigments for types II and III, to medium and high value sienna hues for types IV and V, and a high value umber for type VI. Within the text of the paper, Fitzpatrick (1988: 870) insists that the scale was developed to determine patients' sensitivities to UV radiation, where their 'phenotype' may not always accurately predict the

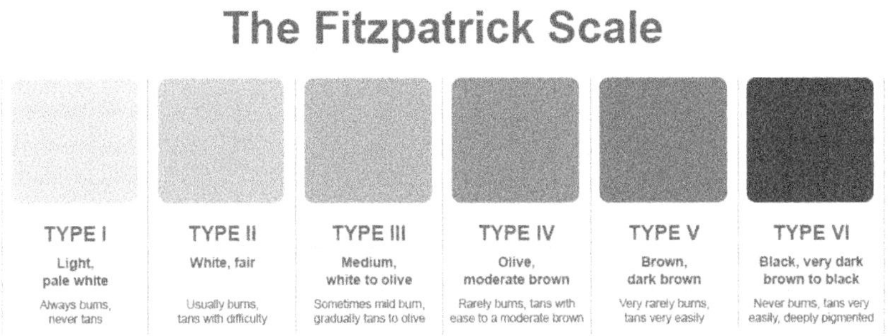

FIGURE 6.2 *The Fitzpatrick Scale, c.* 2016.

skin's response, and that 'ethnicity or "race" is only a cultural and political term with no scientific basis'. Yet the figure flattens any nuance, instead forging direct connections between skin colour and phototype.

Over time, even more schematic versions of the scale began to circulate, especially within media directed at popular audiences. In his op-ed calling attention to the systemic racism that permeates dermatology, for example, Neil Singh (2020) appended a spare diagram to his discussion of Fitzpatrick to help illustrate this thread of dermatological history (Figure 6.2). This diagram's title centres Fitzpatrick, evoking the hagiographic tone of the histories of medicine Singh seeks to counter. The formal properties signalling temporality – and, thus, the scale's relationship to how skin responds to sunlight – have been eliminated. Instead, each phototype has been illustrated with a single representative colour tile. Text connects each tile to a specific phototype and descriptive language, which alternately invokes skin colour ('fair', 'moderate brown') and race ('white', 'Black') without acknowledging any differences between these categories. While textual labels also describe each phototype's capacity to 'burn' or 'tan', the use of smaller font, here, diminishes this information's importance. Despite Fitzpatrick's original emphasis (1988: 870) on the ways patients' appearances, including skin colour, may or may not match clinicians' assumptions about the skin's response to UV radiation, and despite the complex relationship between skin colour and the social categories of race and ethnicity, the diagram collapses any distance between a patient's phototype, skin colour, and perceptions of their race or ethnicity. The diagram's horizontality, too, refigures the conceptual space between phototypes as a spectrum, suggesting that the scale covers the entire range of possible skin tones, and that every patient might find representation within these options. This particular diagram has appeared across diverse kinds of media marshalled to myriad ends: from public-facing publications (Singh 2020) critiquing the scale, to materials physicians (Sutton 2016) have developed to educate patients, and specialized medical literature (Charlton et al. 2020: 3), where authors deploy the diagram uncritically as an illustration.

Despite its prominence, the scale has not escaped critique. Among the most important points raised is the scale's primary focus on light to medium skin tones; it was both formed within and continues to assert a white hegemony. As Fitzpatrick himself emphasized (1988: 869), he developed the phototypes 'to classify persons *with white skin*'. Unsurprisingly, the scale's efficacy in cancer prevention diminishes (Erickson et al. 2023) when used to evaluate patients with darker skin tones, a clinical failure compounded by systemic racism and the underrepresentation of darker skin tones in medical education. It is thus within a framework where dermatology *fails to imagine* caring for patients with darker skin tones and/or patients of colour that the scale came into existence, an issue that the scale and the larger medical systems from which it emerged continue to exacerbate. Indeed, many projects developed to address systemic racism in dermatology, whether activist led, such as 'Brown Skin Matters' (Buchanan Weiss 2019), or physician led, such as Jenna Lester's (2018) 'Skin of Color Program', emphasize representation – particularly the overrepresentation of bodies with lighter skin tones and the underrepresentation of bodies with darker skin tones – as just one symptom of the ways systemic racism shapes dermatological research, education, and care. This is especially significant given skin pigmentation affects how signs and symptoms of all kinds – and not just of dermatological diseases – *look* (Ebede et al. 2006: 687; Alvarado et al. 2021: 1427; Everett et al. 2012: 496). Recent studies of dermatology textbooks (Adelekun et al. 2021: 194–96; Alvarado et al. 2021: 1427–31; and Porras Fimbres et al. 2023) reveal that depending on the sources consulted, anywhere from 5.6–11.5 per cent of images picture what authors primarily describe as 'dark' skin or 'skin of color', a proportion consistent with a study (Ebede et al. 2006: 687–90) conducted fifteen years prior.

Yet the very methods of the studies cited here betray another crucial point of critique: researchers and clinicians' use of the Fitzpatrick phototypes as proxies for the social categories of race and ethnicity. As even the earliest visual diagrams of the phototypes seemed to presage, over time the scale became detached from its origins in cancer prevention research. Physicians increasingly deployed the phototypes in research, education, and clinical practice as a way to signpost patients' skin tone, race and/or ethnicity, where these three categories are frequently confused or conflated. In their 2020 survey of dermatologists, Ware et al. (2020: 79) found that between one-third and half of those surveyed used the scale to indicate patients' 'race/ethnicity' and/or their 'constitutive skin color'. As Everett et al. emphasize (2012: 499), this phenomenon extends beyond dermatology across diverse spheres of medical practice. Phototype designations in clinical documentation are largely determined by clinicians' scopic assessment – what Erickson et al. term a 'visual inspection' (2023: 678) – of patients' appearances rather than any discussion with patients about their skin's response to sunlight. The Fitzpatrick scale's entangled relationship with 'information, imagination, and insight' in 'physical and psychic space', and behaviours such as 'categorizing and defining' performed to seem 'right and aesthetic' (Mirzoeff 2011: 3) are here apparent.

Indeed, within many of the studies cited above critiquing the overrepresentation of light skin tones in research and education, the Fitzpatrick scale was *itself* core to the methodology of determining whether or not representations pictured 'dark skin' or 'skin of color'. The methods sections of these papers (Adelekun et al. 2021: 195; Ebede et al. 2006: 688; Alvarado et al. 2021: 1427; and Porras Fimbres et al. 2023: 2463) describe a similar process: one or several authors reviews each image, 'rates' it on the Fitzpatrick scale, and subsequently classifies it as a 'dark skin image' or an image of 'skin of color' (or not). Far from signalling a risk of cancer, phototypes here come to stand for skin colour and, through the language of 'skin of color', race and ethnicity. Thus, even as critics problematize the scale's development for and within a dermatology which centres light skin tones, the scale continues to constitute *the* baseline for accounting for the diversity of skin tones represented in dermatological teaching and research. What's more, the majority of authors (Ebede et al, 2006: 688; Adelekun et al. 2021: 195; Porras Fimbres et al. 2023: 2463) actively privileged their *own* capacities for skilled looking in doing this work while dismissing diverse kinds of text – some of which may have referenced patients' self-reported relationships to race or ethnicity. In Adelekun et al.'s phrasing: 'To *limit bias* from the reporting of race/ethnicity in figure captions, skin phototypes were assessed *only visually*' (emphasis my own). While these authors recognize text as possibly inhering the original textbook authors' subjective viewpoints, or as something requiring interpretation, they conversely position looking and visual assessment outside the realm of interpretation. Their diction betrays a kind of surety about looking and the relationship between looking and knowing that recalls Lorraine Daston and Peter Galison's (2010: 46) conception of 'trained judgement', an epistemic virtue wherein 'experts relied explicitly on unconscious intuition to guide them'. Or art historian Sarah Archino's (2024) recent observation that in higher education today, administrators, faculty, and staff that would forcefully defend close and critical reading as core objectives of a liberal arts education often fail to recognize close and critical looking as skills to cultivate. Or, to return to Campt, the ways unexamined gazes scrutinizing bodies for evidence – even when such gazes are motivated by efforts to visibilize systemic oppression or marginalization – can easily slip into the reinscription of essentialisms.

That researchers were studying photographs, as opposed to other media, warrants particular scrutiny. As Sarah Lewis (2019) and Lorna Roth (2019) have argued, photography is a 'technology of subjective decisions' developed to most effectively picture lighter skin tones. Within twentieth-century analogue processes, technicians standardized colour correction by working against a test-strip: a photograph of a woman with light skin and hair known as a Shirley card (after the name of the first model). Such processes efficaciously picture subjects and bodies with lighter skin and hair. But they actively fail to picture subjects and bodies with darker skin and hair, producing images with little to no detail, or which flatten subjects' features so as to render them indistinguishable. Transitions to digital technologies witnessed a transformation of the colour-balancing process, and yet photographs continue to misrepresent subjects with darker skin. To offer just one example of this digital echo: to help photographers track and picture human subjects, many digital cameras have built-in algorithmic technologies (Lewis 2019), such as facial recognition software. These algorithmic technologies encode hegemonic whiteness and often do not detect people with darker skin tones. In some ways, these algorithms' very technopolitical comings-into-being comprise a reverberation of photography's origins, or the Fitzpatrick scale's. It's worth noting, too, that the lack of clarity within photographs of darker skin tones likely contributed to their underrepresentation in teaching materials alongside the same systemic racism and hegemonic whiteness shaping *each* of these technologies.

Yet even as medical researchers increasingly critique the Fitzpatrick scale and the manifold ways it has been used, the larger mechanism and value of skin colour classification generally remains unquestioned. Most argue (Coleman et al. 2023: 727–30; Ware et al. 2020: 80; Everett et al. 2012: 499–500, 507–11) that solutions should include the development of more 'precise', 'objective', or 'broad[er] rang[ing]' scales for documenting skin tones. This is the case even among the most ambivalent medical researchers. For example, Ware et al. (2020: 80), writing in collaboration with the Skin of Color Society, write: 'We acknowledge that the conundrum of how to classify individuals with nonwhite skin or skin of color is not simply answered', and conclude their paper by emphasizing how the addition of skin colour to patient charts frequently does more harm than good. And yet the question posed is *how*, not *whether*, to 'classify'. Researchers here demonstrate a faith in more capacious scales, more data, and increasingly 'objective' measurement tools, such as spectrophotometers, that evokes Ruha Benjamin's (2016: 2) powerful assertion that in the face of systemic anti-Black racism, 'the facts, alone, will not save us'. Anthony Hatch (2022: 9) recently brought Benjamin's thinking to bear on the spheres of health and medicine, incisively revealing how 'racial health inequalities data science participates in a form of structural gaslighting that keeps scientists in an endless search for *more and more refined measurements* of racism's harms' even as 'the political and economic systems that comprise the fundamental causes of those harms are given a pass until all the data are counted' (emphasis my own). (Tellingly, Mirzoeff [2011: xiv] has made a similar argument around 'the banality of images', where, contrary to expectations, efforts to spur action by way of more and more images evincing spectacular violence largely led not to change, but complacency.) As thinkers like Sylvia Wynter (1994; 2003) have emphasized, classification and categorization by way of 'descriptive statements' have been core to projects of racialization, the upholding of white supremacy, and the wielding of colonial power – they can never be liberatory. Anthropologist Yesmar Oyarzun (2024) has recently made just such an argument about skin colour scales, including Fitzpatrick's as well as more recent interventions, emphasizing that however precise or capacious, efforts to categorize will always first and foremost reinscribe difference. Even when well intentioned, in their very making, efforts to devise systems of classification most frequently position what Oyarzun terms 'dark bodies' – the 'depersonalized bodies of people with dark skin' – as pathological or, drawing on the research of Deirdre Cooper Owens (2018: 7), a 'superbody', impervious to pain and harm.

Here, artist Byron Kim's ongoing project, *Synecdoche*, is instructive (Figure 6.3). Kim (2020: 197–200) began the project, which remains in-progress, in 1990, when he began painting monochrome panels whose colouring matched aspects of his friends' skin tones. Over time, he expanded the number of portraits/panels to include friends-of-friends, acquaintances, and strangers. When installed, preparators organize the panels into a tight grid, their edges nearly touching. Panels are arranged alphabetically by the first name of the individual represented – information supplied textually beside the paintings. *Synecdoche* fundamentally disrupts the epistemic frameworks driving physicians to develop more and more minute scales of classification for describing, categorizing, and communicating patients' skin tones. Relating the series' originary moment, Kim describes the *impossibility* of choosing a combination of pigments that matched his friend's skin tone, which was flushing as they consumed alcohol together. Indeed, the skin covering every body is *always* multicoloured: its hues and values change

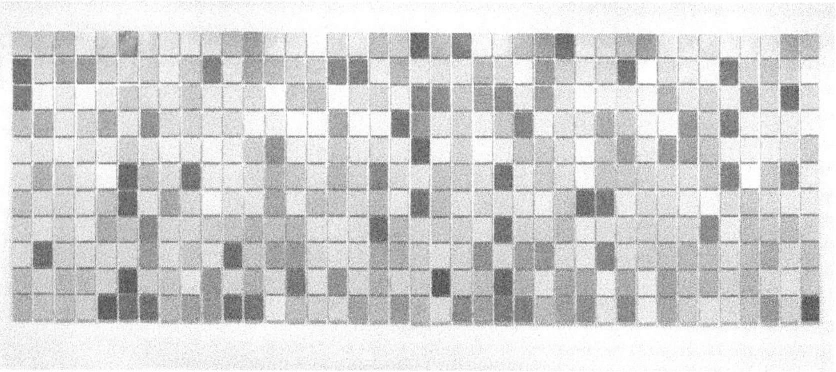

FIGURE 6.3 Byron Kim, *Synecdoche*, 1991–present. Oil and wax on panel, 265 panels, each: 10 × 8" © Byron Kim 2024. Courtesy the artist and James Cohan, New York. Photograph by Dennis Cowley.

not only across diverse parts of the body, but also with activity, age, and time (Kim [2020: 200] notes how differences in his own skin tone between summer and winter mark questions about categorization 'irrelevant'). Even when practitioners agree on a precise location – such as the inner upper arm, an area many dermatologists use to determine so-called baseline constitutive skin colour (Everett et al. 2012: 498) – close looking reveals a multi-hued surface. By actively producing a monochrome image, Kim spotlights the impossibility of precise categorization and reminds viewers that each panel is only a *synecdoche*, a single part *made* to stand for the whole. Such a process, he insists, will always be an abstraction. While the grid evokes precision, measured attention, and the aesthetics of both high modernism and scientific knowledge production, its self-conscious ordering by first name obliterates the organizing principles of the catalogue or the monograph (indexed by surname), the clinical database (databased by date of birth), or, to draw connections to its closest visual referents, the skin colour scale (whether devised to serve physicians or the commercial interests of cosmetic companies, arranged by colour value). Far from rational, Kim's arrangement by given or chosen name centres the recognition of *personhood* as its organizing principle – a counter to Oyarzun's depersonalized 'dark bodies'. Where recent calls (Coleman et al. 2023: 728) for colour scales representing a 'broader range' of skin tones desire precision and certainty, the term *synecdoche* instead emphasizes ambiguity, ephemerality and open-endedness.

To be clear, I in no way seek to dismiss calls for increased representation of manifold skin tones within dermatological education and research. On the contrary, as Singh (2020) and others have emphasized, broad representation across the range of possible skin tones can mean the difference between life and death, or between care and dismissal. Yet the project of increasing representation – of helping students and clinicians understand how symptoms look on all kinds of bodies – need not be tethered to projects of classification. Indeed, in their repeated framing of 'skin of color' or 'nonwhite skin' as a central classificatory problem (Ware et al. 2020:80) – even when such studies are motivated by anti-racist efforts – physicians and medical researchers risk reinscribing darker skin tones as, in Rana Hogarth's phrasing (2019: 837), 'a "problem" to be solved'. What kind of care becomes possible to imagine if medical researchers and practitioners embraced Kim's argument about the impossibility of chromatic categorization? What might medicine become if the energy driving quests for more minute scales could be transmuted, allocated instead to the disentangling of classification, social organization, and naturalization by way of aesthetics? What if, in the place of instrumentalized programs that position art, art history, and visual studies as something to serve medicine in its current iteration, students of dermatology were invited to consider seeing as a situated, multivalent and contested act by thinking with Campt, or Mirzoeff, or Kim? Without classification, what might looking in the context of care hold, do, or be?

References

Adelekun, A, G. Onyekaba, and J. B. Lipoff (2021), 'Skin color in dermatology textbooks: An updated evaluation and analysis', *Journal of the American Academy of Dermatology*, 84 (1): 194–96.

Alvarado, S. M. and H. Feng (2021), 'Representation of dark skin images of common dermatologic conditions in educational resources: A cross-sectional analysis', *Journal of the American Academy of Dermatology*, 84 (5): 1427–31.

Archino, S. (2024), 'Looking at the pictures: Using art history to teach visual literacy across the curriculum', in the session *The Politics of Relevancy: What is the value of art history today?*, College Art Association 112th Annual Conference, Chicago, IL.

Benjamin, R. (2016), 'Racial Fictions, Biological Facts: Expanding the Sociological Imagination through Speculative Methods', *Catalyst: feminism, theory, technoscience*, 2 (2): 1–28.

Buchanan Weiss, E. ([2019]/2024), 'Brown Skin Matters', *Instagram*, available at: https://www.instagram.com/brownskinmatters/ (accessed 9 May 2024).

Callen, A. (2018), *Looking at Men: Anatomy, Masculinity and the Modern Male Body*, New Haven: Yale University Press.

Campt, T. (2012), *Image Matters: Archive, Photography, and the African Diaspora in Europe*, Durham: Duke University Press.

Charlton, M., S. A. Stanley, Z. Whitman, V. Wenn, T. J. Coats, M. Sims, and J. P. Thompson (2020), 'The effect of constitutive pigmentation on the measured emissivity of human skin', *PLoS ONE*, 15 (11).

Coleman, W., K. Mariwalla, and P. Grimes (2023), 'Updating the Fitzpatrick Classification: The Skin Color and Ethnicity Scale', *Dermatologic Surgery*, 49 (8), 725–31.

Cooper Owens, D. (2018), *Medical Bondage: Race, Gender, and the Origins of Medical Gynecology*, Athens: University of Georgia Press.

Daston, L. and P. Galison (2010), *Objectivity*, New York: Zone Books.

Ebede, T. and A. Papier (2006), 'Disparities in dermatology educational resources', *Journal of the American Academy of Dermatology*, 44 (4): 687–90.

Erickson, T., K. Daftary, V. L. Quan, and R. Chovatiya (2023), 'Capturing the Diversity of Dermatology – What's in a Name?', *American Journal of Clinical Dermatology* 24 (5): 675–80.

Everett, J. S., M. Budescu, and M. S. Sommers (2012), 'Making Sense of Skin Color in Clinical Care', *Clinical Nursing Research*, 21 (4): 495–516.

Fanon, F. ([1952] 2008), *Black Skin, White Masks*, trans. Richard Philcox, New York: Grove Press.

Fitzpatrick, T. B. (1975), 'Soleil et peau', *Journal de médecine esthétique*, 2: 33–4.

Fitzpatrick, T. B. (1988), 'The Validity and Practicality of Sun-Reactive Skin Types I Through VI', *Archives of Dermatology*, 124 (6): 869–71.

Fitzpatrick, T. B., A. Z. Eisen, K. Wolff, I. M. Freedberg, and K. F. Austen, eds. (1993), *Dermatology in General Medicine*, 4th ed., vol. 1, New York: McGraw-Hill.

Foucault, M. ([1963] 1973). *The Birth of the Clinic: An Archaeology of Medical Perception*, trans. A. M. Sheridan Smith, New York: Vintage Books.

Hatch, A. (2022), 'The data will not save us: Afropessimism and racial antimatter in the COVID-19 pandemic', *Big Data & Society*, 9 (1): 1–13.

Hogarth, R. (2019), 'Of Black Skin and Biopower: Lessons from the Eighteenth Century', *American Quarterly*, 71 (3): 837–47.

Johnstone, F. (2018), 'Manifesto for a Visual Medical Humanities', *BMJ Medical Humanities Blog*, 31 July. Available online: https://blogs.bmj.com/medical-humanities/2018/07/31/manifesto-for-a-visual-medical-humanities/ (accessed 9 May 2024).

Johnstone, F. (2023), 'Collaborations in Art and Medicine: Institutional Critique, Patient Participation, and Emerging Entanglements', *Leonardo*, 56 (4): 424–29.

Jordanova, L. (1989), *Sexual Visions: Images of Gender in Science and Medicine Between the Eighteenth and Twentieth Centuries*, Madison: University of Wisconsin Press.

Kim, B. (2020), 'The Local Color of Shadow', in C. R. Snorton and H. Yapp (eds), *Saturation: Race, Art, and the Circulation of Value*, Cambridge, MA: MIT Press.

Lester, J. ([2018] 2024), 'Skin of Color Program', *University of California San Francisco*, available at: https://dermatology.ucsf.edu/skin-of-color-program, (accessed 9 May 2024).

Lewis, S. (2019), 'The Racial Bias Built Into Photography', *The New York Times*, 25 April.

Mihm, M. C., Jr. and A. J. Sober. (2004), 'Melanoma Before and After Thomas B. Fitzpatrick', *Journal of Investigative Dermatology*, 122 (2): xxxii–xxxiii.

Mirzoeff, N. (2011), *The Right to Look: A Counterhistory of Visuality*, Durham: Duke University Press.

Pierce, K. (2020), 'Photograph as Skin, Skin as Wax: Indexicality and the Visualisation of Syphilis in Fin-de-Siècle France', *Medical History*, 64 (1): 116–41.

Pierce, K. (2025), '"Typical Cases": Representation, Racializing Medicine, and the Politics of the Case Study in the Moulages Collections of the Hôpital Saint-Louis', *Histoire, Médecine et Santé*, 27, (Summer, 2025): 31-52.

Ott, K. (2010), 'Contagion, Public Health, and the Visual Culture of Nineteenth-Century Skin', in D. Serlin (ed.), *Imagining Illness: Public Health and Visual Culture*, 85–107, Minneapolis: University of Minnesota Press.

Oyarzun, Y. (2024), '"All You See Is White Skin": Race and Dermatology in the United States', PhD dissertation, Rice University.

Pathak, M. A., K. Jimbow, G. Szabo, and T. B. Fitzpatrick (1986), 'Sunlight and Melanin Pigmentation', in K. C. Smith (ed.), *Photochemical and Photobiological Reviews*, 211–39, New York: Plenum Press.

Porras Fimbres, D. C., J. Jacobs, C. Diamond, C. W. Rundle, L. Rodriguez-Homs, C. Presley, and C. Stamey (2023), 'Representation of Fitzpatrick skin phototype in dermatology surgical textbooks', *Archives of Dermatological Research*, 315 (8): 2463–65.

Robertson, A., W. Magdy, and S. Goldwater (2021), 'Black or White but Never Neutral: How Readers Perceive Identity from Yellow or Skin-toned Emoji',

Proceedings of the ACM on Human-Computer Interaction, 5 (CSCW2): 350:1–350:23.
Roth, L. (2019), 'Making Skin Visible through Liberatory Design', in R. Benjamin (ed.), *Captivating Technology: Race, Carceral Technoscience, and Liberatory Imagination in Everyday Life*, 275–307, Durham: Duke University Press.
Singh, N. (2020), 'Decolonising dermatology: Why black and brown skin need better treatment', *The Guardian*, 13 August.
Sutton, M. K. (2016), 'What's Your Type?', *Sutton Dermatology + Aesthetics*, 17 October. Available online: https://suttonderm.com/whats-your-type/ (accessed 8 May 2024).
Vyas, D. A., D. S. Jones, A. R. Meadows, K. Diouf, N. M. Nour, and J. Schantz-Dunn (2019), 'Challenging the Use of Race in the Vaginal Birth after Cesarean Section Calculator', *Women's Health Issues*, 29 (3): 201–4.
Ware, O. R., J. E. Dawson, M. M. Shinohara, and S. C. Taylor (2020), 'Racial Limitations of Fitzpatrick Skin Type', *Cutis*, 105 (2): 77–80.
Wynter, S. (1994), '"No Humans Involved": An Open Letter to My Colleagues', *Forum NHI: Knowledge for the 21st Century*, 1 (1): 42–73.
Wynter, S. (2003), 'Unsettling the Coloniality of Being/Power/Truth/Freedom: Towards the Human, After Man, Its Overrepresentation—An Argument', *New Centennial Review*, 3 (3): 57–337.

CHAPTER SEVEN

Punchlines and power: visual humour as a disruptive tool for the critical medical humanities

Katie Snow, Christine Slobogin and Laura Cowley

Humour helps us to navigate, negotiate and know our place in the world. Exploring what a given community finds funny, and why, has the potential to both clarify and disrupt the power structures that scaffold everyday experiences. What we find 'funny' about bodies, and how they feature in visual jokes or humour, can reveal much about how particular groups or identities are prioritized or devalued. Bodily humour takes on different valences depending on the perceived normativity of the joke's featured body and contextual factors such as who is joking about it, and from what relational position. Jokes often serve to signify or assert power in a relationship; when that relationship operates within a medicalized context, those points of power are typically even more fraught.

Our research on art and medicine is anchored in different periods, spaces and mediums, but has common convictions in the potential of visual humour to disturb medicalized power structures and articulate struggles over agency, hierarchy and representation. In the examples that follow, we draw from our own research to show various ways in which hierarchies have been and can be subverted through apparently funny artistic representations of bodies and the medical sphere.

The powerful art of bodily caricature

The power of caricature rests on unsettling. Its disruptive potential is immense and interminable; coloured by controversies, contradictions, absurdities and vulgarities, it sets out to shock and sway from within a mode whose very existence raises questions about the nature of art itself. Bodily caricature, marked by the comic, debased, hyperbolic and grotesque, provides particularly fertile ground for critical investigations – and interventions – in the critical medical humanities. Caricaturists are attentive to the frustrations, longings, joys, tragedies and transgressions which influence corporeal – and especially pathologized – existence, but they are also quick to mock them and the power dynamics that shape them. Take, for example, Charles Williams's *Mr Lambert in Miniature or Master Wybrants, the modern Hercules* from 1806 (Figure 7.1), which confronts us with a body shocking in its defiance of expectations.

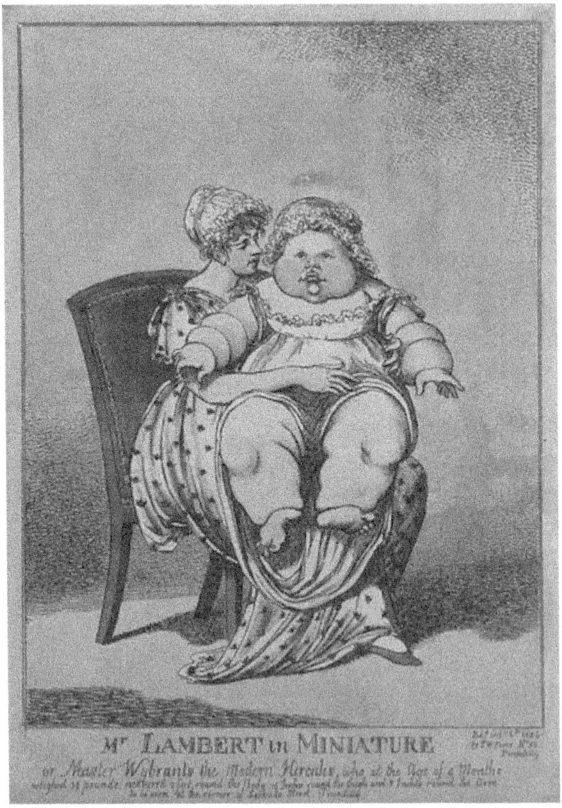

FIGURE 7.1 Charles Williams, *Mr Lambert in Miniature or Master Wybrants, the Modern Hercules,* 1806. Wellcome Collection 8521.

With 'enormous' (George 1952) limbs bulging out from a flimsy chemise, 'Master Wybrants' is a caricatured miniature of Daniel Lamberts, a man whose corpulency gained him notoriety in the early 1800s. Said to eat a 'normal' diet, abstain from alcohol, and to be regularly physically active, Lambert's size – he weighed upwards of fifty stone – attracted both medical and public interest. Medical journals published investigations into his bodily functions, presentations and pathologies (they found few), and caricature matched this medical gaze with visceral visions of his larger body, presenting him as a figure of fun, an object of pity and a challenge to cultural and medical ideas about body size.

In 1806, Lambert entered into Britain's show-circuit of pathologized bodies when he began exhibiting his body to paid viewers. Achieving celebrity status – and some wealth – through his perceived anatomical oddity, Lambert's vexed representation across culture – including in caricatures like *Mr Lambert in Miniature* – raises questions at the heart of critical medical humanities investigations into humour and health. Why are some differences pathologized and others celebrated? Why is difference sometimes the object of laughter or mockery? Is there power in representation, even if ostensibly negative? Is humour a response to fear?

The infant's robe in *Mr Lambert in Miniature* is pulled back to reveal excess rolls of skin gathered at the legs. This uncloaking makes the pathologized body knowable, forcing viewers to bear witness to its truths and thus displacing them to the public sphere. This approach mapped onto wider contemporary medical-moral frameworks, which sought to 'strip away ornament and artifice in order to expose reality, to see things as they really were' (Wagner 2013: 96–97). However, as the British Museum's catalogue points out, the drawn dimensions of Master Wybrants' body 'far exceed' the claims of the inscription, which tell how he 'weighed 39 pounds, measured 2 feet round the Body, 15 Inches round the thigh and 8 Inches round the Arm' (George 1952). Contradicting this empirical account, the caricature shows the infant's great mass barely contained by his mother. This playful discordance between art, humour and science reminds us of the futility of looking for definitive answers in caricature. To do so, Mark Philp warns, is to 'misread the nature of satire', overlooking 'the plurality of possibilities' within each frame (2017: 189).

Questions have abounded around caricature's value as a historical artefact due to its characteristic exaggeration and invention. This is especially acute when it comes to bodily representation, with caricatures drastically departing from alternative imagery such as anatomical drawings and medical photographs and models. Caricatures draw upon, but do not aspire to represent, 'reality'. Ian Haywood writes that caricature provides a window into society that is filled with 'distorting and kaleidoscopic glass', and it is precisely within this altered vision that its power lies (2012: 437). Turning to reality in order to turn away from it, caricature visualizes new 'truths': alternative ways of being in the body, moving within institutions and negotiating pathologies. The world which caricature plunges us into is colourful, disorientating, fractured, fluid and above all, playful; alike, in many ways, to the aspirations of the critical medical humanities.

Subverting hospital power relations through cartoons

As graphic satire playfully unsettled social and bodily realities and power relations in the eighteenth and early nineteenth centuries, so cartoons unsettled hospital hierarchies in the twentieth century. Women working in a myriad of different roles during the Second World War used cartoons in order to express the ridiculousness of their positionality (Lewis-Smith 2006; Schaap 2015). This is particularly apparent within the medical space, where illustrators used their pens and pencils to conceptualize their own role within the hospital, draw attention to their needs and bring their superiors down a notch.

Two female surgical artists working in mid-twentieth-century Britain, Dickie Orpen (1914–2008) and Dorothy Davison (1889–1984), made cartoons that pointed out masculine disregard for their work within the operating theatre. At a very basic level, these artists needed to *see* the patient in order to draw them. And yet this did not always happen. In *Artist at Work* (Figure 7.2), Orpen draws herself contorting comically, bending her body to an impossibly small size in order to peer between the legs of others gathered around an operating table. We know that she is trying to draw what they are all looking at, but it is exceedingly clear that she has no way to see it. In a similar cartoon, Davison also depicts herself as an exaggeratedly diminutive figure (about half the size of a surgeon) standing on her tiptoes atop a whimsical set of stairs in the operating theatre (Palfreyman 2022: 136). Peering over the surgeon's shoulder, she seems to have pointed out that she cannot see the body she is meant to depict, but he dismisses her concerns by saying that *he* can feel and therefore 'see' the body part of focus. Both artists played with size in these cartoons, making their bodies small in comparison to the other clinical staff. By poking fun at their lack of power within the operating theatre at the site of their own bodies, they advocated for their professional needs within this medical space.

In addition to highlighting the ridiculous difficulties of their jobs, women such as these two depicted their superiors in portraiture or in caricatures. At least in Orpen's hospital, the surgeons were aware of these visual jokes; there is evidence that Orpen's sketchbooks were passed around convivially (Slobogin 2023). Sometimes she used the captions at the bottom of her caricatures to subvert their seemingly innocuous, portrait-like presentations. For instance, she labelled a drawing of the surgeon Grey-Turner as if he

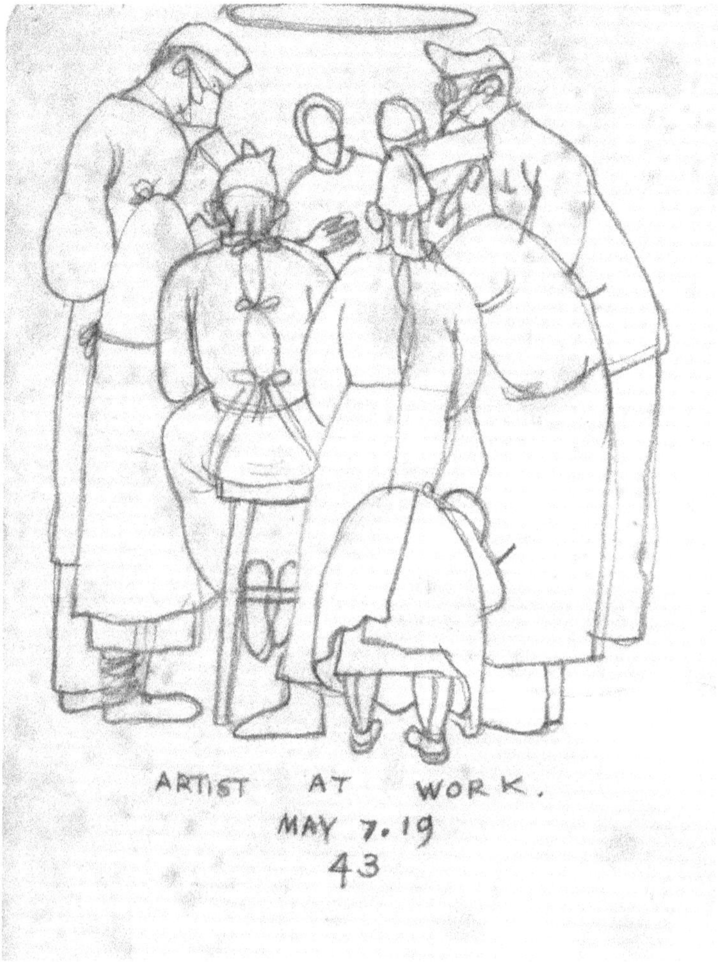

FIGURE 7.2 Dickie Orpen, *Artist at Work*, 1943. From Dickie Orpen's personal papers, courtesy of Bill Olivier and the British Association of Plastic, Reconstructive, and Aesthetic Surgeons.

were a creature in a zoo or a textbook: *Homo Sapiens. Species Chirurgo-Leprechanus*. 'Chirurgo' refers to surgery, and 'Leprecaunus' refers to his abnormally large ears, made more noticeable in the drawing because of the added caption. By representing these surgeons with pencil and paper, women like Orpen claimed power over these men's images and reputations – which could be altered with humour in many ways.

This type of artwork helped to upset the immediately assumed hierarchy within the hospital in this period. The men had medical degrees, ran the wards, held the power. By humorously depicting their own bodies alongside those of their male colleagues, these women claimed some of that power for themselves.

Scatological humour and disability aesthetics

Finding humour in the body is itself a bodily enterprise, and laughter is sometimes as involuntary and as inappropriate as any other bodily function or malfunction. Scatological humour trades in such embarrassments. In the disability arts movement of the United Kingdom (c. 1976–), humorous references to toileting were urgently political, alchemizing pity and shame into provocative pride. The slogan 'Piss on Pity' became a rallying cry after police officers proved its potential to offend by confiscating a placard in 1990 (Lisicki 2018). There was a political utility to scatological swearing; the language was particularly transgressive in the mouths of infantilized disabled people (Cameron 2009: 385). Shock humour repudiated condescension from the charity sector and curative medicine, while forcing the practical difficulties of the disorderly body into public consciousness, critiquing a disempowering lack of disabled access to public toilets and therefore public spaces.

This humour can also be enduringly funny, if culturally specific. I once laughed aloud in the archive at a self-caricature by artist and disability activist Steve Cribb (1944–1995), captioned *Introducing the Bad Spastic, Keeper of the Key* (Figure 7.3). Cribb's key is a 'radar key', from a charity scheme which, since 1981, has managed locks on adapted public toilets in the United Kingdom, keeping them accessible to people who have purchased a key. Cribb depicts himself as a powerful and sinister wheelchair-using figure, possessing horns, spiky shoulders and a fancy tie, with an absurd penchant for hoarding access to accessible bathrooms. Cribb was indignant at needing to cross extra hurdles to access something so fundamental, and the illustration pokes fun at the absurdist structures that contain and create disability. There is also a defiant acknowledgement of taboo functions of the body and a rejection of the associated vulnerabilities.

Pissing logistics became a repeated topic for Cribb. He depicted his recurring characters, Mrs Pennington and her guide dog Bonzo, the latter drawn propped like a teddy-bear in a wheelchair, confronting an 'inaccessible lamppost', and getting neatly to the repressed animality revealed and satisfied by vulgar humour (Cribb 1991). Cribb's cartoons differ from the other images in this present text, joking from the positionality of the disabled body, an often-overlooked perspective (Shakespeare 1999: 49). Analysis of Cribb's work shows how visual humour, from artists who resist medicalization, reveals absurdity in biological hierarchies and seemingly rational responses to disability. This deconstruction is furthered by the proffered opportunity to laugh with – and not at – the medicalized body.

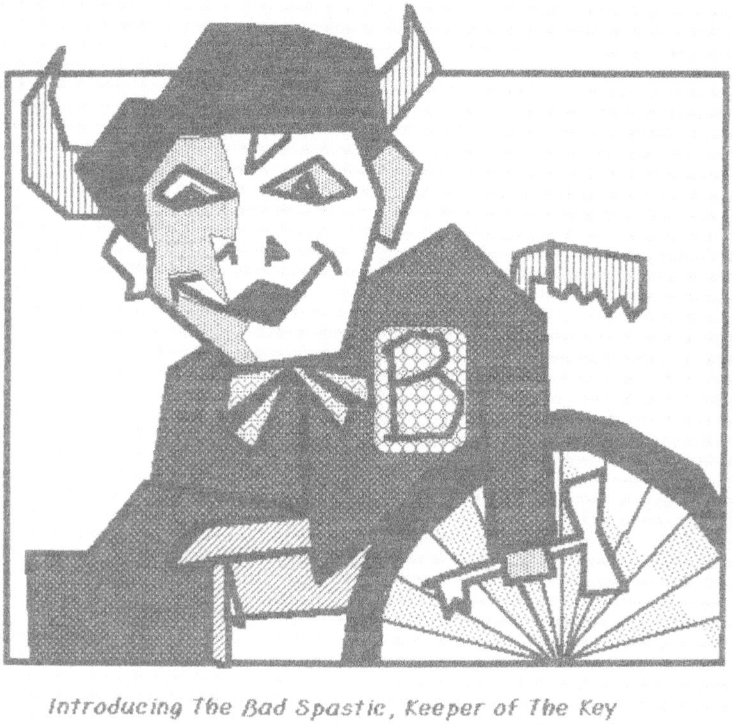

FIGURE 7.3 Steve Cribb, *Introducing the Bad Spastic, Keeper of the Key*, 1990. Courtesy of the National Disability Arts Collection and Archive, https://the-ndaca.org.

Conclusion

As these three examples show, analyzing visual culture at the intersection of humour and medicine reveals how unstable power relations can be disrupted and resisted through imagery. The edited volume that the three of us are working on together, which focuses on visual histories of humour, health and the body, brings in other examples to further elucidate the disruptive power of the humorous visual medical humanities. Humour can act as practical research intervention into the ever-uncomfortable matter of being a body and having a body, because humour contains within it the invitation to laugh. Laughter, like illness and injury, can contort the body. Esther Leslie (2016) calls laughter a shattering of words and thoughts, reflecting that as things break, there is the opportunity to reflect and replace. Humour might then be described as a productive tool for a discipline that strives towards critical engagement, as an embodied antidote to rationality in medical spaces that aim towards the reasonable and the curative.

Although we have set out historically specific examples that treat the visual body as a source of entertainment, academic writing practices which rely on close analysis can feel – at times productively – undermining to the substance of humour. The degree to which this research should be or even can be funny continues to be a source of debate amongst us, and sometimes we work on pieces that we don't personally find funny at all. For example, caricature 'goes low' in dark ways; rife with racism, misogyny, homophobia, transphobia, ableism and classism, it punches down as a comedic tactic, perpetuating harmful stereotypes and reinforcing marginalization. Part of the power of historical analysis is in confronting these harmful narratives and extracting lessons from them. Investigations into art and humour within the critical medical humanities have the potential to generate micro-interventions that can disrupt dangerous legacies and suggest new ways of representing and inhabiting the body in all its comic glory.

References

Cameron, C. (2009), 'Tragic but Brave or Just Crips with Chips? Songs and Their Lyrics in the Disability Arts Movement in Britain', *Popular Music* 28 (3): 381–96.

Cribb, S. (1991), 2 *Cartoons*, National Disability Arts Collection and Archive. Available online: https://the-ndaca.org/collection/?uniqueID=ARC1260 (accessed 24 September 2024).

George, M. D. (1952), Catalogue of Political and Personal Satires in the Department of Prints and Drawings in the British Museum. Vol. 8. London: BMP.

Haywood, I. (2012), 'Rude Britannia: New Perspectives in Caricature', *Eighteenth-Century Studies* 45 (2): 437–40.

Leslie, E. (2016), 'Those in Glass Houses Laugh', Verso Books [blog], 27 September. Available online: https://www.versobooks.com/en-gb/blogs/news/2855-those-in-glass-houses-laugh (accessed 14 November 2023).

Lewis-Smith, A. (2006), *Off Duty!: Bletchley Park Outstation Gayhurst Manor WW2*, Newport: Traeth Publications.

Lisicki, B. (2018), 'Block Telethon 1992 - the day we "pissed on pity"', @theNDACA [Blog], 16 February. Available online: https://medium.com/@theNDACA/block-telethon-1992-the-day-we-pissed-on-pity-69117b03825a (accessed 14 February 2022).

Palfreyman, H. (2022), 'Material Images: Flesh on Paper in Twentieth-Century Surgical Drawing', in J. Nott and A. Harris (eds), *Making Sense of Medicine: Material Culture and the Reproduction of Medical Knowledge*, 232–44, Bristol and Chicago: Intellect.

Philp, M. (2017), 'Nervous Laughter and the Invasion of Britain 1797–1805', in M. Knights and M. Morton (eds), *The Power of Laughter and Satire in*

Early Modern Britain: Political and Religious Culture, 1500–1820, 173–89, Woodbridge: Boydell & Brewer.

Schaap, T. (2015), '"Girl Takes Drastic Step": Molly Lamb Bobak's W110278–The Diary of a CWAC', in M. Kadar and J. Perreault (eds), *Working Memory: Women and Work in WWII*, 171–90, Waterloo: Wilfrid Laurier University Press.

Shakespeare, T. (1999), 'Joking a Part', *Body and Society* 5 (4): 47–52.

Slobogin, C. (2023), '"'E's a Funny Doctor": Dickie Orpen and the Visual Humour of the Second World War Reconstructive Surgery Ward', 111–35, in J. Pattinson and L. Robb (eds), *British Humour and the Second World War: "Keep Smiling Through"*, London: Bloomsbury.

Wagner, C. (2013), *Pathological Bodies: Medicine and Political Culture*, Berkeley: University of California Press.

CHAPTER EIGHT

Two faces of the same object: borderline bodies in art and visual culture

Natasha Ruiz-Gómez, Tania Cleaves (née Woloshyn) and Keren Rosa Hammerschlag

What is a borderline body? To explore this question, we take as a case study the *Ataxic Venus* (c.1880, Figure 8.1), one of the most extraordinary 'scientific artworks' to survive the nineteenth century (Ruiz-Gómez 2024). The *Ataxic Venus* is a polychrome wax cast of a sixty-year-old patient at Paris' Hôpital de la Salpêtrière named Berthelot, a woman whose effigy acquired a certain fame after her death. The cast highlights Berthelot's ataxic joints, a symptom of locomotor ataxia. A complication of tertiary syphilis, this devastating illness typically resulted in loss of coordination and the degeneration of the joints, among a host of other painful symptoms, and could eventually lead to paralysis, amputations and even insanity. Berthelot's body and those distended and deformed joints are challenging to look at and evoke a visceral response of discomfort and even repulsion.

It is unclear who gave the wax cast its moniker, though it was likely intended to establish its lineage with anatomical 'Venuses' – the *Venere dei Medici* by Clemente Susini (1754–1814) at La Specola foremost among them – which sit uneasily at the juncture of the 'high' art tradition of the female nude and medical images of sick, disabled, anatomized and dead female bodies (Stephens 2010; Ebenstein 2017; Ruiz-Gómez 2013). But the *Ataxic Venus* is

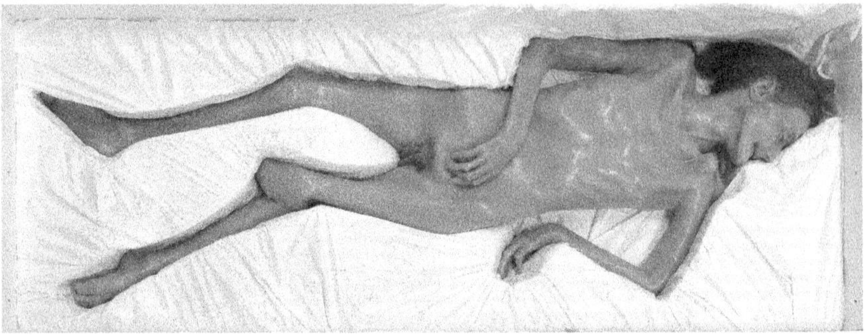

FIGURE 8.1 Louis Loreau, *Venus ataxique*, polychrome wax cast, *c.* 1880. Musée de l'Assistance publique – Hôpitaux de Paris, inv. AP 2001.0.4.3.1 Photo © AP-HP/musée – F. Marin

the macabre partner (elderly, decrepit, distorted, barren) to the aestheticized and sexualized young, beautiful, usually pregnant, women more regularly portrayed in anatomical imagery and modelling and in paintings of medical subjects (Jordanova 1989; Hunter 2016; Ruiz-Gómez 2024).

The *Ataxic Venus* was cast by a photographer and *mouleur* at the Salpêtrière named Louis Loreau (1846–1907), about whom almost nothing is known. (We know substantially more about the patient than we do about the technician.) Loreau was one of the many collaborators who worked with Jean-Martin Charcot (1825–1893), *medecin en chef* of the Salpêtrière Hospital and one of the founders of modern neurology, thanks in part to the patients under his care whose illnesses progressed, sometimes over the course of decades, under his watchful eye. By the time Loreau had cast Berthelot's body around 1880, Charcot had established at the hospital a photography and casting studio, a consulting room for ophthalmology, an amphitheatre for his internationally renowned lectures, and a museum of pathological anatomy (the so-called Musée Charcot, where the *Ataxic Venus* would be the star attraction).

The *Ataxic Venus* was intended as a medical specimen, to be studied by (future) clinicians at the Musée Charcot; a photograph of the sculpture takes centre-stage in the only known photograph of the museum (Levillain 1894). But the fact that the hospital's clinicians, as well as the international coterie of doctors and esteemed politicians, artists and celebrities who attended Charcot's famous lessons at the Salpêtrière, might have seen Berthelot during her lifetime highlights the recognizable features of the cast that also make it a portrait. In other words, they would not have failed to recognize the patient Berthelot, the woman who was studied, if not treated, at the Salpêtrière because of her incurable illness. This sculpture, then, is both medical specimen *and* portrait and should thus be considered at the porous and messy border of the histories of medicine and of art (Jordanova 2000 and 2013; Hammerschlag 2013a).

Charcot facilitated the photographing of Berthelot during life and the casting of her body after death, an attempt to preserve her decomposing corpse so that it could be studied in the future, compared to her excised skeleton (also exhibited in the museum), and contribute to the glory of the clinician whose innovative diagnosis remains attached to her affliction. The *Ataxic Venus* might therefore be associated with other cast bodies and body parts from the eighteenth and nineteenth centuries that were used for instruction and entertainment, including death masks of famous and notorious individuals (Pointon 2014; Ruiz-Gómez 2021). The turning of Berthelot's corpse into the *Ataxic Venus* also bares uncanny and disturbing similarities to the story of Sarah Baartman, whose body was also cast after death and exhibited in a Parisian museum so that the 'Hottentot Venus' could continue to be gawked at (and groped) in death as in life (e.g., Qureshi 2004; Lyons 2018). 'Charcot joint' is still the nomenclature used for the kind of deformed joints (arthropathy) evidenced by the *Ataxic Venus*. Significantly, the International Medical Congress in 1881 named it so after Charcot presented the material traces of Berthelot: a photograph of her while alive, the polychrome cast of her body, her actual skeleton and microscopic sections of her bones (Charcot 1881). For Charcot, Berthelot and her diagnosis became a kind of possession: he wrote proudly to his wife from London, 'my wax lady has made a sensation' (quoted in Goetz, Bonduelle and Gelfand 1995: 147).

Not only a key material remnant of the Salpêtrière School's engagement with the history of art and contemporary artistic practices, Charcot's 'wax lady' is also a borderline body. Julia Kristeva deploys the concept of the border in her definition of abjection, writing that it is 'what disturbs identity, system, order. What does not respect *borders*, positions, rules. The in-between, the ambiguous, the composite' (emphasis added; Kristeva 1982: 4). The *Ataxic Venus* exists in a liminal conceptual space, created at a hospital as well known for its (medical) studies of art as for its innovative neurological diagnoses, exhibited in a curated medical museum that included commissions by a contemporary artist (Ruiz-Gómez 2024). As Charcot and his collaborator Dr Paul Richer (1849–1933) would write in their popular book *Les Difformes et les malades dans l'art (The Deformed and the Ill in Art,* 1889): 'Science and art are nothing more than two manifestations of the same phenomenon, two faces of the same object' (Charcot and Richer 1889: iii).

The *Ataxic Venus*, moreover, was crafted from a material which too can be considered borderline: while wax is especially suited for representing skin, its use in fine art has always been problematic and contested. This ability to represent flesh accurately makes it both uncanny and extremely useful in documenting medical illness, especially dermatological (Hunter 2008; Fend

2018). Coloured wax in particular can give the impression of life-likeness, yet the *Ataxic Venus* shows us a life stilled by death. This wax cadaver is a pale sandy colour all over, but Charcot and Loreau decided to implant hair on the scalp, in the eyebrows and in the *mons veneris* to create a more 'realistic' figure. While casting is traditionally considered indexical (i.e., created without human intervention), the *Ataxic Venus* gives the illusion of objectivity even as it displays the results of myriad artistic decisions. In this too it is borderline.

Artists and doctors: these professions rely on being *intimate with* the human body, including marginalized and vulnerable bodies (Hammerschlag 2013b; Woloshyn 2017; Ruiz-Gómez 2019). As art historians working within the medical humanities, our attending to these bodies involves related processes of close looking to 'flesh out' and substantiate (give 'substance' to) things which are often overlooked or taken for granted, i.e., the visual and material representations through which we encounter such bodies. Berthelot may be the origin for the *Ataxic Venus* but the sculpture is not Berthelot. It is a material presentation of her body, and yet as we follow its contorted, jarring contours – its bodily borders – it is so easy to conflate body and representation, even to refer to the sculpture as 'she'.

The three authors of this paper have considered similarly confounding borderline bodies in their work at the intersection of the histories of medicine and art. Working within the medical humanities has taught us how to be interdisciplinary art historians, working within, between and across borders of different disciplines (Biernoff and Johnstone 2024). Drawing inspiration from Marco Mogiani's conception of borders as '"meeting points", that is, places of encounter, interaction/clash, and reassessment/redefinition of different epistemological and empirical processes', we decided to bring together scholars from around the world working in different disciplines to consider the visual and material representations of 'borderline' human bodies (Mogiani 2023: 1324). The result is *Borderline Bodies in Art and Visual Culture: Unsettling Identity and Place Since 1800* (Manchester University Press, 2026).

Contributors to *Borderline Bodies* consider representations of bodies across a range of geographies and media that move across borders and/or embody indefinite or multiple racial, religious, gender, physical, social or political categories. As well as carrying geographical and political meanings, the concept of the 'borderline' is used, of course, in medical practice to describe diagnostic ambiguity, even failure. In medicine, the 'borderline case' is a term which characterizes uncertain diagnosis, qualities or conditions, here between the normative and the pathological. It is the 'not quite' of medical diagnosis, defying labels and, for better or worse, what those labels could enable or disable (e.g., access to medication, to rights, to care). It is both disruptive and generates conflict because it undermines the clarity of a definitive diagnosis.

But borderline bodies are remarkable precisely because they do not conform to a norm or to a known or desired standard. Instead they disrupt, misbehave and mark out those norms through their difference and their refusal. They are complex, often frustrating and potentially destructive. A borderline can only exist if there are categories or an infrastructure through which to traverse. In other words, if there were no borders, walls or fences, we would never cross territories. This is why we understand the borderline as a *threshold*: one which can literally and figuratively mark out divisions or limits but can also signal new beginnings. Moreover, the act of border crossing is rarely simple or painless: it often involves passing through a 'no man's land' or state of transition – a liminal space – which can be fraught and conflicted. Hence, *Borderline Bodies* considers the ways art and visual culture can reveal the unbounded, vulnerable, permeable and mobile nature of human corporeality. It explores representations of 'borderline bodies', such as the *Ataxic Venus*, their questionable boundaries and capacity to breach boundaries. Above all, it examines the relationship between borders and identity formation in order to throw into focus the 'two faces of the same object'.

References

Biernoff, S. and F. Johnson (2024), 'What can art history offer medical humanities?', *Medical Humanities*: https://mh.bmj.com/content/early/2024/05/30/medhum-2023-012763# (accessed 11 September 2024).

Ebenstein, J. (2017), *The Anatomical Venus: Morbid Anatomy Presents*, London: Thames & Hudson.

Charcot, J.-M. (1881), 'Demonstration of Arthropathic Affections of Locomotor Ataxia', *British Medical Journal* (August 13): 285.

Charcot, J.-M. and P. Richer (1889), *Les Difformes et les malades dans l'art*, Paris: Lecrosnier & Babé.

Fend, M. (2018), 'Order and Affect: The Museum of Dermatological Wax Moulages at the Hôpital Saint-Louis in Paris', in J. Grave, C. Holm, V. Kobi, and C. van Eck (eds), *The Agency of Display: Objects, Framings and Parerga*, 79–98, Dresden: Sandstein Verlag.

Goetz, C. G., M. Bonduelle, and T. Gelfand (1995), *Charcot: Constructing Neurology*, New York: Oxford University Press.

Hammerschlag, K. R. (2013a), 'The Gentleman Artist-Surgeon in Late Victorian Group Portraiture', *Visual Culture in Britain* 14: 154–78.

Hammerschlag, K. R. (2013b), 'Identifying the Patient in George W. Lambert's *Chesham Street*', *Medical Humanities*, 39: 20–28.

Hunter, M. (2008), '"Effroyable réalisme": Wax, Femininity, and the Madness of Realist Fantasies', *RACAR*, 33 (1-2): 43–58.

Hunter, M. (2016), *The Face of Medicine: Visualising Medical Masculinities in Late Nineteenth-Century Paris*, Manchester: Manchester University Press.

Jordanova, L. (1989), *Sexual Visions: Images of Gender in Science and Medicine between the Eighteenth and Twentieth Centuries*, Madison: University of Wisconsin Press.

Jordanova, L. (2000), *Defining Features: Scientific and Medical Portraits, 1660–2000*, London: Reaktion.

Jordanova, L. (2013), 'Portraits, Patients and Practitioners' (editorial), *Medical Humanities*, 39: 2–3.

Kristeva, J. (1982), *Powers of Horror*, trans. L. S. Roudiez, New York: Columbia University Press.

Levillain, F. (1894), 'Charcot et l'École de la Salpêtrière', *Revue encyclopédique* 10 (March 1): 108–15.

Lyons, A.P. (2018), 'The Two Lives of Sara Baartman: Gender, "Race," Politics and the Historiography of Mis/Representation', *Anthropologica* 60 (1): 327–46.

Mogiani, M. (2023), 'Studying Borders from the Border: Reflections on the Concept of Borders as Meeting Points', *Geopolitics*, 28: 1323–41.

Pointon, M. (2014), 'Casts, Imprints, and the Deathliness of Things: Artifacts at the Edge', *Art Bulletin*, 96(2): 170–95.

Qureshi, S. (2004), 'Displaying Sara Baartman, The "Hottentot Venus"', *History of Science* 42(2): 233–57.

Ruiz-Gómez, N. (2013), 'A Hysterical Reading of Rodin's *Gates of Hell*', *Art History*, 36 (5): 994–1017.

Ruiz-Gómez, N. (2019), 'The Model Patient: Observation and Illustration at the Musée Charcot,' in A. Graciano (ed.), *Visualizing the Body in Art, Anatomy, and Medicine since 1800: Models and Modeling*, 203–232, London and New York: Routledge.

Ruiz-Gómez, N. (2021), 'Of Sculptural and Corporal Remains', in N. Abdel Nabi, C. Ariot and A. Borchardt-Hume (eds), *The Making of Rodin*, 46–53, ex. cat., London: Tate.

Ruiz-Gómez, N. (2024), *Pathology and Visual Culture: The Scientific Artworks of Dr. Jean-Martin Charcot and the Salpêtrière School*, University Park, Pennsylvania: Pennsylvania State University Press.

Stephens, Elizabeth (2010), *Anatomy as Spectacle: Public Exhibitions of the Body from 1700 to the Present*, Liverpool: Liverpool University Press.

Transactions of the International Medical Congress. Seventh Session held in London, August 2nd to August 9th, 1881. (1881), Vol. 1, London: J. W. Kolckmann.

Woloshyn, T. (2017), *Soaking Up the Rays: Light Therapy and Visual Culture in Britain, c.1890–1940*, Manchester: Manchester University Press.

CHAPTER NINE

Between mania and melancholy: Thomas Lawrence's *Mad Girl*

Anna Jamieson

In 1786, the celebrated painter Thomas Lawrence submitted a series of pastels to the Royal Academy's summer exhibition. Of the seven artworks exhibited by the seventeen-year-old British artist, all went unnoticed by the day's periodical press. In recent years, however, Lawrence's pastel number 184 has captured scholarly attention (Kromm 2002: 150–52). Lawrence, titling the pastel *Mad Girl*, presents a woman looking skyward, expressing intense passion and melancholic despair. Tears fill her eyes and roll down her cheeks, her right breast is exposed and wisps of straw crown her flowing hair. Situated in a bleak cell-like interior with chained wrists, her raised hand calls upon the viewer's sympathy. On the back of the frame reads an inscription taken from a popular folksong titled 'A Maid in Bedlam':

Madsong
One Morning very early
One Morning in the Spring,
I heard a Maid in Bedlam,
Who mournfully did sing;
Her chains she rattled in her hands
While sadly thus sung she,
I love my Love, -because
I know my Love loves me!

Bethlem Hospital was London's most notorious asylum, having been opened to visitors since around the beginning of the seventeenth century. By 1770, a new ticketing system meant that only the privileged few were able to access the asylum, via the permission of a governor (Andrews 1997: 189–91). Though Bethlem's doors had been closed to the general public for sixteen years, Lawrence's 1786 pastel invited the Royal Academy's crowds back into Bedlam. Despite its lack of contemporary attention, the pastel's inclusion at the Royal Academy, situated amongst a selection of significant late eighteenth-century artworks, highlights an important cultural phenomenon: the feminization of madness.

Elaine Showalter's *The Female Malady* argued that women became *the* cultural archetype for madness in the latter half of the eighteenth century, a sensation often described as its 'feminization' (1987). These years saw all manner of cultural offerings which spectacularized female insanity. Stories

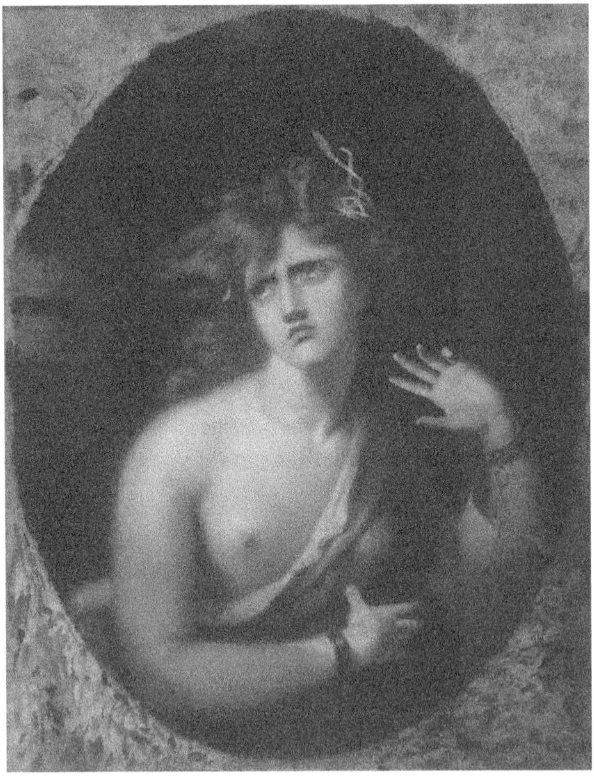

FIGURE 9.1 Thomas Lawrence, *Mad Girl*, 1786. Pastel on brushed vellum, 46 × 36.5 cm. Philadelphia Museum of Art: Purchased with the SmithKline Beckman Corporation Fund, 1985-51-1

of fictional and living 'madwomen' were shared in newspapers, reproduced in chapbooks, performed in theatres and, as with Lawrence's pastel, displayed in galleries. Typically, these depictions fell into two categories. The first of these tropes was the maniacal, raving madwoman, a violent, and transgressive force. Incarcerated and chained within a gloomy cell, she was depicted with straw-like hair, bulging eyes and bare breasts. The second was the melancholic love-mad woman. With tearstained cheeks, downcast eyes and dishevelled clothing, these women were portrayed as young and beautiful, hopelessly wandering nondescript settings in search of their lost loves. Art historians, literary critics and historians have shown how this particular construction of madwomen took on unprecedented significance within the dynamics of sensibility (Small 1996; Kromm 2002; Gerard 2005). At a time when it was fashionable to display one's emotions and be responsive and sensitive, the melancholic was well placed to prick the pity of the viewer, thus demonstrating the extent of their feeling and refinement.

Whether shared in broadsides or prints, periodicals or chapbooks, the ubiquity of images that drew upon these tropes suggest that individuals across classes were literate in the visual paradigms of women's madness. As Sander L. Gilman has stated, a dualistic conception of mental illness was integral to the cultural characterization of madwomen in this period (1996: 12). But viewing the madwoman purely in binary terms runs the risk of glossing over the rich texture of responses, interpretations and experiences from which these archetypes stray. And while maniacal and melancholic modes of madness can be understood as widely recognizable representational strategies, these stereotypes were not necessarily indicative of experience. True, mania and melancholy were real illnesses that were often viewed as polar opposites. Robert Burton's seventeenth-century *Anatomy of Melancholy* had peddled a distinct characterization of the morose melancholic; in contrast, mania was viewed as the most 'turbulent and extreme' of the mental disorders, its external markers of wildness and passion making it a 'common source of uncivil behaviour' (Kromm 2004: 346; Kromm 2002: 146). Most medical writers believed the two to be interconnected, with melancholy being the primary disorder, and mania its augmentation (Porter 1987: 46). Though the cultural feminization of madness perpetuated a visual language that set melancholy and mania up as opposites, it is important to remember that these were *reference* points upon which to represent illness and match behaviour, rather than distinct behavioural modes. Someone could experience both manic or melancholic symptoms, and there were a whole host of pathologies which did not fall into these two camps.

These tensions surface in *Mad Girl*. While the inscription on the back of the canvas identifies the love-mad symptomology of Lawrence's figure, the heavy-set brow, fleshy arm and strong nose is distinctly masculine. The manic markers, such as the bare breast, chains, cell and sprig of straw (commonly used for asylum bedding and therefore a signifier for mania and incarceration) mingle with the melancholic features: tears, flowing locks, flushed cheeks and rosebud lips. In *The Art of Frenzy*, art historian Jane Kromm argues that the melancholic iconography in *Mad Girl* overrides the more manic aspects of the pastel: 'Not only is the impact of maniacal agitation reduced to an assumed role, but the condition's traditional symptomology, the threat to persona or public safety, is thereby rendered inconsequential' (2002: 150–52). Though eloquently put, when assessing whether one or the other trope dominates, the answer relies on the viewer's own subjectivity. Only they can decide which set of schema proves unthreatening, and rendered insignificant. Perhaps more interesting is how Lawrence goes against the artistic grain by grafting markers of *both* manic disorder and sensitive delicacy to his emblem of female insanity. Unlike most other artists, printmakers, playwrights and poets who tended to stick to one convention and its associated iconography, Lawrence assembles love-mad features alongside chains, straw and nudity. In doing so, he makes love's madness dangerous.

We can read the fluidity of this representation as a nod to a more complicated understanding of women's mental illness during these years. Indeed, if we look beyond mainstream and familiar examples from within visual cultures of madness, other works gesture to this fluidity. Inspired by William Cowper's poem *The Task* (1785), which introduced readers to the impoverished, lovelorn Crazy Kate, artist Henry Fuseli's painting *Mad Kate* (1806) combined wide-eyed Gothic intensity with a coastal setting and red-trimmed bonnet. In Fuseli's retelling, the meek and modest Crazy Kate becomes dangerous. Likewise, when penning his image for the frontispiece of Charles A. Somerset's *Crazy Jane* in 1824, Robert Cruikshank borrowed markers from both tropes; pairing a neo-classical dress and flower garland with electrified hair and an intense stare. As I have argued elsewhere, love's madness was not a straightforwardly sentimental, harmless or mild malady, but could be transgressive, dangerous or deviant (Jamieson 2023), and this is certainly visualized with these more subtle and complex representations of women going mad. Just because dualistic frameworks of female madness existed and proliferated widely across culture does not mean that these were the only way that contemporaries could understand living madwomen, or that women experienced madness. The reality was messy, blurry and perhaps closer to modern conceptions of mental illness and health than we might assume. *Mad Girl* articulates these ideas in a small but significant way.

References

Andrews, J., and A. Briggs, R. Porter, P. Tucker, K. Waddington (1997), *The History of Bethlem*, London; New York: Routledge.

Gerard, W. B. (2005), '"All that the heart wishes": Changing Views toward Sentimentality Reflected in Visualizations of Sterne's Maria, 1773–1888', *Studies in Eighteenth-Century Culture*, 34: 197–269.
Gilman, S. L. (1996), *Seeing the insane: A cultural history of madness and art in the western world*, Nebraska, NE: University of Nebraska Press.
Jamieson, A. (2023), 'Crazy Jane Hats and Maria Medallions: Consuming, Collecting and Containing Love's Madness', in D. Woolley, P. Chambers, E. Sampson and F. Johnstone (eds), *Wearable Objects and Curative Things: Materialist Approaches to the Intersections of Fashion, Art, Health and Medicine*, 315–38, Basingstoke: Palgrave Macmillan.
Kromm, J. (2002), *The Art of Frenzy: Public Madness in the Visual Culture of Europe, 1500–1850*, London: Continuum.
Kromm, J. (2004), 'Olivia Furiosa: Maniacal Women from Richardson to Wollstonecraft', *Eighteenth-Century Fiction*, 16(3): 344–72.
Porter, R. (1987), *Mind-Forg'd Manacles: A History of Madness in England from the Restoration to the Regency*, London: Athlone Press.
Showalter, E. (1987), *The Female Malady: Women, Madness and English Culture, 1830–1980*, London: Virago.
Small, H. (1996), *Love's Madness: Medicine, the Novel and Female Insanity, 1800–1865*, Oxford: Clarendon Press.

PART III

Making and remaking medicalized bodies

CHAPTER TEN

Dissecting 'mental pictures': revisiting twentieth-century surgical illustration

Ashley Lazevnick

A swelling form emerges from the parted veils of glistening flesh, amid a crowd of hovering tractors and grooved dissectors. The instruments effortlessly, magically, parse an intestine from the surrounding viscera while stylized letters hint at some purpose beyond the scene's velvety realism (Figure 10.1). A barely noticeable signature indicates that this image was produced by Lillian Sternberg.

Sternberg's drawing of an 'Operation for Strangulated Oblique Inguinal Hernia' was included within Warren Stone Bickham's ambitious six-volume textbook *Operative Surgery* (1924). First issued in 1905, the 1924 edition featured a significantly expanded text and image program. In the preface, Bickham credits forty-six artists, mostly women, for the unprecedented execution of 6,300 drawings: a result of 'painstaking labor' and 'cleverness in interpreting… subjects often hard to understand'. His narration continues:

> At times, as many as ten Artists were working in the home of the Author, simultaneously—some coming at eight in the morning—and some not leaving until eight in the evening—and many a night passed and daylight came upon the uninterrupted and sleepless labor of text-writing, for the progress of the work—or of picture-preparation and planning, for the Artists—to be followed by days of shoulder-hovering, from chair to

> chair, to aid in explaining—or unraveling—or correcting—or remaking some difficult picture-problem.
>
> (Bickham 1924: viii)

In this frenetic scene, Bickham places artistic effort in a symbiotic relationship with that of the author's, recalling a long tradition of intimate partnerships between artist and anatomist. But he strategically glosses over

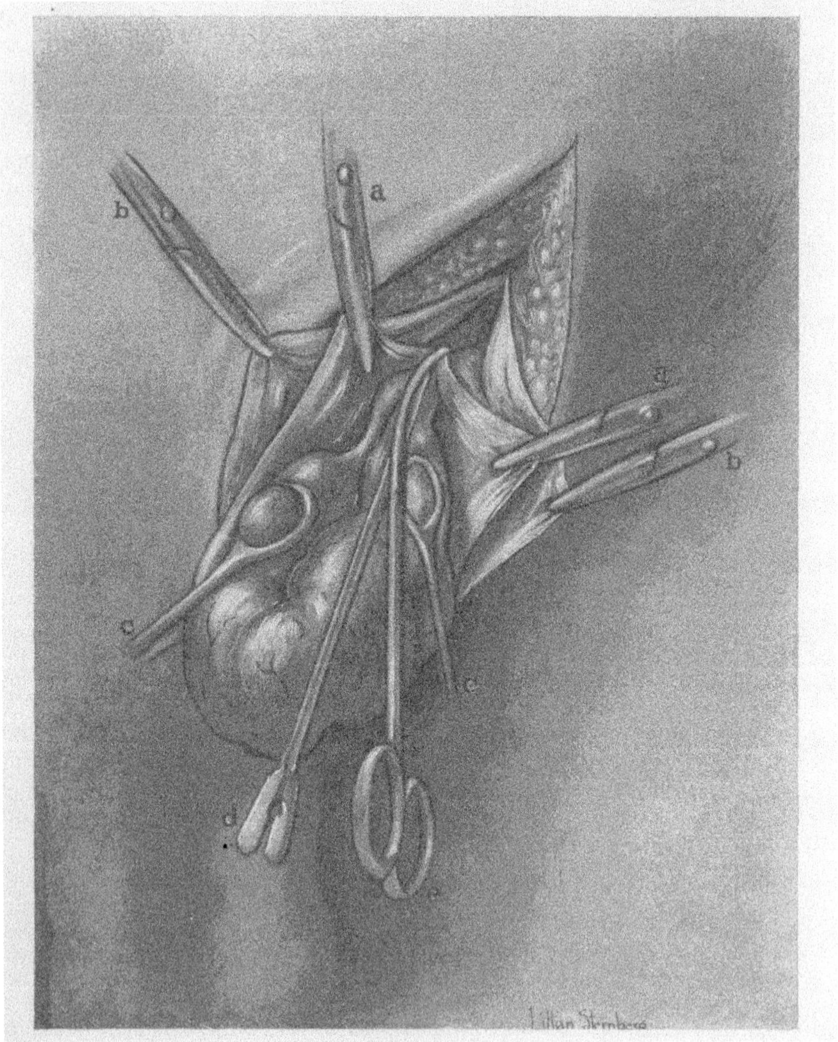

FIGURE 10.1 Lillian Sternberg, 'Operation for Strangulated Oblique Inguinal Hernia' in Warren Stone Bickham, *Operative Surgery*, vol. 4 (Philadelphia: W.B. Saunders Co., 1924), 187.

the details of how these illustrations were produced. While some were based on artists' observations from a cadaver or a live operation, many were derived from previous illustrations, photographs or verbal descriptions. The resulting pictures feature everything from axiomatic views of a steam-pressure sterilizer to suturing techniques and limb amputations. As one might expect, the quality of this encyclopedic undertaking was mixed. Alongside fully rendered demonstrations of operations and pulsating anatomical cross sections, one finds schematic line drawings and clumsy attempts at rendering the figure.

Almost every artist commissioned for this project has been lost to history, though a few, including Lillian Sternberg, published their work regularly in medical journals and textbooks. Sternberg was one of several illustrators employed by Bickham who had trained in the Department of Art as Applied to Medicine at Johns Hopkins University under the tutelage of the German émigré Max Brödel. In fact, Bickham's at-home atelier was becoming obsolete as the professional field of medical illustration expanded in the twentieth century. Between 1911 and 1940, Brödel trained over two hundred students, many of whom started their own departments across the United States. This effort culminated in 1945 with the founding of the Association of Medical Illustrators, an organization devoted to promoting the work of artists and ensuring standardized methods for teaching medical illustration (Demarest 1995). During the same period, the technique pioneered by Brödel began to dominate journals and textbooks, profoundly changing the aesthetics of medical imagery. Borrowing materials from lithography, Brödel's style was highly tactile, blending anatomical accuracy with a seductive beauty (irrespective of the gritty details of the procedure underway). In his images, the body of the patient was typically eliminated from the visual field, replaced by sanitized and isolated surgical specimens. Sternberg's depiction contains all of the hallmarks of this new approach in its mastery of three-dimensional modelling, its imitation of living flesh, and its re-commitment to the materiality of drawing.

In the literature on anatomical illustration, the early twentieth century is largely a neglected period, overshadowed by the lavish anatomical atlases of previous centuries and the computer-generated imaging technologies, such as CT scans and MRIs, that emerged in the 1960s and 1970s (Ackerman 2006). I open with Bickham's anecdote because it suggests that this moment was in fact pivotal, as *Operative Surgery* points backwards and forwards at once, clinging to romantic notions of anatomical illustration while profiting from photo-reproductive technologies that afforded an unprecedented glut of images. By placing drawings from Bickham's text in the wider context of operative surgical manuals, and in conversation with Brödel's philosophies on illustration, I will show how this was a crucial time of transition, shaped as much by nostalgia as by technological promise, in which the hand-drawn image held epistemological prestige and functioned as a connective device between surgeon, illustrator and student. What links these disciplines are somatic techniques deployed in the procedures of surgery, drawing and reading. I uncover an attentiveness to embodied action first by examining Brödel's pedagogy, then by showing how a single image was placed within a sequence, creating a presentation which mimics cinema and aims to bring to life the haptic encounter of a surgical operation.

* * *

Biographical details on Warren Stone Bickham are slim, if tantalizing. The son of Jefferson Davis' doctor, Charles Jasper Bickham, Warren Stone completed his medical training at Tulane University and joined the College of Physicians and Surgeons at Columbia University in 1887 ('Warren Stone Bickham' 1925: 98–99). Despite Bickham's anonymity, *Operative Surgery* was generally well received. Published by the Philadelphia-based company W. B. Saunders Press, the six-volume set sold 18,312 volumes in ten months and was singled out for the scale of its execution (ibid.). Over nearly sixty thousand pages and ninety-seven chapters, the volumes move from general procedures to subdivisions based on individual systems and anatomical parts. At least a few reviewers found the text gratuitous: one noting that over fifty-three options for partial rhinoplasty left too much choice to the reader ('Operative Surgery' 1925: 238). The illustrations occasionally came under the same scrutiny, since they were characterized as at once schematic and overly complex, perhaps because they too were so copious, overflowing in their depiction of each step of a procedure (more on this later).

Though quite a bit longer than previous examples, *Operative Surgery* conforms to the format of operative textbooks, which provided practical advice for conducting a variety of procedures and were geared predominately towards students of surgery, interns or general practice physicians. By the turn of the twentieth century, a typical format emerged, wherein a series of chapters were devoted, first, to preparatory steps – the inventory of operating room and the assembly of necessary instruments – followed by chapters divided by successive regions and parts of the body, covering one or multiple operations for each ailment. The pragmatic rather than theoretical outlook of such texts is reflected in the overwhelming emphasis on concision in the description of operations and in the occasional self-reference to the text as a 'training manual' for the student.

On its surface, the brief would appear quite simple. Yet, most authors painfully acknowledged the shortcomings of their medium. Astley Paston Cooper Ashhurst expressed the common sentiment that a textbook is, necessarily, a supplemental object. 'Every text-book... has limitations. At best it can but teach the student to *know*; it cannot teach him to *do*. And though knowledge is power, much practical experience in laboratory, dispensary and hospital wards must supplement didactic instruction'

(Ashhurst 1920: vii). Note Ashhurst's firm division between *knowledge* gained passively, through reading, and *experience*. This was hardly a new issue. The celebrated anatomist Andreas Vesalius believed whole-heartedly in the value of live dissection, even though he issued one of the finest books of anatomical illustration in the early modern period: a text which, in practice, served as a proxy for the absent cadaver (Kornell 2022: 3).

The importance of illustration to medical texts from the medieval period to the present has been well documented (Kemp and Wallace 2000; Kemp 1993; Herrlinger 1970). Though the pre-eminence and power of images was not without its detractors, most anatomists since Vesalius's *Fabrica* (1543) agreed with his insistence that illustrations would 'place a subject before the eyes more precisely than the most explicit language' (Vesalius 2014: 8). Anatomical images have always adopted a visual vocabulary that prioritized *seeing* as a path towards knowing (Kemp and Wallace 2000: 13), though they hardly presented unbiased depictions of the human form. Highly stylized illustrations, such as the idealized plates of Vesalius and Bernhard Siegfried Albinus – wherein skeletal or muscled figures are set within refined landscape and assume poses reminiscent of classical sculpture – responded to trends in both the fine arts and the philosophy of science. As Martin Kemp has argued, however, 'style' was no less important in the 'flesh-and-blood school' adopted by eighteenth-century anatomists such as John Bell or William Hunter, who, informed by Enlightenment theories of observation, emphasized an accurate reportage of that which is seen and insisted on first-hand encounter with a specific body (Kemp 2010: 198).

From Vesalius to Hunter, the scale and expense of illustrated medical publications indicate the role that such books and plates held in practice; as Ludmilla Jordanova and others have noted, these didactics were activated by students who, alone or in groups, consulted the images in the midst of a dissection or surgical operation ('William Hunter's Atlas'). Like previous atlases, operative textbooks carried a conflicted purpose: to supplement but also, ultimately, to stand in for the direct encounter of the operating room. Perhaps even more so, since it was unlikely that surgeons were consulting texts like Bickham's *Operative Surgery* during an actual procedure. Accordingly, the images within were charged not only with re-presenting a body but by making it freshly present to the reader.

Despite evolutions in surgery, the questions facing early twentieth-century illustrators remained largely unchanged: should the image highlight the individual subject or strive for a 'typical' presentation? Should the artist eliminate excessive information, or include everything in the visual field? Should a surgical procedure be portrayed at each stage or in a synthetic overview? Around the turn of the century, authors no longer favoured a unified visual atlas that supported a coherent ideological agenda but rather presented a jumble of incongruent images: from diagrammatic renderings of equipment, photographic case studies, X-rays and drawings. Even Bickham's text, which strived for better uniformity and is mostly absent of photographs, featured a bizarre diversity of drawing styles. It was precisely this cluttered and confused visual experience that inspired the revisionary efforts of Lillian Sternberg's teacher, Max Brödel.

~

Brödel trained at the Academy of Fine Arts in Leipzig and arrived at Johns Hopkins University in 1894 with the explicit mission of illustrating the first edition of Dr. Howard Kelly's *Operative Gynecology* (Crosby and Cody 1991: 23–25; for an interpretation of Kelly's textbook within a history of gendered and racial codifications of the female body in gynaecological texts, see Snorton 2017: 44–53). To understand the virtuosic flair that Brödel developed early in his career, let us consider an image from William Halsted's *The Operative Story of Goitre* (Figure 10.2). Demonstrating the removal of a thyroid gland, Brödel presents a moment when the isthmus is divided, cropped and decontextualized. Soft highlights and careful shading create a glistening effect that heightens the texture of skin and muscle. The drawing achieves an integrated and uncluttered presentation with diffuse lighting, as the viewer surveys the scene at a middle distance (as though enveloped *within* the field of dissection). Characteristic of Brödel's art, this illustration showcases his ability to convey anatomical detail with some modest fictional moments, blending artistic techniques of illusionism and perspective with the prosaic information needed to communicate how bodily parts relate to one another. This combined effect was not so much new as forgotten; it suggests a return to the aspirations of a refined realistic eighteenth-century style of Hunter no less to the luxurious quality of engravings used by Vesalius or Albinus. And Brödel's own writing supports this notion of a romantic return: 'It is an error to think there is no beauty or charm in medical work. The outlines of the various organs of the human body and their detail always possess a certain grace and an interesting character all their own' (Brödel 1907: 139).

An eager and fastidious worker, Brödel quickly became a fierce advocate for the reform of medical illustration. Surveying the field in 1907, he complained of rampant plagiarism (artists who merely copied from previous illustrations rather than studying surgical techniques from life) and conceded that the problem was a matter of seemingly unbridgeable expertise, since only a surgeon has the 'knowledge of the operation' while the artist has the 'knowledge of drawing'. He explained:

> There is no doubt to my mind that the most valuable impression, such as would crystallize itself into a picture without undue labor and experimentation on paper, is the one possessed by the scientist. The person whose hands have palpated or felt of the object which is to be

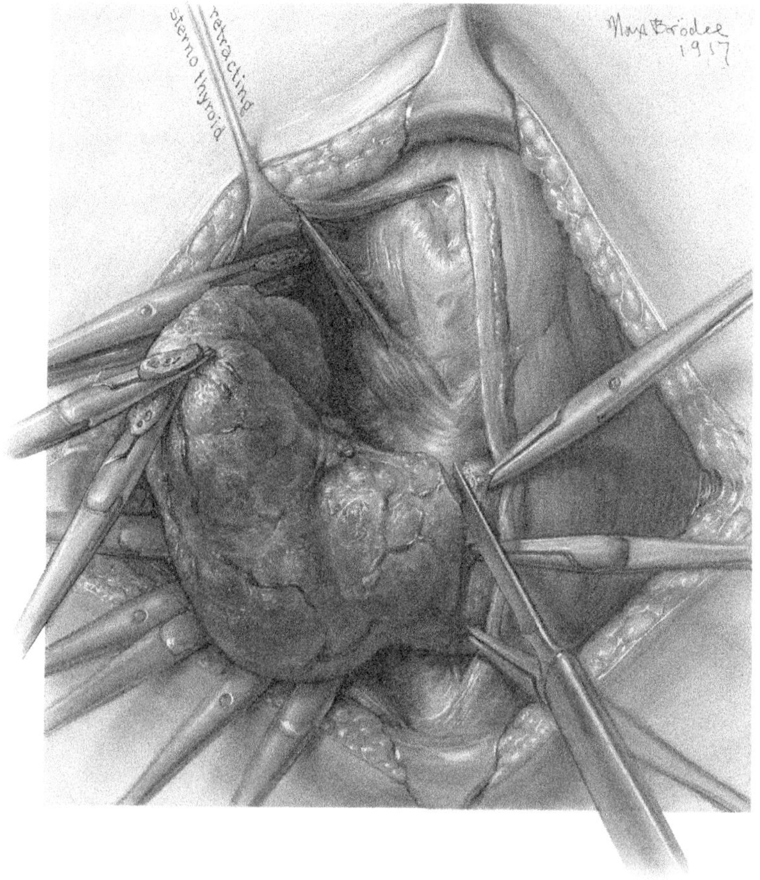

FIGURE 10.2 Max Brödel, 'the act of dividing the isthmus' for William Halsted, *The Operative Story of Goitre: The Author's Operation* (1919). Illustration courtesy of the Max Brödel Archives, Department of Art as Applied to Medicine, Johns Hopkins University School of Medicine.

> pictured and whose mind has passed through the various stages of the evolution of a mental picture, that person is best fitted to preserve that picture on paper.
>
> (Brödel 1907: 139)

For the medical illustrator to correct for their deficiency in this regard, he too, like the scientist, needed to study his objects 'with eye and mind' in order to achieve a valid 'mental picture' which would equal that of the operator's. Just as the scientist should learn about art, he reasoned, so too should the medical illustrator adopt the methods of surgical training by attending dissections and autopsies (Brödel 1907: 139). Thus, for Brödel, the mental image is wholly dependent upon – and constructed from – the physical experience of *both* dissecting and drawing.

In 1911, Brödel was appointed director of a new Department of Art as Applied to Medicine: the first academic department devoted to the field of medical illustration. Established with a short-term stipend and a later endowment funded by railroad tycoon and art collector Henry Walters, the department grew slowly within the first few years. Illustrators were first taught to copy anatomical studies alongside the 'fresh material from autopsies' and preserved pathological specimens. Through this process, the student studied each organ individually, in full, then its pathological variations and its microscopic structures. 'The most important part of the student's work in the dissecting room, however, is sketching and drawing', Brödel wrote. 'Everything revealed by the student's eye and hand is put on paper immediately, while the impression is fresh. The sketches are made boldly and rapidly… Thousands of such sketches are made. They are the test that the student has grasped the subject' (Brödel 1941: 670).

Only once they mastered the principles of dissection did students go on to study live treatments, examinations, and operative procedures (Brödel 1911–1926). Typically, students were paired with doctors, under an apprenticeship model through which (in Brödel's ideal dynamic) doctor and artist would work reciprocally to develop an accurately rendered illustration. An overwhelming majority of Brödel's students were women within the first decades of the program, indicative of a larger trend in the profession of medical illustration (recall that most of the illustrators for Bickham's textbook were also women). Though it is outside the scope of this discussion, I wish to acknowledge this gendered division of labour and suggest that a careful study of the work of female illustrators might alter the conventional writing on the topic, which so predominantly focuses on the intrusion of voyeurism into the site of anatomical depiction.

Just as important as the curriculum that Brödel put in place was the new process that he created and taught to successive generations of students: the 'Carbon Dust Technique'. Devised to evoke the sensation of living flesh and inspired by lithography (which Brödel had been familiar with from his training in Germany), the technique involved a two-step transfer of an initial sketch to transparent paper and finally to a stippled carbon-coated paper, using dry stable brushes dipped in carbon dust, watercolour and lamp black. To achieve passages of pure white, Brödel used a blade, preferably from an engraving needle, to incise highlights into the soft and absorptive surface of the paper. His notes explain how to guide the needle from the broadest part of the ellipse to the sharpest, to create wide scratches, narrow ones, then thin lines: all by varying the tilt of the instrument (Crosby and Cody 1991: 311).

It is significant that the materials that Brödel used approximate both a flesh-like surface and a scalpel-like instrument, for the manner in which he manipulated the brushes and blades echoes the kind of instruction found in operative surgical texts. Bickham, for instance, advises the surgeon on how to prepare for surgery and how to carry the scalpel: 'Preceding the actual cut, the Surgeon should have very definitely determined in his own mind_What he intends to do_How he intends to do it_What he is likely to encounter_and_How he is going to get into the body' (Bickham 1924: 219–20). After describing how the scalpel enters at a right angle with a 'controlled stab', moves along the surface in a single sweep and is swiftly removed, a diagram demonstrates how the scalpel may be held like a dinner-knife, pen or violin bow. This was, in fact, an older trope: the positions of the knife, pen and violin bow were repeated and recirculated in operative texts over the course of the nineteenth century (Bryant 1887: 18–19; Treves 1892: 50–51).

Whether holding an engraving needle or a scalpel, the directions offered by Brödel and Bickham share a common emphasis on instrumental control: the cognitive analysis, then the deliberate motions of the hand, that allowed for efficient incisions or precise lines. This was no accident. Metaphors of surgery and diagnosis had long infiltrated artistic circles, deployed since the mid-nineteenth century in reference to Realist painting, photographic portraiture and even abstraction (Fried 1987; Sheehan 2011; Lazevnick 2023). At the same time, following the developments in anesthetics and asepsis, which allowed for more careful and intricate operations, the surgeon's work was beginning to be considered an artform comparable to the skill of an accomplished musician or a graceful writer. Considering this analogic relationship between surgeons and artists, Thomas Schlich has argued that surgical skill required the coordination of 'corporeal and mental qualities', learned through repeated practice (Schlich 2015: 385). Evoking Michael Polanyi's concept of 'tacit knowledge' – a form of knowing that is forged through first-hand, iterative experiences – Schlich explains how surgical skill is transmitted primarily through 'performance', with each surgeon or era of surgery cultivating its own style of performativity. Recent scholars have also compared surgery to scripted plays and choreography, arguing that each field has a prescriptive structure in which '[e]very step in this task has been broken down into steps that need to be undertaken in a predictable fashion' (Reid, Rauch and Numanoglu 2024: 159). Like surgery, medical drawing depends upon tacit knowledge. If the 'style' of anatomical illustrations comes at the end, then the performative 'style' is revealed in the process of creation: in Brödel's insistence that the artist link the eye and mind or Bickham's description of shoulder hovering, unravelling and correcting an illustration.

~

The importance of making a 'mental picture' through repetitive, embodied engagement is what distinguishes a medical drawing from taking a photograph. Medical illustration has always required *more* than what can be empirically captured by mechanical vision, but the tension between drawing and photography was particularly acute in the early twentieth century, especially after the fanatical adaptation of X-rays to medical research (Kelves 1997). The allure of photography had to do with its perceived veridical power – its seemingly faithful representation of the world, uninterrupted by human fallacy – which caused some scientists to flatly reject any images produced by the human hand (Sappol 2017; Daston and Galison 2001; Ackerman 2006). Ironically, the staid and serious reputation of photography often collided with the domain of entertainment; this occurred especially in medical portraiture, wherein subjects may be staged in a theatrical manner that uncomfortably recalled the conventions of pornography or circus exhibitionism (O'Connor 1999; Sappol 2017; Sheehan 2011).

For all its popularity, Brödel and others were sceptical of photography's service to medical illustration. To paraphrase Brödel, only the medical *drawing* can clarify elements of the anatomical field that are understood through direct encounters. Unlike the partial and particular view of the photograph, the drawing is a composite picture that becomes most vivid in in recollection: 'To make such a picture the artist must know his subject so thoroughly that he can shut his eyes and coax into existence a mental picture of great clarity' (Brödel 1941: 668). This is why Brödel considered the action of continuous sketching more important than the mere spectatorship of a dissection, for it was only by putting the hand in motion while the procedure is itself unfolding that a student might acquire a full understanding of what she was confronting. For him, a successful illustration – one which gathers and then conveys knowledge about the object – begins as an image in the mind that has been formed over time, through this labour-intensive (and embodied!) process of observation and synthesis.

Almost always, the photographs that appear in early twentieth-century textbooks – of operating rooms, X-rays, or pathological specimens – were complemented by drawings that recreated the operation (Curtis 2012b: 73). In other words, photography was essential to the epistemic claims made by textbook authors – just as it was frankly useful for draftsmen who might have trouble accessing a live or dissected body – but it was ultimately the *transformation* of photograph into drawing that elicited the uncanny sensation of vitality (Sawchuk 2012: 123). This preference for drawing fits within what Lorraine Daston and Peter Galison have labelled the domain of 'Trained Judgement'; in examples from later decades, they show how surgeons began to favour 'interpreted' images that required the intuitive knowledge of a viewer to be deciphered and understood. Without being a naïve return to representations in the atlases of Vesalius or Albinus, such drawings presented a composite view that even incorporated intentional exaggerations for the purpose of aiding classifications or giving procedural cues (Daston and Galison 2001: 347). Like Brödel, most practitioners recognized photography's constraints: not only that it was unable to indicate depth or texture but also that its insistent flatness could never recreate the three-dimensional interaction with a real body (Sappol 2017: 5–7).

If photographs as *illustration* were becoming less favorable, then another aspect of photography was on the insurgence. New modes of photo-reproduction fuelled a growing market of inexpensive mass-market textbooks. Publications such as Bickham's overflowed with an extraordinary number of images due to the widespread embrace of offset printing. Replacing earlier modes of woodblock or engraving, offset printing allowed for the inclusion of halftones which the publishers derived from the 'cut' of the original drawing (Sawchuk 2012: 126). With this increase in quantity came a precipitous decrease in the quality of reproductions, which often appeared grainy and blurred. Acutely aware of these issues, Brödel began his 1907 article by lamenting the 'inadequate character' of cuts in medical textbooks and articles, especially in comparison with well-illustrated magazines and novels (Brödel 1907: 138). Typically, cuts used for one publication would be recycled in others, and some volumes were composed entirely of cuts taken from previous publications. Thus, while photography was undoubtably useful for the illustrator, it was inadequate in at least two respects: first, because it could not conjure the detail nor the tangible experience of a surgical operation and, second, because photo-reproduction rendered an original drawing – however painstakingly produced – flat and imprecize. Within this standoff between drawing and photography, I propose we analyze another medium, one that is better suited the performative and somatic activities that linked the illustrator and surgeon: cinema.

The use of film within medical education was indeed a new attraction. Lisa Cartwright has traced the codependence of cinematography and physiology in the late nineteenth and early twentieth century through a range of examples, showing how medical cinema was used as a tool of bodily surveillance and control (Cartwright 1996). Film technology was also promoted by Frank Gilbreth, in time-motion studies of surgeons, and by Eugène Louis Doyen, who employed it in his surgical teaching, celebrating its 'vividness' of presentation, which he considered superior to that of textbooks (Curtis 2012a). Doyen singled out film's ability to show how 'various stages of the procedure succeed one another without precipitation or interruption' (Doyen 1917: 7). Yet, textbook authors *did* increasingly aspire to the same uninterrupted multi-step procedure, to the same 'vivid' presentation, by minimizing written instructions. In a 1944 manual, for instance, Thomas J. Orr writes that '[a] clear visualization of the steps in an operation is many times more instructive than the descriptive text. The text has purposely been made as brief as is consistent with step-by-step description of each operation' (Orr 1944: v). This 'step-by-step' process is precisely where the logic of cinema guides the illustrative endeavour.

Turning back to Bickham's *Operative Surgery*, we find countless examples of this process-based method. Take Helen Babbitt's illustrations of a partial thyroidectomy for the removal of a goitre. In nine separate images, the series accounts for the significant moments of the Kocher technique as it moves from the initial cut to the ligations, removal of capsules and suturing. Across each of the illustrations, the neck of the anonymized patient is presented with the head tilted back and cropped at the chin. Crucially, the pictures themselves are centrally positioned on the page: so that, for the reader who flips through without dwelling on the text, it is as if the operation unfolds in a staccato manner before one's eyes. One image in the sequence displays the instruments used to cut through the surgical capsule to expose the goitre but, on either side of the central action, Babbitt has used a before-and-after strategy to illustrate the division of the sternothyroid muscle. The temporal components to this series are therefore layered: meant to be understood consecutively but also containing within the images themselves a compression or expansion of time as an action is performed.

This tells us something about how an author imagined the textbook might be used, as a reader must choose either to toggle between text and image or to simply flip through the images while sidelining the text. Since Bickham provides captions that act as stand-alone explanations of the operation's individual steps, it is likely that he acknowledged a full textual description was optional. And Brödel provided a similar possibility in his images for Halsted's report, since the figure discussed earlier was a 'before' image, paired with an 'after' view of the divided isthmus and placed within a series of twelve drawings that highlighted key moments in the operation. Included as an appendix to Halsted's lengthy report, they effectively recreated a stand-alone visual account of the operation.

Such a strategy, which puts forth the superiority of the image and presents a sequential progression, was perfected in George Schwartz's *Illustrative Operative Surgery for Students and Practitioners*, where the reader was promised a picture on every page. 'The best way to learn an operation is to see it', Schwartz wrote, 'I have taken all of the standard operations on the neck, chest, and abdomen, and have shown these operations in graphic form from the primary incision until the closure of the skin' (Schwartz 1928: 7). In a series of fourteen drawings, Ann Coles isolates the individual moments of Dr. Andre Crotti's technique for a thyroidectomy (Figure 10.3). Only the briefest explanation of the surgical technique is provided prior to the series of images. Each illustration occupies the entire expansive of the page. As with Babbitt's drawings, the patient is shown affixed in an unmoving central position, with hands and instruments manipulating the muscles, vessels and tumour with graceful ease.

It was no longer enough to 'place a subject before the eyes' (*pace* Vesalius); the author had to *mobilize* the images. Profiting from the ease of photo-reproduction, a single operation was now presented through nine,

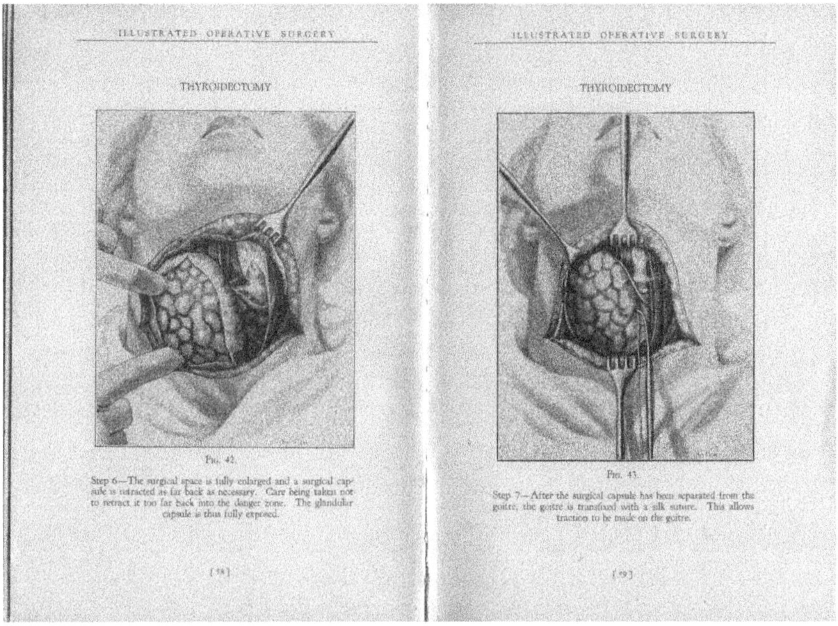

FIGURE 10.3 Ann Coles' illustrations of a Thyroidectomy in George Schwartz, *Illustrated Operative Surgery for Students and Practitioners* (New York: Dartmouth Publishing Corp., 1928), 58–59.

twelve or fourteen separate steps. Devised to overcome the challenge posed by Ashhurst (that a text could only teach one how to *know*, but not to how to *do*), the 'step-by-step' progression invited a reader to participate in the surgical operation as it moved through sequential actions. This method did not emerge in a vacuum; it was prefigured by the formulaic structure of operative texts as well as the task-based predictive logic that suggested surgery's affinity to 'performances' of various kinds. It also built upon historical attempts to simulate dissection through life-sized anatomical tables, moulages and flap books that beckon the user to explore the successive layers of the body's infrastructure through sight and touch (Gensler 2022: 83–94; Sperling 2021). Like those interactive technologies, the operative surgical textbooks became the site of an active encounter.

The goal was not only to make the text cinematic but to visually reconstruct an iterative, haptic enterprise, one that recalls the visual and tactile practices that Brödel found so essential for the illustrator as well as the performative actions that were central to surgical instruction. No illustration, no textbook, could adequately recreate the feel of a surgery or dissection. But – by pairing a step-by-step illustration of the (virtual) procedure with the (actual) manual act of flipping through the book – authors and illustrators increasingly sought to overcome the textbook's limitations and aspired, instead, to recreate the tacit knowledge of the operating room.

~

I have been suggesting that the analogy between surgery and drawing crystallized in the somatic modes of working that involved coordination of eye and mind that came together in the operating room and the drawing studio. While active learning has been prized since the invention of the clinical model, recent developments in surgical simulation expand upon that psychological-physical connection through virtual reality technologies that require a sophisticated blend of medical understanding, computer programming and engineering to approximate the physical sensations of an operation (Prentice 2012: 277–308). The authors and illustrators studied here were precursors to this virtual revolution, and their aspirations were the same. In a more modest manner, the step-by-step cinematic strategy employed by illustrators invited a reader to engage physically with the page. With varying degrees of illusion, such illustrations sought to make a scene fantastically present to a reader and thus to dissolve the layered process of representation, which required the transfer from body to illustrator to image to viewer.

References

Ackerman, M. (2006), 'Anatomy in the Digital Age' in B. Rifkin, M. J. Ackerman and J. Folkenberg (eds), *Human Anatomy: Depicting the Body from the Renaissance to Today*, 319–29, London: Thames & Hudson.

Ashhurst, A. P. C., and G. Wantz (1920), *Surgery: its principles and practice for students and practitioners*, Philadelphia: Lea & Febiger.

Bickham, W. S. (1924), *Operative Surgery: Covering the Operative Technic Involved in the Operations of General and Special Surgery*, 6 vols, Philadelphia: W.B. Saunders Co.

Brödel, M. (1907) 'How May Our Present Methods of Medical Illustration be Improved?' *Journal of the American Medical Association (JAMA)*, 49 (2): 138–40.

Brödel, M. (1911–1926), Annual Reports, 1911–1926, Max Brödel: Student art, personal papers, Art as Applied to Medicine Archives, Johns Hopkins University.

Brödel, M. (1941), 'Medical Illustrations', *Journal of the American Medical Association (JAMA)*, 117 (9): 668–72.

Bryant, J. D. (1887), *Manual of operative surgery, With about eight hundred illustrations*, New York: D. Appleton and company.

Cartwright, L. (1996), *Screening the Body: Tracing Medicine's Visual Culture*, Minneapolis: University of Minnesota Press.

Crosby, R., and J. Cody (1991), *Max Brödel: The Man Who Put Art into Medicine*, New York: Springer-Verlag.

Curtis, S. (2012a), 'Dissecting the Medical Training Film', in M. Braun, C. Keil, R. King, P. Moore, and L. Pelletier (eds), *Beyond the Screen: Institutions, Networks and Publics of Early Cinema*, 161–67, Bloomington: Indiana University Press.

Curtis, S. (2012b), 'Photography and Medical Observation', in N. Anderson and M. R. Dietrich (eds), *The Educated Eye: Visual Culture & Pedagogy in the Life Sciences*, 68–93, Hanover: Dartmouth College Press.

Daston, L., and P. Galison (2001), *Objectivity*, New York: Zone Books.

Demarest, R. J. (ed.) (1995), *The History of the Association of Medical Illustrators, 1945–1995*, Atlanta, GA: The Association of Medical Illustrators.

Doyen, E. (1917), *Surgical Therapeutics and Operative Technique*, vol. 1, New York: William Wood and Co.

Fried, M. (1987), *Realism, Writing, Disfiguration: On Thomas Eakins and Stephen Crane*, Chicago: University of Chicago Press.

Gensler, T. (2022), 'Interior Visions: Representing the Body in Three Dimensions', in M. Kornell (ed.), *Flesh and Bones: The Art of Anatomy*, 83–94, Los Angeles: Getty Research Institute.

Herrlinger, R. (1970), *History of Medical Illustration from Antiquity to 1600*, G. Fulton-Smith (trans.), New York: Editions Medicina Rara.

Kelves, B. H. (1997), *Naked to the Bone: Medical Imaging in the Twentieth Century*, New Brunswick: Rutgers University Press.

Kemp, M. (1993), '"The Mark of Truth": Looking and Learning in Some Anatomical Illustrations from the Renaissance and Eighteenth Century', in W. F. Bynum and R. Porter (eds), *Medicine and the Five Senses*, 85–121, Cambridge: Cambridge University Press.

Kemp, M. (2010), 'Style and Non-style in Anatomical Illustration: From Renaissance Humanism to Henry Gray', *Journal of Anatomy*, 216: 192–208.

Kemp, M., and M. Wallace (2000), *Spectacular Bodies: The Art and Science of the Human Body from Leonardo to Now*, Berkeley: University of California Press.

Kornell, M. (2022), 'The Illustration of Anatomy', in M. Kornell (ed.), *Flesh and Bones: The Art of Anatomy*, 1–14, Los Angeles: Getty Research Institute.

Lazevnick, A. (2023), 'Chapter 3: Weapons and Scalpels: The Surgical Art of Georgia O'Keeffe and Marianne Moore' in *Fantasies of Precision: American Modern Art, 1908–1947*, 115–68, Minneapolis: University of Minnesota Press.

O'Connor, E. (1999), 'Camera medica: Towards a morbid history of photography', *History of Photography*, 23 (3): 232–44.

'Operative Surgery' (1925), *The Indian Medical Gazette*, 6 (2): 238–9.

Orr, T. G. (1944), *Operations of General Surgery*, Philadelphia: W.B. Saunders Co.

Prentice, R. (2012), 'The Anatomy of a Surgical Simulation: The Mutual Articulation of Bodies in and through the Machine', in N. Anderson and M. R. Dietrich (eds), *The Educated Eye: Visual Culture & Pedagogy in the Life Sciences*, 277–308, Hanover: Dartmouth College Press.

Reid, S., L. Rauch and A. Numanoglu (2024), 'The Performance of Surgery', in G. Bouchard and A. Mermikides (eds), *The Routledge Companion to Performance and Medicine*, 157–65, New York: Routledge.

Sappol, M. (2017), 'Anatomy's Photography: Objectivity, Showmanship and the Reinvention of the Anatomical Image 1860–1950', *REMEDIA*: 1–14.

Sawchuk, K. (2012), 'Animating the Anatomical Specimen: Regional Dissection and the Incorporation of Photography in J.C.B. Grant's *An Atlas of Anatomy*', *Body & Society* 18 (1): 120–50.

Schlich, T. (2015), '"The Days of Brilliancy Are Past": Skill, Styles and the Changing Rules of Surgical Performance, ca. 1820–1920', *Medical History*, 59 (3): 379–403.

Schwartz, G. (1928), *Illustrated Operative Surgery for Students and Practitioners*, 2nd ed., New York: Dartmouth Publishing Corp.

Sheehan, T. (2011), 'Making Faces and Taking off Heads: The Operations of Photography and Medicine', in *Doctored: The Medicine of Photography in Nineteenth-Century America*, 48–80, University Park: Pennsylvania State University Press.

Snorton, C. R. (2017), *Black on Both Sides: A Racial History of Trans Identity*, Minneapolis: University of Minnesota Press.

Sperling, J. (2021), 'Modeling Maneuvers: Anatomical Illustration and the Practice of Touch', in M. Brückner, S. Isenstadt and S. Wasserman (eds), *Modelwork: The Material Culture of Making and Knowing*, 191–212, Minneapolis: University of Minnesota Press.

Treves, F. (1892), *A manual of operative surgery*, Philadelphia: Lea Brothers & Co.

Vesalius, A. (2014), *The Fabric of the Human Body: An Annotated Translation of the 1543 and 1555 Editions of 'De Humani Corpis Fabrica'*, D. H. Garrison and M. H. Hast (eds), Basel: Karger.

'Warren Stone Bickham' (1925), *New Orleans Medical and Surgical Journal*, 78 (1): 98–99.

'William Hunter's Atlas of Human "Gravid Uterus": The Production and Uses of Atlases', Paul Mellon Centre for Studies in British Art, June 20, 2021, https://www.youtube.com/watch?v=ILhIhKdZjEk&t=618

CHAPTER ELEVEN

Becoming an image: photography, ownership, language and power in the clinical encounter

Fiona Johnstone and Liz Orton

Fiona Johnstone (FJ): This conversation focuses on your artist's book, *Every Body is an Archive* (published in 2019 in an edition of 300), which developed out of your five-year Wellcome Trust-funded project *Digital Insides* (2015–20), a major art-led investigation into photography and contemporary medical images. What was your starting point for this work?

Liz Orton (LO): I'd been teaching medical students for a number of years, using the photographic image as a way of thinking about power within the doctor–patient relationship. Photography can work as a useful metaphor to explore concepts like consent, trust, privacy and ownership, and the idea of the gaze is key to both photography and medicine. In my artistic practice I often take up the photographic image as a way to question institutional values and practices.

FJ: I read your work as a form of institutional critique (Johnstone 2023); you take the medical image as a site of enquiry for interrogating questions around power in both clinical relationships and artist–participant relationships.

LO: Yes, although I was mindful throughout the project not to reproduce clinical power relationships in the way I engaged participants. I'm interested in how medical images shape our knowledge of the body. For example, the X-ray, developed at the turn of the twentieth century, enabled a radical shift in the way the human body was conceptualized and defined, undermining the established notion of a contained subject by collapsing the inside and the surface of the body into an image. Medical technology plays a formative part in our understanding of what the body actually is (see Cartwright 1995; Kevles 1997; van Dijck 2005; Lippit 2005).

FJ: You have written that 'being a patient today increasingly means being an image' (Orton 2018: 6). Can you expand on that sentence?

LO: In hospitals, images are now the single most important diagnostic tool in medicine. And almost every medical intervention is preceded by, enabled by, and verified by the image. This increasing reliance on images at least in part reflects the promise of visual evidence. This dominance of vision means that the patient can become marginalized from the process of diagnosis. The image can stand in for the body and enable its absence from clinical decision-making. For example, radiologists almost never meet patients, and patients rarely see their own images. Images produce gaps and disconnections.

FJ: How did you work with patients and other participants? Were you working with a specific clinical group, or perhaps people who had experienced a particular type of imaging technology?

LO: My project was in partnership with Professor Steve Halligan, a radiologist at University College London Hospital, and I was a visiting artist at the hospital for about three years. I worked with a number of radiologists, observing their clinics and following up with patients who were interested in becoming further involved in the project. The idea was approved by the hospital's Governance Committee which, along with the Wellcome Trust and others, helped me put together a consent procedure for patients. There was no template for this and it took two years to define a process that was artistically, ethically and clinically viable. It was never about a particular clinical group or one technology more than others. I was interested in individual patient experiences but also in broader questions about image systems. I was seeking to bring some light to the black-box of medical-image processing, by listening to and learning from a variety of bodies, both fleshy and theoretical, analogue and digital.

FJ: Why did you feel this topic could be addressed in an interesting way by an artist; what did you think that you could offer that another discipline could not?

LO: I think being an artist gives you certain privileges, to see things as an outsider, to ask difficult questions, and to be curious without having to necessarily solve anything. Medicine tends to treat images as a window onto the body, whereas I am interested in how the image makes possible certain material approaches or interventions. Historically, for example, the representation of the body in medical illustration as dry, bloodless, passive and fragmented facilitated quite risky surgical experimentation. The medical image is not just a reflection of a pre-given body but is formative of the body's various realities (see Armstrong 1983).

FJ: Could you say a bit about why the project resulted in a book, as opposed to another format?

LO: Although screens now dominate medicine, the book as a form is such an important part of medical history, and I was interested in taking up the material problem of how to translate the depth of the body onto the surface of the page.

FJ: Let's describe *Every Body is an Archive* as a material artefact. It's a small book, measuring approximately 15 × 18.5 × 1 cm, with lay-flat sewn binding. The covers are in a gently shimmering medium-weight off-white card. The front cover is printed with a black-and-white photograph of woman wearing a hospital gown; a sense of performance is conveyed by her pose as she twists her body away from the camera, her day clothes crumpled in a disorderly pile at her feet. The image is overlaid with a yellow circle; the title of the book and the artist's name are typed in thin yellow capitals. The main body of the 165-page book consists of black-and-white photographs which fall into three broad categories: re-appropriated pictures from old medical imaging textbooks; contemporary photographs of collaborators re-enacting the poses typically assumed for medical scans; and computational software-generated medical images. Throughout, images are in dialogue with enigmatic fragments of text printed in yellow font.

LO: The re-appropriated photographs come from old copies of *Clark's Positioning*, an X-ray manual for radiographers. I was amazed the first time I saw these images, where the body is so graphically subordinated to the machine, as a quantifiable object made up of axes and angles.[1]

---

[1]*Clark's Positioning* is the definitive text for radiographers, first published in 1939 and now in its 13th edition. The photographs used by Orton are from edition 10 published in paperback in 1984.

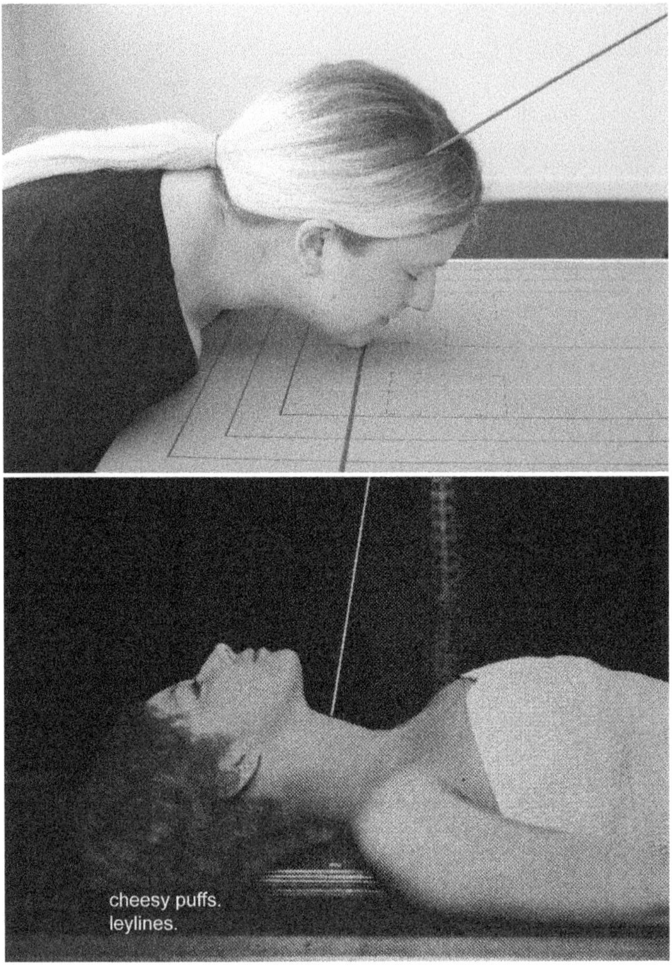

FIGURE 11.1 Liz Orton, selected images from *Every Body is an Archive*, 2019. Courtesy of the artist.

FJ: The images are curious in that they're often very aesthetic: the women are wearing make-up, they look like fashion shoots, and some are quite Surrealist.

LO: I agree, they completely exceed their scientific designation. They can't be contained by science; not only do we see cultural influences but also broader prejudices around gender, age, ableism and race.

FJ: Have you altered the images at all?

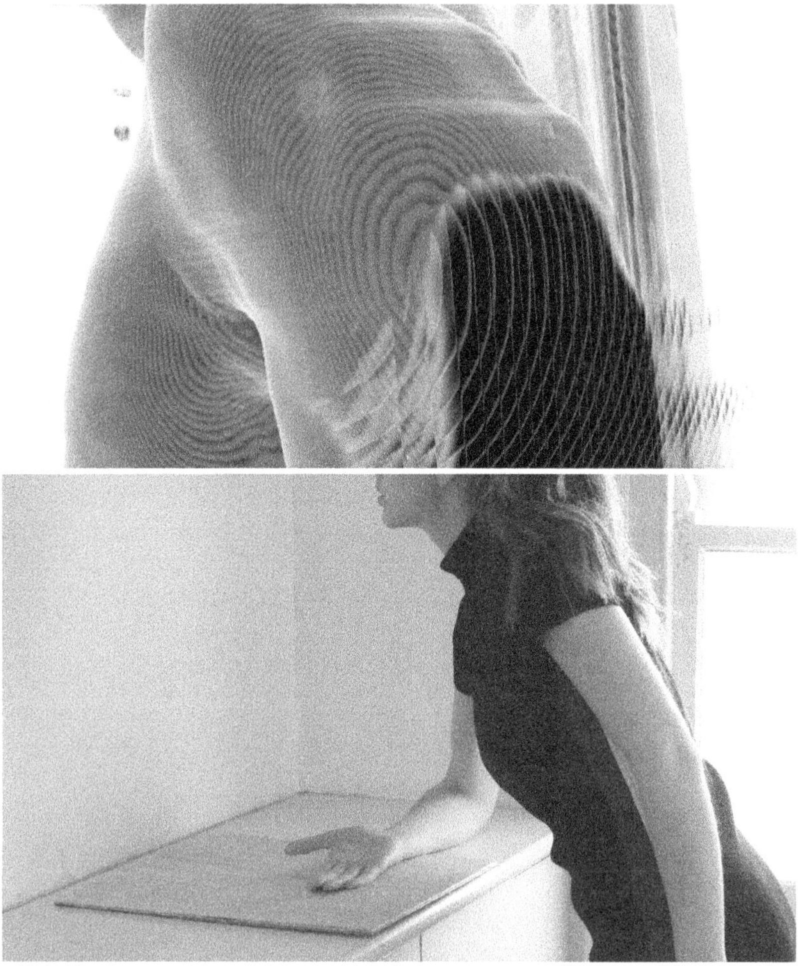

FIGURE 11.2 Liz Orton, selected images from *Every Body is an Archive*, 2019. Courtesy of the artist.

LO: No, I selected some and re-photographed them. I'm interested in the idea of re-exposure that happens as part of appropriation. The act of re-printing an existing image in a different context opens it up to new forms of cultural and ethical enquiry.

FJ: It strikes me that the whole project is about appropriation. How did you go about making the re-enactment photographs, and what was the impetus to do this?

LO: I developed the framework of restaging patients' descriptions of their experiences of being scanned. I worked with models, rather than the patients, because I was interested in reproducing some of the gaps between experience and image. I'm not trying to accurately show something, but to work with the idea of an imagined observer, who is both inside and outside of the imaging event. I make a long sequence of still images and select one, much like the radiographers do when reviewing patient images.

FJ: It's not just about individual personal experience, it's about layering all these experiences into something richer.

LO: Yes, although I worked with many individuals, some over long time periods, the project is more about the body as a clinical category that emerges through encounters with imaging systems.

I did, however, think deeply about the risks of working with participants in this context. Illness makes us very vulnerable and I didn't want to exploit it. I spent two years on a participant selection process that included a long consent procedure. I am clear about my boundaries as an artist and didn't seek to work directly with people's trauma, though some participants described the process as therapeutic.

FJ: We sometimes refer to the primal scene of the medical humanities as the encounter between clinician and patient, but I think you have identified a different primal scene, which is the patient-image encounter.

LO: I think where others are interested in the vulnerability of the patient, you might say I am interested in the vulnerability of the representation.

FJ: Can we discuss the pictures you made using medical imaging software?

LO: I co-opted a professional medical viewing software, called Osirix, which was given to me (in error, I think) by St Thomas Hospital. The software is used by radiologists and other clinicians to view and interpret patient images, including MRI, CT and PET scans, in both 2D and 3D. Working with patient data that had already been shared with me, I used – or rather, misused – Osirix, to generate images of patients' bodies as seen from the outside: not only was this a refusal of the usual spectacle of the interior body, but an attempt to show something of the capacity and audacity of the machine gaze. The images have been misread as photographs (even by clinicians), but they are actually visualizations of data not directly accessible to human vision. There is no real or embodied reference for digital skin, which is a sampling that also includes hair, water, tissue, blood and air. And the machine can't distinguish between the body and artefacts such as zips and clasps, even the bed on which the body lies: everything is seen.

FJ: It doesn't understand what a body is.

LO: Exactly. It's just data, it's just pixels. There is no judgement, only calculation. It's a machine aesthetic which is purely mathematical.

FJ: There is something exciting about disassembling and reassembling the body from the data; there is a sculptural quality to the process that really comes across in your images.

LO: I think the sense of sculpture arises from medicine's use of image slices, which means surfaces are not seamless. It is also due to the way the software simulates lighting: we can read these bodies having depth and form because the software adds highlights and shadows. And the reference for that is the photographic body: the images are constructed not only from the raw material of data but from cultural traditions of representing the body.

FJ: Can we talk about language? The book contains brief slivers of text printed in yellow ink, sometimes superimposed on an image, sometimes printed on a white page so that the words are barely visible; each phrase is set in dialogue with one or more images.

LO: The colour is sampled from something called the Repulsor Tool in the medical image software. It's bright on screen but much paler on paper. I like how it challenges the viewer and draws attention to the act of looking. The text felt like the riskiest element of the book, because it's not explained, and is completely different in tone and meaning from the images. I enjoyed the uncertainty of that and the playfulness of these almost nonsensical passages. But the text is attributed at the back of the book. It was really important to me that the reader can understand those words have bodies, that they have a documentary basis.

FJ: These phrases are intriguing and often quite cryptic! Examples from the first few pages of the book include 'an island'; 'rave graphics'; 'wallpaper'; and 'stigmata'. Did these come out of your conversations with patients?

LO: Yes, they came out of long dialogues with patients. I anatomized individual words and phrases, lifting them from the dialogues. I wondered if this gesture was too surgical but the different words and phrases immediately began to converse with each other.

FJ: We are invited to understand these phrases as metaphors for experience.

LO: Yes, because as patients we don't have a visual language to describe our insides, so we have to invent one, and in doing this we reach for other images. The result is a highly subjective glossary of words, almost the opposite of medical language which is uniform, the same for everybody. Language is a really big part of what separates a patient from their body in medicine, because it's exclusive, and belongs to the clinicians.

FJ: You're working with the patient voice, but in a way that suggests shared, rather than strictly personal experience; I find that exciting, given ongoing debates in the medical humanities on the limitations of individual illness narratives (e.g., Woods 2011).

LO: I wanted to work with the tension between medical and vernacular language, and to experiment with ideas of a collective voice. Similarly, the software-generated images are more about the interface between bodies and technology than about any single individual.

FJ: Given your pedagogic work with medical students, perhaps we could end on a constructive note by considering the productive potential of images for communication in clinical contexts?

LO: I've talked about the separation of bodies from images, and bodies from patients but I did see glimmers which suggested a different possibility. In some instances, I observed clinicians using images to talk to patients about their illness, using the screen to diffuse the intensity of the medical gaze and open up the clinical space. In this triangle of engagement, the image can be generative, pulling the patient and doctor towards a common object, momentarily aligning their views. Perhaps there is nothing inherently divisive about the medical image, and it has the capacity, with different practices, to become an agent of dialogue and inclusivity.

References

Armstrong, D. (1983), *Political Anatomy of the Body: Medical Knowledge in Britain in theTwentieth Century*, Cambridge: Cambridge University Press.

Cartwright, L. (1995), *Screening the Body: Tracing Medicine's Visual Culture*, Minneapolis: University of Minnesota Press.

Johnstone, F. (2023), 'Collaborations in art and medicine: institutional critique, patient participation, and emerging entanglements', *Leonardo* 56 (4): 424–29.

Kevles, B. (1997), *Naked to the Bone: Medical Imaging in the Twentieth Century*, New Brunswick: Rutgers University Press.

Lippit, A. M. (2005), *Atomic Light (Shadow Optics)*, Minneapolis: University of Minnesota Press.

Orton, L. (2018), *Becoming Image: Medicine and the Algorithmic Gaze*, London: Digital Insides.

Orton, L. (2019), *Every Body is an Archive*, London: Digital Insides / self-published artist's book.

van Dijck, J. (2005), *The Transparent Body: A Cultural Analysis of Medical Imaging*, Seattle: University of Washington Press.

Woods, A. (2011), 'The limits of narrative: provocations for the medical humanities', *Medical Humanities* 37 (2): 73–78.

CHAPTER TWELVE

Engraving the fetal subject: William Smellie, *A Sett of Anatomical Tables*

Rebecca Whiteley

This image (see Figure 12.1) appears to be, to modern viewers, a mass of contradictions: elegant and violent; dynamic and static; medical and aesthetic. How are we to interpret it? What is this surprisingly conscious-looking fetus, staring us dead in the eye, trying to say?

Table 16 is an illustration from William Smellie's midwifery manual of 1754, *A Sett of Anatomical Tables*, drafted by Petrus Camper and engraved by Charles Grignion. It represents, therefore, a collaborative effort between those with medical and those with artistic expertise. Indeed, all medical imagery requires creativity in its production and aesthetic training in its interpretation. Today, these elements are often obscured by a fantasy of medical imagery as truthful, acultural, objective (Daston and Galison 2010). In the eighteenth century, the links between art and medicine were more obvious and more highly valued, understood to inform and enrich each other. *Table 16* is simultaneously a technical image of the application of forceps in an obstructed labour and a commentary on the changing nature of midwifery and the rise of the 'man-midwife'.

Smellie was a Scottish surgeon who built a career in London attending labours, publishing books and teaching both male and female midwifery students. He was a key figure in the contested shift towards professionalization and masculinization in midwifery that occurred in Britain (as well as elsewhere) in the eighteenth century (Fissell 2018). A

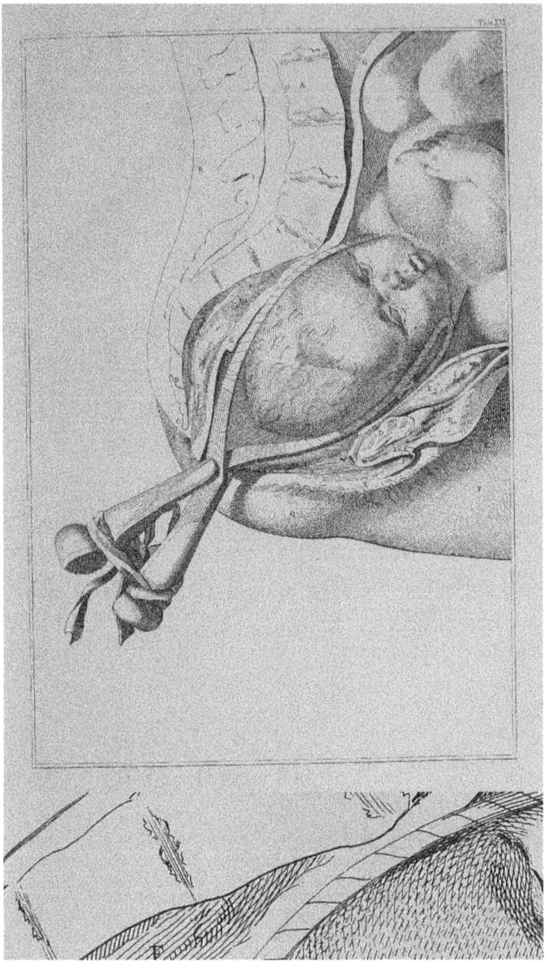

FIGURE 12.1 Petrus Camper (draftsman) and Charles Grignion (engraver), *Table 16* [and] *Detail from Table 16*, etching, 46.3 × 32.7 cm (plate). From William Smellie, *A Sett of Anatomical Tables, with Explanations, and an Abridgment, of the Practice of Midwifery, with a View to Illustrate a Treatise on that Subject, and Collection of Cases* (London: [n. pub.], 1754). RG93.S57 1754, Claude Moore Health Sciences Library. Courtesy of Historical Collections & Services, Claude Moore Health Sciences Library, University of Virginia.

previously largely female and communal affair, childbirth attracted the interest of trained surgeons in this period, who used their education and gender to assume control over the lucrative parts of practice: emergency cases, wealthy clients, and lecturing and hospital positions. The forceps, a tool only recently made public, was crucial to the 'man-midwife's' project.

The advantage they offered in delivering obstructed fetuses fell largely to men because women were officially forbidden the use of all surgical tools. Yet forceps were by no means uncontroversial: critics noted that women were terrified of them, and that in anything but the most skilled hands they could *cause* more harm than they prevented (Whiteley 2023: 137–78). It is in this context of professional and public controversy over the safety and propriety of man-midwifery that Smellie commissioned his illustration.

Some midwifery manuals in this period were published for a broad readership. However, the expense and technicality of Smellie's books indicates that his prospective audience was more educated: successful professionals, and wealthier students and lay readers. This audience was not exclusively male, but the epistemology the book presents is certainly that of a masculine, elite, academic medicine. This audience was expected not only to have an existing knowledge of the physiology of birth and use of tools, but also of the interpretation of print as a medium.

By the mid-eighteenth century, essentially everyone had some experience interpreting prints. Illustrations and single sheet prints proliferated and catered to diverse interests and budgets. Among elites, the collecting and appreciation of fine prints was a popular pastime (Nenadic 1997). These viewers were trained to analyze the skill with which an engraver transformed black lines on white paper into the representation of form, tone, texture, movement, even colour (MacGregor 1999). They were also sensitive to the hierarchy of media. 'Engraving' was a catchall term for printed images but also referred to a specific technique where grooves are cut into the prepared copper plate using a fine chisel called a burin. It was the most time-consuming and demanding print technique, and was used in elite reproductive prints and book illustrations. Mezzotint was largely for single sheet portraits, and etching and woodcut for cheaper productions. *Table 16* is an etching, where the grooves are scratched into a wax surface added to the plate, before being 'bitten' into the copper using an acid bath (Stijnman 2012). This technique produced sketchier and more fluid lines and was easier to learn, but stood lower down the hierarchy. *Table 16* is entirely etched, but large portions are done in a convincing imitation of engraving, in a convoluted stylistic exercise that makes an argument for the status of the author and his profession.

It is largely the skin that is rendered in the style of engraving, with smooth, even, tapered lines arranged in regular hatches. The use of cross-hatched meshes interspersed with dots was an established technique in engraving associated with the almost-miraculous ability of the engraver to use lines to evoke the complex contours, softness and beauty of the idealized human form. Martin Kemp suggests that such skill produced in viewers of this period 'a delight in the improbability that such overt artifice could function to imitate nature' (Kemp 1994: 235). By the mid-eighteenth century, this mesh technique had also come to be associated specifically with portraits of elite men and classical sculpture, creating 'associations of permanence, nobility, and authority' (Chuong 2022: 70).

Grignion at once demonstrates an attention to the specifics of the fetal body – the facial features, the unsutured plates of the skull – and associates this body with the idealized adult classical body. The torso, arms and legs are modelled in the classical style, the hand assumes the rhetorical gesture 'compello' which connotes invitation (B. [John Bulwer] 1644: 570). The fetus invites the educated viewer in, encouraging examination and understanding, and perhaps also indicating consent for the application of the forceps which were so often criticized for being used *without* invitation. The eyes of the fetus are blank, making direct reference to the rendering of classical sculptures in reproductive engraving. This is a remarkable move on the artists' parts away from the anatomical rhetoric of close observation. It renders this fetus not an individual, but an ideal, a rhetorical fetus. They look both directly at us, exhorting us with their crooked finger to learn the lesson of their deliverance, and beyond us, to more elevated and abstract thoughts.

If we look to the maternal body, very different kinds of line are evident. Particularly in the sectioned view of the maternal spine and pelvis, more space is left blank, and the lines are sketchier, freer and more varied. This style is not just more typical of etching, but also imitates the quality of a pen and ink drawing. Framing the elevated representation of the fetal body, we have anatomical elements of the maternal body rendered in the style of the observational drawings undertaken by artists and students in the dissection room. The relative blankness of these sections not only frames the heavily worked fetal skin, it also lays out in visual terms the line between observed and idealized truth, between the specifics of the body studied directly and the aggregate knowledge of the medical expert about the body *in principle*. The image demonstrates how the learned, elite medical professional could balance high culture and medical knowledge. The sketchy anatomical elements of the maternal anatomy are contrasted with the smooth pseudo-engraved skin of buttock and leg. The presence of pubic hair on the woman's body makes a statement about the importance of observation and accuracy in medical illustration; its neatness, sparsity, and the way it is largely hidden by the shadows of the modelled skin, demonstrate how that knowledge can be tempered, made elegant.

One other body is present in this image, but only by implication. While the forceps have been carefully inserted and secured around the fetal head, the skilled hands that have done this, and that will shortly exert traction to deliver the obstructed fetus, are absent. This absence takes three interlinked bodies at work and stills them, rendering them atemporal and tensionless. By flicking through the following tables in the book, viewers experience the twisting, squeezing, traumatic process of birth, but here it is made safe. The absence of the practitioner's hands defuses much of the fearsomeness of the forceps, refusing the actual force of traction that made them useful but also dangerous. The same absence also reinforces the message of the medium. The 'man-midwife' is legitimized through his work, but that work is rendered intellectual, *almost* immaterial. By turning a medical image into a fetal portrait, Smellie, Camper and Grignion construct a new elegant and enlightened kind of midwifery.

References

B. [John Bulwer], J. (1644), *Chirologia: Or the Naturall Language of the Hand*, London: Tho. Harper.

Chuong, J. Y. (2022), 'Engraving's "Immoveable Veil": Phillis Wheatley's Portrait and the Politics of Technique', *The Art Bulletin*, 104 (2): 63–88.

Daston, L., and P. Galison (2010), *Objectivity*, New York: Zone Books.

Fissell, M. E. (2018), 'Man-Midwifery Revisited', in N. Hopwood, R. Flemming and L. Kassell (eds), *Reproduction: Antiquity to the Present Day*, 319–32, Cambridge: Cambridge University Press.

Kemp, M. (1994), 'Coming into Line: Graphic Demonstrations of Skill in Renaissance and Baroque Engravings', in J. Onians (ed.), *Sight & Insight: Essays on Art and Culture in Honour of E.H. Gombrich at* 85, 221–44, London: Phaidon.

MacGregor, W. B. (1999), 'The Authority of Prints: An Early Modern Perspective', *Art History*, 22 (3): 389–420.

Nenadic, S. (1997), 'Print Collecting and Popular Culture in Eighteenth-Century Scotland', *History*, 82 (266): 203–22.

Stijnman, A. (2012), *Engraving and Etching 1400–2000: A History of the Development of Manual Intaglio Printmaking Processes*, London: Archetype Publications.

Whiteley, R. (2023), *Birth Figures: Early Modern Prints and the Pregnant Body*, Chicago: University of Chicago Press.

CHAPTER THIRTEEN

Re-mythologizing the (re)productive body: Wangechi Mutu's *Cervical Hypertrophy*

Arya Thampuran

How do we draw the boundary between myth and reality? Myth is often shelved in the realm of the fictive, something without the validity or veracity of 'reality'. But what if we begin to see what we consider 'reality' itself not as what *is*, but a collagic construction of multiple mythologies about how we *should* see, know, and relate to the world? As Peter Fryer poignantly reminds us, English racism was rooted in 'the development of a strident pseudo-scientific mythology of race that would become the most important ingredient in British imperial theory' (1984: 165). What Kenyan-American visual artist Wangechi Mutu's aesthetic enmeshment of the old and new, nonhuman and posthuman reminds us, however, is that this colonial scientific racism is not simply a relic of the past, but roots and reifies racist structures now. Mutu uses collage to powerfully probe how multiple sociobiological myths have been woven together, over time, to form – and *naturalize* – a particular reality, filtered through a Western heteropatriarchal gaze.

Science has been used to intellectualize and institute value-laden ideas of racial difference; specifically, the measurement of physical anatomy – from cranial capacity to nose shape and hair type – mapped onto sociocultural ideals; as Anne McClintock powerfully asserts, 'the features of the face spelled out the character of the race' (1995: 50). The eighteenth-century work of Dutch anatomist, obstetrician and artist, Petrus Camper exemplifies this impulse. He mapped 'facial angle' (the degree to which the jaw protrudes from skull) onto beauty, intellect and psychosocial development; in this sliding scale across Africans, Indians and Europeans, European (colonizers) had the highest degree and hence superiority. Unsurprisingly, Camper found an 'amusing' resemblance in the skulls of 'Monkies' and 'Blacks'. This 'scientific' rationality of racial difference took different guises, but fundamentally sought to demonstrate the developmental deficiencies of the colonized by endowing them animalistic, subhuman status, thereby rationalizing the intervention of colonial civility and reifying racism.

Mutu reclaims this scientific register, turning it on its own head to deconstruct its fetishistic fallacies: she evocatively asserts that her 'lab is the female body' (2011). Mutu's twelve-part mixed media series, *Histology of the Different Classes of Uterine Tumors* (2004–5) overlays nineteenth-century medical diagrams depicting uterine cancer with contemporary magazine cuttings, packing tape, faux fur, glitter and Mutu's own pencil drawings.[1] Mutu picks apart, mis-places, and pastes these textual layers – the multiple mythologies of womanhood from medicine to mass media – onto the skin, which morphs into an alien-esque embodiment of female sexual, reproductive and domestic objectification. Indeed, Mutu describes her collaging process as 'dissecting things in order to understand them', then 'reconfiguring them into a new solution' (Barber, Naimou and Mutu 2016: 356). Her art refracts the medical gaze, mapping how the biologized female body becomes the site onto which sexual desire, racial derision, and reproductive labour are projected.

One collage in this series, *Cervical Hypertrophy* reproduces anxieties over biological and political futurity, and captures this slippage between the natural and naturalized, myth and reality. Mutu's experimentation with biological form invokes the fraught history of medical experimentation on the bodies of the racialized and enslaved – human bodies rendered in service of a Western medical body of knowledge. Reproductive medicine is rooted in racial malpractice and continuing mistreatment from contraceptive trials to corrective surgery. J. Marion Sims, a nineteenth-century physician, for example, developed a surgical remedy for vesicovaginal fistulas by operating 'openly and publicly on nude African American women, when to do so with white and middle- and upper-class women patients would have caused severe repercussions' (McGregor 1998: 61; Holloway 2011: 31–32).

Cervical hypertrophy, or the infection of cervical mucus, is often caused by sexually-transmitted infections, symptomatized by inflammation and an enlargement of the cervix. Mutu transplants enlarged reproductive organs prominently across the face, making visible the invisibilized bodies of racial

[1]Wangechi Mutu, *Histology of the Different Classes of Uterine Tumors*, 2004–5. We were unable to obtain permission to publish an image of either the full work, *Histology of the Different Classes of Uterine Tumors*, or of the detail *Cervical Hypertrophy*, in this volume; at time of writing, both can be viewed on the website of the National Galleries of Scotland, who acquired the work for their collection in 2020 (accession number GMA 5725).

minorities who 'tend to be simultaneously underrepresented in medical research and historically exploited in experimentation' (Schiebinger 2017: 6). This is a vexed tension in the case of the Black female body: on one hand, issues of female sexual and reproductive health are met with silence and shame; on the other, the Black female body has always been hyper-visible as sexual and reproductive object. The seeds of the sexualized 'Jezebel' or maternal 'Mammy' mythological figures were sown during periods of enslavement, the carnal, libido-driven antithesis to white Victorian femininity and the Black domestic help 'embrac[ed]' simultaneously (White 2007: 125–27). Deirdre Cooper Owens also notes the dissonance in how white medical men appraised Black women's superior fecundity, hypersexuality, and physical strength relative to white women – as what she terms 'medical superbodies' capable of gynaecological experimentation. Yet, they denied Black women the very qualities seen as 'natural' to white women, a particular construction of femininity and a more fundamental humanity (2017: 109). These myths have morphed and mutated under different guises over time, but still fundamentally speak to anxieties over the Other, whose embodiment must remain ontologically and ethically distinct from that of the imperialist imaginary.

In the same stroke, then, Mutu draws on the trope of enlargement to expose what has been effaced. The enlarged reproductive organs from medical diagrams occupy space in dissonant ways; on an exposed brain, hanging by the ears and hair. An animal's nose is nestled between human nostrils, its ears fanning out across lipstick-ed lips, which, like the eyes heavy with glittery shadow, are presumably cut from contemporary magazines. Stripped bare in this confounding composition of material and biological elements, this embodied form exposes the subjection of the body to a capitalist and heteropatriarchal gaze – at once a consumer and to be consumed, a site of desire and derision. The cut-and-paste method also gestures towards the reductive appraisal of women as a sum of biological parts; the subject of critique is the cultural construction of the biologically female body through reproductive functionality and sexual fetishization. Toying with the colonialist and medical conflation of animal and racialized (sub)human, Mutu's boundary-crossing art radically disrupts the bedrock of this scientific body – its classificatory schemas – and by extension, the very logic of racial hierarchies themselves. In the seeming arbitrariness of collagic construction and (mis)placement, Mutu calls to attention the constructed quality of biological boundaries, unsettling the very structural mythologies that structure society.

Mutu de-forms through her collagic forms. The grotesquely exaggerated misplacement of biological organs generates unease – to me at least, and I read this unease as Mutu's way of relocating disease from the biological body to the social, a kind of structural malaise in the systemic scientific racism and sexualization of Black womanhood. To the (white) heteropatriarchal gaze, it is at once an object of desire and disgust, even derision; it becomes a site onto which this conflictual discomfort of duality is projected. The hyperbole evokes the overwhelm of being objectified as a Black woman: how the female body is structured, silenced and surveilled. Here, the viewing gaze is turned inward, forced to reckon with the naturalization of a particular essentializing *form* of the biologically female body.

But Mutu's fragmentary approach is also a potent means to re-form; the female body in her rendering embodies a curative potential to both expose and remedy, to re-imagine alternative expressions which exceed existing sociobiological scriptings. This makes it at once, and perhaps paradoxically, thoroughly embodied and disembodied; in its collagic quality, these multiple layerings of metaphorical and material 'skins' and anatomically-defiant placements of reproductive organs, create an alternative 'wholeness' to the female body beyond a medicalized conception of biological unity. This is not an attempt to redress animalistic dehumanization, subhuman enslavement or the equally pernicious 'superhumanization' of the Black body as magical or mechanistic (Waytz, Hoffman and Trawalter 2014: 243). Instead, what is reconfigured from the dis-figured female body is a material form which exists outside these politico-ontological imaginaries, which transcends the essentialist categories serving a Western scientific, spiritual and/or sexual fantasy. Here, fragmentation invokes a fissure with a received, reductive rationality that reproduces racism. The female body becomes a barometer for social malaise, but the dis-ease produced by it becomes a generative space for imagining differently. In its unboundedness, its spillage beyond the boundaries of existing scripts, Mutu's work can be seen as a form of what Walter Mignolo terms 'border thinking' (2013: 134): a decolonial de-linking from Eurocentric myths of identity.

References

Barber, T., A. Naimou and W. Mutu (2016), 'Between Disgust and Regeneration', *ASAP/Journal* 1(3): 337–63.

Cooper Owens, D. (2017), *Medical Bondage: Race, Gender, and the Origins of American Gynecology*, Georgia: University of Georgia Press.

Curtin, P. D. (1960), '"Scientific" Racism and the British Theory of Empire', *Journal of the Historical Society of Nigeria* 2(1): 40–51.

Fryer, P. (1984), *Staying Power: The History of Black People in Britain*, London: Pluto Press.

Holloway, K. F. C. (2011), *Private Bodies, Public Texts: Race, Gender, and a Biocultural Ethics*, New York: Duke University Press.

Holmes, C. M. (2016), 'The Colonial Roots of the Racial Fetishization of Black Women', *Black and Gold* 2(2): 1–11.

McClintock, A. (1995), *Imperial Leather: Race, Gender, and Sexuality in the Colonial Contest*, New York: Routledge.

McCulloch, J. (1995), *Colonial Psychiatry and the 'African Mind'*, Cambridge: Cambridge University Press.

McGregor, D. K. (1998), *From Midwives to Medicine: The Birth of American Gynecology*, New Brunswick: Rutgers University Press.

Mignolo, W. (2013), 'Geopolitics of sensing and knowing: On (de)coloniality, border thinking, and epistemic disobedience', *Confero* 1(1): 129–50.

Mutu, W. (2011), 'My Lab is the Female Body', *African Voices: Interview with CNN.*

Schiebinger, L. (2017), *Secret Cures of Slaves: People, Plants, and Medicine in the Eighteenth-Century Atlantic World*, California: Stanford University Press.

Waytz, A., K. M. Hoffman, and S. Trawalter (2014), 'A Superhumanization Bias in Whites' Perceptions of Blacks', *Social Psychological and Personality Science* 6(3): 243–359.

White, D. G. (2007), 'Jezebel and Mammy: The Mythology of Female Slavery', in *Race, Ethnicity, and Gender: Selected Readings*, ed. by J. F. Healey and E. O'Brien, 123–32, New York: SAGE Publications.

PART IV

Reproducing reproduction

CHAPTER FOURTEEN

In living colour: realism and abstraction in anatomical models of the female reproductive body, 1880–1900

Jessica M. Dandona

'It has been 18 years since all of Europe echoed the Germans in stating that France was a nation in a state of decadence,' lamented sociologist Arsène Dumont in his 1890 study of population decline, adding, 'it would be only wise to ask ourselves if the wound healed on the surface is truly healed deep down' (1890: 1–2). Reflecting fears of 'degeneration' first voiced after France's defeat in the disastrous Franco-Prussian War (1870–71), Dumont's warning is located at the intersection of medical discourse, nationalism, and debate over the rights of women and infants. In referring to a hidden wound, Dumont evokes both potential weaknesses lurking beneath the nation's apparent prosperity *and* the frailties of the human body, here cast as essential to the perpetuation of French political, financial, and even intellectual excellence.

A new generation of physicians and scientists in the field of medicine would seek answers to these challenges in the study and regulation of the female reproductive body. Their theories circulated widely in the professional pamphlets, journals, and medical treatises that proliferated in this period, many illustrated through new processes such as colour lithography. As research and teaching in fields such as midwifery and gynaecology expanded, so did the need for pedagogical objects employed in the lecture theatre and the anatomy museum. By the late nineteenth century, the individual experimentation and handcrafted techniques employed by makers of early anatomical models had largely given way to quasi-industrial forms of production. Four makers dominated the market for wax models – Tramond, Deyrolle and Jules Talrich in Paris and Adolf and Friedrich Ziegler in Freiburg. Durable and highly detailed papier-mâché models by the French firm of Louis Auzoux, meanwhile, offered students a more interactive encounter with the body's structures and systems. While plaster casts continued to be made in-house in many anatomy programmes, the Leipzig firm of Bock-Steger advertised a range of colourful, painted models depicting both internal and external structures. By 1900, serially produced models appeared in catalogues printed in multiple languages, featured in exhibitions at World's Fairs, and were employed in lecture theatres around the world.

At the same time, emerging cultural anxieties regarding the replication, dissemination, and function of images and objects, especially those picturing the female body, lent urgency to the task of establishing an anatomical lexicon of reproduction deemed both effective and appropriate in its depiction of human sexuality. In France, the passage of a new censorship law in 1852 intensified surveillance, creating a system whereby works could be submitted to the Paris Minister of Police or local prefects for approval. Both the Comstock Act of 1873 in the United States and the Obscene Publications Act 1857 in Britain were similarly employed to limit public display and sale of 'obscenities', including anatomical models and texts discussing birth control. In 1868, the ruling in the British trial *R. v. Hicklin* further fuelled debate when it defined 'obscenity' based not on intent but on distribution, opening the door to the prosecution of popular medical works discussing matters related to sexuality and reproduction (Bull 2017: 714–15). Such attempts to regulate the use, display and sale of works related to human reproduction rendered imperative the need to secure the authority of anatomical models and atlases.

The three works discussed in this chapter existed at the intersection of professional and popular discourse, made use of new technologies of production and diffusion and presented the female reproductive body according to the emerging conventions of anatomical realism. Yet each work – a plaster cast by Deyrolle, a wax model by Tramond, and an anatomical atlas by Witkowski – also functioned in dialogue with long-standing histories of making and pictorial conventions for depicting the body in both art and medicine. These works mark a pivotal moment of transition in the study of reproduction and anticipate the multiple forms of simulacra that map the body today, from durable plastic models to high-tech virtual reality platforms. In their appeal to bright colour, detail and serial reproduction, they defined a new style for picturing the body – an enduring 'anatomical aesthetic' pairing abstraction and realism. In the process, they also asserted medicine's authority over the body, supporting physicians' attempts to recast human sexuality and reproduction as medicalized spheres of knowledge.

Deyrolle

On 1 February 2008, dozens of French firefighters struggled to contain a raging inferno engulfing one of the oldest and most illustrious shops in Paris – Maison Deyrolle. Founded in 1831 by Jean-Baptiste Deyrolle, the venerable institution housed an array of natural history collections dating back to the early nineteenth century. It was Jean-Baptiste's grandson, Émile, who secured the firm's international reputation: a naturalist and dealer in natural history specimens, in the 1880s he expanded Deyrolle's holdings to include charts, wall displays, and anatomical models for use in both primary and secondary schools. By the time of the Paris World's Fair of 1889, the Deyrolle workshops in Auteuil functioned like a small factory, employing 'Preparers, taxidermists, osteologists and anatomists, moulders, colourists, designers, locksmiths, turners, carpenters, printers, [and] mechanics' alongside 'twelve machines powered by a 25-horsepower steam engine' (Picard 1891: 432).

Among the works produced by Deyrolle is a brightly-coloured plaster model of the female reproductive organs (Figure 14.1), entitled *Bassin de femme* (Female Pelvis). The original paper label, which references Émile's heirs, 'Les Fils d'Émile Deyrolle', dates the works to 1893 or later. *Female Pelvis* represents the right leg and half of the abdomen of a female figure, reducing the body to those areas most clearly associated with reproduction. When viewed from the front, the left side of the model is composed of a smoothly curving line that follows an incision from the spine to just above the *mons pubis*. Individual organs and structures are vividly painted and textured to provide both description and differentiation. The heavy plaster model is mounted on a brass rod atop a black wooden box, suggesting its function as an object of display and visual study.

The model exhibits a high degree of realism, including many superfluous details such as the depiction of pubic hair and smoothly painted buttocks. The use of vivid colour further intensifies the model's verisimilitude, as does its life-sized scale and status as an indexical cast of the body. The figure appears in cross-section along the sagittal plane as if neatly bisected in two, implying that the absent half is the mirror image of the structures presented. The uniform surface created by this cut may originate in the contemporary practice of sawing through frozen cadavers, which allowed anatomists to view the body as a succession of flat planes. The clearly delineated organs, absence of viscera, and fragmentary quality of the figure similarly suggest the model's origins in anatomical dissection.

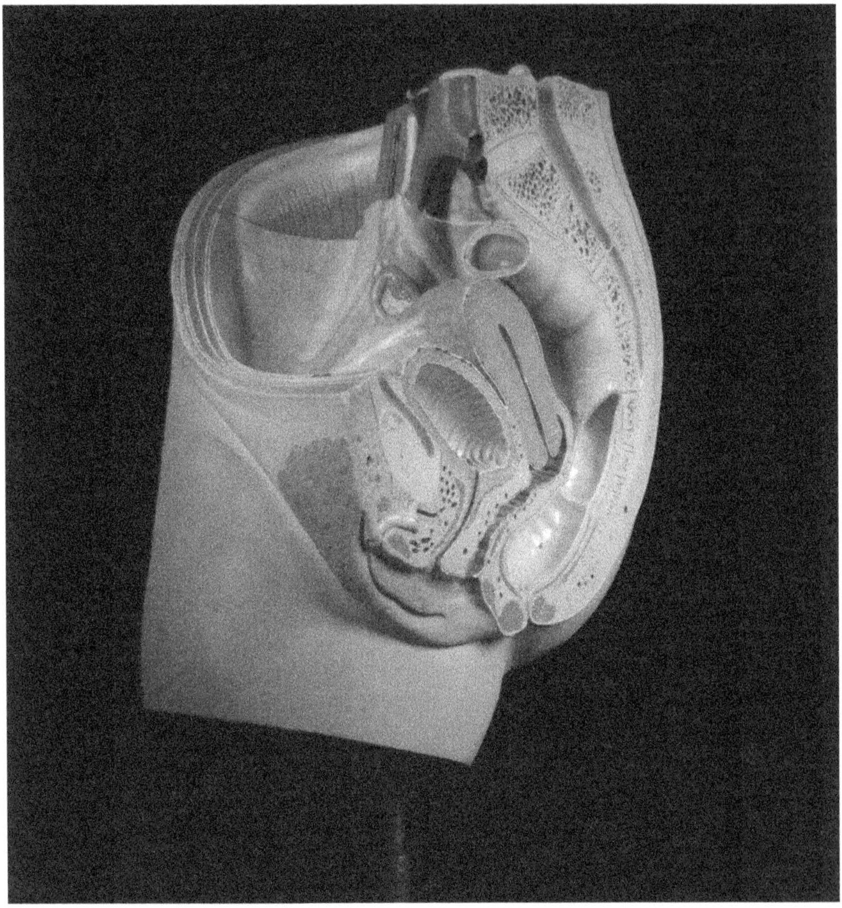

FIGURE 14.1 Deyrolle, *Anatomie Humaine / Bassin de Femme* (Human Anatomy, Female Pelvis), *c.* 1890s. Painted plaster mounted on a metal rod and black wooden box. Photograph by Sophie Haldane. Collection of the Centre for Anatomy and Human Identification, University of Dundee.

In its subject matter, materials, and incomplete presentation of the body, Deyrolle's figure recalls plaster casts created by Scottish man-midwife William Hunter in the eighteenth century. Recent conservation efforts have confirmed that Hunter's casts were intended to be viewed in the same prone position as the bodies they depicted (Campbell 2018: 249). Whereas Hunter's works underscore the deathliness of his subjects, however, Deyrolle's model signals a new aesthetic at play. In its upright pose, glossy surfaces, and use of bright, saturated hues – including canary yellow, celadon green, and a fleshy pinkish-red – the plaster creates the impression of a living body.

Plaster models were not uncommon in medical teaching collections: many were made on-site, and anatomical treatises often included instructions for creating simple casts from human remains. Casts could be made directly from the cadaver or the living body by creating a plaster mould, which was allowed to dry before being removed, oiled, and filled with liquid plaster to create the final model. Such works often appeared alongside another category of plaster model commonly found in anatomical museums, art academies and medical schools – classical casts reproducing ancient Greek and Roman sculptures. In art classes, these classical casts served primarily to suggest the outward appearance created by underlying structures, including muscle and bone. Their presence in the lecture theatre and dissecting room, meanwhile, helped associate the practice of anatomical investigation with the elevated ideals of Greek art, establishing a precedent for anatomy's intensive exploration and partitioning of the corporeal form.

The white hue of classical casts emulated the appearance of marble, which had long been a privileged material for the creation of sculpture. Despite evidence that classical statues were in fact polychrome, by the late eighteenth century the writings of Johann Joachim Winckelmann and others had come to associate marble's white hue with notions of purity, immortality, clarity of form, and above all disavowal of the abject qualities of 'flesh' (Blühm 1996: 12). The use of white marble also functioned as a 'supposedly universal abstraction' that suppressed notions of racial difference (Nelson 2007: 68). In contrast, polychrome sculpture has historically been viewed as deceptive, a mere distraction from the ideal form (Syson 2018: 18).

Through its bold, vivid hues and partial presentation of the body, Deyrolle's plaster model disrupts this classical ideal, reasserting the cast's proximity to the anatomical subject and provoking associations with the sensuality, vulnerability, and even messiness of 'real' bodies. While such realism could suggest objectivity and rationality, in this period it could just as easily be associated with 'scandal, gratuitous detail, and pornography' – especially in matters related to the female body (Hunter 2008: 48).

It is Deyrolle's use of anatomical conventions, including a view in cross-section and incomplete presentation of the body, which mediates the model's heightened realism and reasserts its function as a universalizing and even idealized pedagogical object. Despite the work's origins in anatomical dissection, its clean edges and clearly legible and regular structures suggest the figure was carefully finished to produce an authoritative, generalized depiction of female anatomy. The figure's presentation also recalls black-and-white wood engravings in contemporary textbooks such as a cross-section of the pelvis depicted in Figure 18 of *Manuel pratique de l'art des accouchements* (1883) by Eugène Verrier. Many such texts reprised existing drawings and diagrams, creating an increasingly standardized view of human anatomy. It is also notable that the hues employed in Deyrolle's model depart from strict naturalism, and certain colours follow anatomical conventions such as the use of red to indicate arteries. In a cultural context wherein representations of sexuality and the female body were subject to intense scrutiny and frequent accusations of indecency, models needed to connote both 'art' and 'science'. The imperative to reaffirm the pedagogical nature of these objects was rendered even more acute in the case of wax models, whose uncanny ability to emulate the appearance of the living body often provoked controversy.

Tramond

In a shadowy corner of Philadelphia's Mütter Museum, a startlingly illusionistic depiction of the 'pelvic organs of a woman' lies encased in a nineteenth-century vitrine (Figure 14.2). Created by the French firm Vasseur-Tramond, the wax model rests alongside a range of other curiosities, including a dried specimen of a penis, a wax cast of the scrotum, and a preserved vulva. Maison Tramond and its successors, Vasseur-Tramond and N. Rouppert, were based on the rue de l'École de Médecine, where the

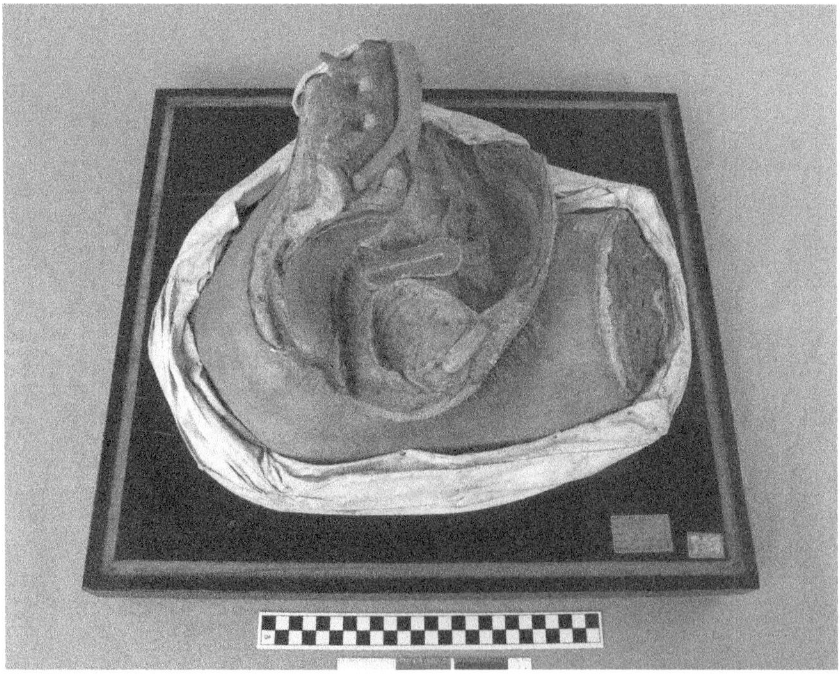

FIGURE 14.2 Maison Vasseur-Tramond, Model showing the pelvic organs of woman, *c.* 1880s. Photograph by Lisa Geiger. Collection of the Mütter Museum, Philadelphia.

company had easy access to both cadavers used in the Paris medical school and a market for their wares.

Tramond's model of the female pelvis most likely functioned in a museum setting – its flat, horizontal presentation and fragility would have rendered it unsuitable for use in the lecture theatre, while its high degree of detail invited study at close quarters. It would have been displayed in conversation with a range of other objects related to human reproduction – a process Elizabeth Hallam has termed 'anatomical intermediality' (2016: 17). At the Lying-In Hospital of New York, for example, models of the pelvis were shown alongside an ovology set by Auzoux, models of human embryos by Ziegler, and a range of preserved specimens (Markoe and Wollstein 1897: 318). Tramond's model no doubt drew upon this context for its authority: proximity to anatomical preparations underscored the model's resemblance to bodies living and dead, while the use of consistent pictorial conventions across a range of media asserted the centrality of anatomy as a system for understanding the corporeal form.

Like Deyrolle's model, Tramond's wax depicts the interior of the female pelvis in sagittal section, focusing attention on those structures most directly related to reproduction – the external genitalia, vagina and uterus. Where Deyrolle employs vibrant, discrete areas of colour, Tramond closely recreates the appearance of an anatomized cadaver: hues range from a rosy pink to shades of reddish-purple, yellow and ivory, with one vivid scarlet section denoting an artery. The use of white fabric around the model simultaneously directs the viewer's eye, alludes to the ragged edges of a dissected cadaver, and given the prone position of the figure, inevitably evokes both medical treatment and the act of coitus.

Tramond's waxes sought to capture delicate structures such as blood vessels and nerves, which were often difficult to dissect and preserve. While the firm's working methods remain a closely guarded secret, it is likely that structures revealed by anatomical dissection were first modelled or cast directly in wax, and then recreated through use of a plaster mould. A combination of wax, solvents, and natural pigments were then heated and poured into the mould, layer by layer. Once complete, wax models were polished and painstakingly painted to match the appearance of the specimen. Fine structures such as nerves were created using thread coated with coloured wax, and blood vessels were formed through a process called *corrosion casting*, whereby natural arteries were first injected with wax and then corroded to reveal the resulting cast (Pastor et al. 2016: 187).

The painstaking detail and rich colour of Tramond's wax models secured their status as extremely lifelike replicas of bodily structures, but their realism extended beyond effects produced by the hand of the modeller. Many of Tramond's models were built upon an underlying structure of preserved bone and also contained other bodily materials, such as hair (Pastor et al. 2016: 188). The combination of human remains with the visual artistry of wax created strangely hybrid anatomical models – part specimen, part invention – what Rebecca Martin has termed 'augmented remains' (2020: n.p.). The resulting works operate on two registers, at once functioning as markers of the 'real' *and* as the products of invention, highly refined skill, and specialized knowledge. In this way, they celebrate the labour of the anatomist, who defines form in the process of revealing it, but also the work of the artist, who transforms mute matter into legible structure.

The fine craftsmanship of these objects is attested by the fact that each model is not only labelled with the maker's name, but often signed as well. Many works bear the inscription 'Tramond fecit à Paris', employing a term more commonly associated with printmaking, *fecit*, or 'he made it', which marks the works as unique copies issued from a single matrix. Tramond's waxes thus assert their accuracy through reference to multiple acts of reproduction – the making of a more or less 'exact' copy of the body, recreated by the hand of the wax modeller. While the model's reproducibility attests to its scientific nature, references to the artistry of its creator affirm its distance from similar representations of the female body considered pornographic in nature.

Indeed, the fine quality of its waxes brought the firm widespread acclaim and recognition in public venues such as the Paris World's Fair of 1889, where Tramond was awarded the grand prize. Summarizing the jury's findings, Alfred Picard writes, 'Tramond ... is an artist, an inventor', whose works 'stand out for their sober and conscientious execution and for faithful execution of the smallest details' (1890–92: 601). In his review of medical exhibits at the Fair, Marcel Baudouin attributes the accuracy of Tramond's works specifically to his use of hybrid materials. 'These pieces are partly artificial, partly natural', he notes, adding, 'The conservation of the natural skeleton... ensures an accuracy... that cannot be obtained on artificial pieces' (1889: 271).

The use of wax in anatomical modelling originated in the Early Modern period. Among the most illustrious examples are those produced in eighteenth-century Florence, where naturalist and anatomist Abbé Felice Fontana commissioned artists such as Clemente Susini to create works for the Royal Museum of Physics and Natural History (La Specola). By the mid-nineteenth century, wax anatomical models also figured prominently in travelling fairs such as Pierre Spitzner's *Grand Musée anatomique et ethnologique*, which featured a so-called Florentine Venus inspired by those produced in Italy. Anatomical models also appeared in popular anatomy museums including those run by the Jordan family in New York, Philadelphia, and other cities. Bearing names such as the Parisian Gallery, these venues devoted considerable space to the topics of conception and pregnancy – and offered visitors free consultations intended to diagnose venereal disease. As a result of their association with the fairground and the popular anatomy museum, by the late nineteenth century anatomical waxes were increasingly viewed by critics as sensational, even pornographic, and many sought to limit their display to medical settings (Bates 2008: 1–22; Maerker 2013: 536).

Whereas early anatomical models were promoted as tasteful alternatives to anatomical dissection, Tramond's *Pelvis* stakes its claim to medical credibility on *directly* referencing the act of cutting into the body in order to reveal its secrets. In contrast to the idealized classical perfection of anatomical Venuses, Tramond depicts not an intact body that can be taken apart and reassembled, but one already broken down into its constituent parts. Whereas eighteenth-century figures were 'highly sexualised by virtue of their conspicuously feminine features: long hair, smooth skin, [and] passive pose' (Jordanova 1989: 50), Tramond's *Pelvis* lacks any such markers of sensuality. Rather than appealing to the aesthetics of beauty and classical refinement to justify representation of the female body, the work offers viewers not a nude, but a body stripped of its enveloping skin.

If Deyrolle's figure presents a somewhat sanitized view of the body, Tramond's wax captures the ragged edges and irregular surfaces of the dissected cadaver. The presence of white fabric around the simulated specimen does little to counteract the impression of violence: a view of the thigh in cross-section strongly recalls the butcher's shop, and the lack of visually distinct organs underscores challenges the anatomist faced in transforming the body into a display of its own structure. Moreover, hooks, strings, and other implements employed during cutting were often included in the firm's models as markers of their verisimilitude (Hallam 2016: 298), effectively commemorating both the body *and* the process whereby it is divided and made legible. Tramond's model thus centres reproduction and acts of making by recreating the body, reproducing it in serial form, and recasting 'sexuality' as 'reproduction' – all strategies also employed by Witkowski in his widely published anatomical atlas.

Witkowski

Today, the physician and popularizer of medical history Gustave-Joseph Witkowski is best-known for abundantly illustrated, humorous, and slightly scandalous books such as *Tetoniana* (1898), a volume on the history of the female breast. Sold in a lockable case to prevent prying eyes from glimpsing its secrets, his 11-part atlas of the human body – published as *Anatomie iconoclastique* in France (1873–78; 1880–84), *Human Anatomy and Physiology* in Britain (*c.* 1878–88), and *A Pictorial Manikin, or, Movable Atlas* in the United States (*c.* 1880s) – was intended for a more professional audience. The complexly layered atlas permitted a kind of virtual, progressive exploration of the body achieved by lifting its printed paper flaps to reveal underlying structures. The earliest anatomical works to employ this approach, such as those by Heinrich Vogtherr, date back to the sixteenth century, but Witkowski's flap anatomies are distinguished by their appeal to intense, luminous colour and heightened realism.

Witkowski spent sixteen years as a provincial physician before returning to the city he termed 'the modern Babylon, the capital of the syphilized world, dominated by Mount Venerian' (1917: 9). It is perhaps not surprising, given his description of Paris as the capital of sex, that his atlas includes a volume dedicated to the 'female genital organs and perineum' (*Organes génitaux et périnée de la femme*, 1874) (Figure 14.3). Witkowski's series achieved remarkably widespread circulation: his work on female reproductive organs also appeared in Japan (*Jinshin senkei*, 1882–83) as well as in his popular medical treatise, *La génération humaine* (Human Generation, 1880), published in at least eleven French and Spanish editions between 1880 and 1927.

The drawings for Witkowski's atlas were made by medical illustrator J.-B. Léveillé, whose designs for Henry Savage's *Illustrations of the Surgery of the Female Pelvic Organs* (1863) may have provided the initial inspiration for *Organes génitaux*. The series was printed using chromolithography, which made possible its brilliant, saturated hues and glossy surface. Like lithography, this process involves drawing on a stone using a greasy crayon. The stone is then dampened and covered with grease-based ink, which is repelled by the water and adheres only to those surfaces marked with crayon. The process of chromolithography dates to 1837, when printers Jean and Godefroy Engelmann invented a system for printing colour images employing a series of separate but nearly identical blocks. After printing, the images for Witkowski's atlases were die-cut and assembled by hand in a complex process of folding, gluing and layering.

As users open Witkowski's atlas, they are confronted with an intimate view of the female anatomical subject, legs spread wide and severed mid-thigh. The flap anatomy is life-sized and conforms to the shape of the body itself, conflating image and referent. Users begin the process of exploration by lifting up the topmost flap to reveal not only subsequent layers of muscle and viscera, but also the *back* of the previous sheet, as if each flap were a thin slice of the body. The verso of the figure includes an illusionistic rendering of the buttocks, underscoring the visual conflation of the body and its representation. This slippage between anatomical subject and paper model is evident in contemporary accounts: advertisements for the New York edition promise, 'An exact counterpart of each organ is presented, and the necessary knowledge of its anatomy and physiology acquired almost as readily as from actual dissections' (Witkowsky [*sic*] 1880: back cover). While Witkowski's atlas appears visually flat, the three-dimensionality of its flaps quickly disrupts any notion of distance between the user and the figure, intensifying the work's eroticism, an effect also produced by the frank depiction of elements such as pubic hair and external genitalia, as well as by the private contemplation its format invites.

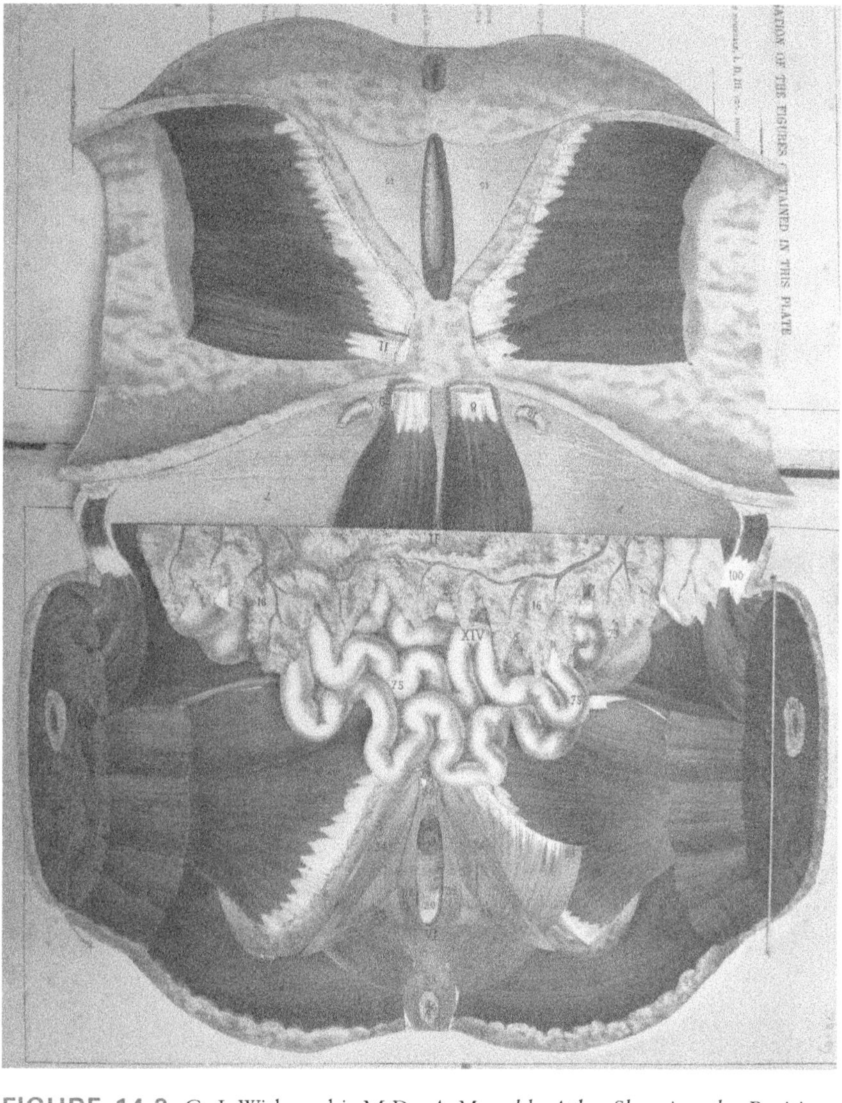

FIGURE 14.3 G.-J. Witkowski, M.D., *A Movable Atlas Showing the Positions of the Female Organs of Generation and Reproduction by Means of Superposed Coloured Plates*, 3rd ed., London: Baillière, Tindall, and Cox, *c.* 1880s. Photograph by author. Collection of the Wangansteen Historical Library, University of Minnesota, Minneapolis.

In its pictorial logic, Witkowski's atlas seeks to create an analogue for anatomical dissection: as users turn the flaps, they penetrate ever deeper into a body organized as a series of discrete, individually labelled structures. One reviewer noted, 'Turning the first page [is] like lifting the skin... and looking behind it' (Meunier 1885: n.p.). While medical touch remained a fraught topic in emerging fields such as gynaecology, here tactile exploration is recoded as pre-eminently scientific as users manipulate the body in the absence of a living subject.

The concept of penetration dominates the spatial organization of the figure: users can peer through the vaginal opening – a literal slit in the paper – to organs below, and muscles appear as silhouetted cutouts that provide glimpses of underlying layers. Following the logic of dissection, flaps are 'cut' so as to reveal the shape of individual structures. By lifting the viscera – an act which recalls the removal of the intestines during anatomical investigation – users reveal the *pubis symphysis* joining the two halves of the pelvis. As intervening layers are folded up, down, or to the side in a complicated manoeuvre, users effect a virtual dissection of the vaginal canal, uterus and rectum, seen first whole and then in cross-section, before arriving at the back of the pelvis.

The colourful, serialized, and affordable format of Witkowski's atlas marked its precarious position on the boundary between popular and professional audiences. The fields of gynaecology and midwifery had long been plagued by association with matters of a sexual nature, and anatomical models in particular were prone to accusations that their heightened realism provoked lurid and spectacular pleasures (Alberti 2009: 33). The presentation of the series at the Paris World's Fair of 1878 thus caught the eye of a visiting physician, who disapprovingly observed that the publisher's display 'invites the curiosity of the public' (*Promenades* 1878: 616).

In *La génération humaine,* Witkowski proffered a cautious justification of his subject matter by affirming the scientific quality of his publication, a strategy commonly employed in sexual health treatises published in this era (Stewart 1997: 383–84). Witkowski bases his defence of the work on the accuracy of its anatomical illustrations, which in some editions appeared in a discrete brown paper envelope tucked inside the back cover, writing, 'The pencil of Mr. Léveillé... guarantees the accuracy and precision of the drawing' (1880: 6). Yet the colourful and richly detailed illustrations that affirmed the series' usefulness, accuracy and even its modernity in the minds of reviewers also rendered it vulnerable to associations with less culturally elevated forms of reproduction.

By the late nineteenth century, the use of steam-driven mechanical presses enabled the production of a range of cheap and colourful commercial products printed using chromolithography, including posters, greeting cards and calendars. The proliferation of trade cards, designed to serve as an inexpensive and attractive form of advertising, helped cement the association of chromolithographs with the worlds of commerce and popular entertainment, and with the female consumers who avidly collected them (Kalba 2018: 156). While it is chromolithography that permitted Witkowski to create his highly illusionistic, vividly coloured simulacra of the human body, his use of this medium risked associating his atlas with the domestic and popular spheres rather than with the male-dominated realm of medicine – an association further strengthened by his publication of popular medical treatises.

Like the producers of fin-de-siècle nude photographs and *tableaux vivants*, Witkowski distances his images from these commercial associations by emphasizing the artistry of his creations (Teukolsky 2020: 6). In *La génération humaine*, his images of the female reproductive body are signed in the fashion of prints: 'Dr Witkowski inv^{t} [invenit] / Léveillé, del^{t} [delineavit]' (1880: n.p.). The Latin term *invenit* signifies that Witkowski provided the initial design for the image, while *delineavit* suggests that Léveillé created the subsequent drawing. The concept of 'invention' might refer to a dissection created by Witkowski, in which case the physician casts his own anatomical labour as artistry, or to the concept for the atlas itself. This notion of translating between multiple, serial forms – body, drawing and print – troubles Witkowski's claims of anatomical truth as the guarantee of his works' scientific, rather than prurient, nature. Yet the association with printmaking also functioned to establish the works' status as artistic productions and thus to mitigate the more 'pornographic' elements of their presentation.

In Witkowski's *Organes génitaux*, the use of colour links the author's work not only to commercially printed images but also to contemporary racial theory. As with many atlases produced in the nineteenth century (Hammerschlag 2021: n.p.), Witkowski depicts his model of the anatomical female body as 'white'. This meaning is secured by references in the accompanying text, which describe racially coded bodies as pathological departures from a universal ideal. These include a description of the purported hypertrophy of the *labia minora* in 'Hottentots' (1880: 6), a characteristic commonly associated with the supposedly heightened sexuality of Black women in this period (Gilman 1985: 212–16).

If Witkowski's description of female anatomy establishes a clear contrast between a 'normal' reproductive body and one marked by racial and cultural difference, his text also reflects widespread anxiety concerning the act of reproduction and its consequences. Echoing neo-Lamarckian notions of genetic inheritance widely accepted in France (Roseman 1999: 156), Witkowski warns readers, 'Conception that takes place under the influence of drunkenness produces epileptics and imbeciles' (1880: 29). Witkowski's *Organes génitaux* thus employs the language of contemporary scientific debate and early eugenic theory to cast his potentially scandalous representation of the female reproductive organs as an ideal anatomical subject – and mother.

Conclusion

Despite their material differences, each of the three works examined in this chapter sought to map, explain and preserve the appearance of the female reproductive body. All three moved between popular and professional realms, disseminating a broad knowledge of anatomy as a system for understanding the body. Each brought into visibility internal and external structures associated with both sexuality and notions of obscenity and worked to inscribe their representation within a medical framework through visual references to the act of dissection. By transmitting and reproducing the conventions of scientific illustration, these works effectively defined a new anatomical aesthetic premised upon the use of vivid, lifelike colour and a subtle interplay of abstraction and realism, which both restored a semblance of life to the anatomical subject and also inevitably evoked the sensuality, fleshliness and even potential abjectness of the female body. At the same time, each of these three works should be understood in the context of the history of artistic media – from plaster to wax and printmaking, the material forms of such representations carried their own shifting meanings in nineteenth-century society. While each would eventually be surpassed in importance by the advent of plastic models and colour photography, this anatomical aesthetic – based on extensive use of colour, serial reproduction, and heightened verisimilitude – continues to inform the creation of medical texts, objects, and images well into the twenty-first century.

Coda

In these works by Deyrolle, Tramond, and Witkowski, it is the insistent physicality of the anatomical models that both confirms their usefulness and invites controversy. In contrast, in her film *As You Were* (2024), Scottish filmmaker Lyndsay Mann revisits the histories of pregnancy and childbirth and their impact on the lives of contemporary women through a dematerialization of the maternal body. By layering the voices of mothers over a series of evocative images which allude indirectly to maternal labour, including a spider spinning its web and a woman's rowing team moving in unison, Mann allows for a multiplicity of perspectives. Those she interviews – new mothers who are also midwives and obstetricians – are cast not as universal anatomical subjects or idealized maternal figures, but multiply situated individuals with shifting, evolving identities. As their voices weave in and through the film's immersive flow, we see motherhood itself as a process of becoming. In place of the absent maternal body, viewers are presented with a series of historical obstetrical instruments such as forceps, which become a stand-in for the bodies they were designed to treat. Although these objects provoke associations with pain both institutional and personal,

Mann gently cradles them in her hands, suggesting the potential for healing through acts of care and remembrance. In this lyrical meditation on the act of giving birth, motherhood is no longer reduced to a physical or biological state but is instead cast as a powerful moment of transformation. In this way, the consequences of an anatomical aesthetic that conflates female identity with reproduction, privileges invasive methods of bodily exploration, and normalizes a view of the pregnant and parturient body as inherently passive are made clear, even as Mann's film restores complexity and indeterminacy to our shared understanding of 'motherhood'.

References

Alberti, S. (2009), 'Wax Bodies: Art and Anatomy in Victorian Medical Museums', *Museum History Journal* 2 (1): 7–36.

Bates, A. W. (2008), 'Indecent and Demoralising Representations: Public Anatomy Museums in mid-Victorian England', *Medical History* 52 (1): 1–22.

Baudoin, M. (1889), *Guide médical à l'Exposition universelle internationale de 1889, à Paris*, Paris: E. Lecrosnier et Babé.

Blühm, A. (1996), 'In Living Colour: A Short History of Colour Sculpture in the 19th Century', in A. Blühm (ed.), *The Colour of Sculpture 1840–1910*, 11–60, Leeds: Henry Moore Institute.

Bull, S. (2017), 'Managing the "Obscene M.D.": Medical Publishing, the Medical Profession, and the Changing Definition of Obscenity in Mid-Victorian England', *Bulletin of the History of Medicine* 91: 713–43.

Campbell, M. (2018), 'The Anatomy of the Human Gravid Uterus', in *William Hunter and the Anatomy of the Modern Museum*, M. Campbell and N. Flis (eds), 248–41, New Haven, CT: Yale Center for British Art.

Dumont, A. (1890), *Dépopulation et civilization: étude démographique*, Paris: Lecrosnier et Babé.

Gilman, S. (1985), 'Black Bodies, White Bodies: Toward an Iconography of Female Sexuality in Late Nineteenth-Century Art, Medicine, and Literature', *Critical Inquiry* 12 (1): 204–42.

Hallam, E. (2016), *Anatomy Museum*, London: Reaktion Books.

Hammerschlag, K. R. (2021), 'Black Apollo: Aesthetics, Dissection, and Race in Joseph Maclise's *Surgical Anatomy*', *British Art Studies* 20. https://doi.org/10.17658/issn.2058-5462/issue-20/khammerschlag

Hunter, M. (2008), '"Effroyable réalisme": Wax, Femininity, and the Madness of Realist Fantasies', *RACAR* 33 (1/2): 43–58.

Jinshin senkei botai zukai (1887), [Japan]: Yo Sonoji.

Jordanova, L. (1989), *Sexual Visions: Images of Gender in Science and Medicine between the Eighteenth and Twentieth Centuries*, Madison: The University of Wisconsin Press.

Kalba, L. A. (2018), *Color in the Age of Impressionism: Commerce, Technology, and Art*, Philadelphia: Penn State University Press.

Maerker, A. (2013), 'Anatomizing the Trade: Designing and Marketing Anatomical Models as Medical Technologies, ca. 1700–1900', *Technology and Culture* 54 (3): 531–62.

Markoe, J. W. and M. Wollstein (1897), 'Report of the Curator', in *Medical Report of the Society of the Lying-In Hospital of the City of New York*, 317–9, New York: D. Appleton.

Martin, R. (2020), 'Normalising Whiteness: The Use of Standardised Anatomical Methods of Teaching, 1800–1910', IAHR Virtual History of Medicine and Health Development Seminar.

Meunier, V. (1885), 'Causerie scientifique', *Rappel* 5541: n.p.

Nelson, C. A. (2007), *The Color of Stone: Sculpting the Black Female Subject in Nineteenth-Century America*, Minneapolis: University of Minnesota Press.

Pastor, J. F., B. Gutiérrez, J. M. Montes and R. Ballestriero (2016), 'Uncovered Secret of a Vasseur-Tramond Wax Model', *Journal of Anatomy* 228: 184–89.

Picard, A., ed. (1890–2), *Rapports du jury international*, Vol. 2, Paris: Imprimerie nationale.

Picard, A., ed. (1891), *Rapports du jury international: Group V*, Paris: Imprimerie nationale.

Roseman, M. J. (1999), *Birthing the Republic: Midwives, Medicine, and Morality in France, 1890 to 1920*, PhD diss., Columbia University, New York.

Stewart, M. L. (1997), '"Science is Always Chaste": Sex Education and Sexual Initiation in France, 1880s–1930s', *Journal of Contemporary History* 32 (3): 381–94.

Syson, L. (2018), 'Polychrome and its Discontents: A History', in *Like Life: Sculpture, Color, and the Body*, L. Syson et al. (eds), 14–41, New York: The Metropolitan Museum of Art.

Tartivel, Dr. A. (1878), 'Promenades d'un medecin à l'Exposition universelle (section française)' *Union médicale* 124: 609–17.

Teukolsky, R. (2020), 'Victorian Erotic Photographs and the Intimate Public Sphere', *Nineteenth-Century Contexts: An Interdisciplinary Journal* 42 (2). https://doi.org/10.1080/08905495.2020.1733321

Witkowski, G.-J. (1880), *La génération humaine*, 1st ed., Paris: H. Lauwereyns.

Witkowski, G.-J. (1917), *Autobiographie*, Paris: n.p. La Roche-sur-Yon: Imprimerie Centrale de l'Ouest.

Witkowsky [*sic*], G. J. (1880), *A Movable Atlas Showing the Positions of the Female Organs of Generation and Reproduction by Means of Superposed Coloured Plates*, trans. James Palfrey, New York: Joseph Christadoro.

CHAPTER FIFTEEN

Making meanings from medicine: visual histories of medicine, race and reproductive health

Anna Arabindan-Kesson and Gabriella Nelson

This conversation was facilitated by the project *Art Hx: Visual and Medical Legacies of British Colonialism*. In it, art historian Anna Arabindan-Kesson and artist, curator and city planner Gabriella Nelson explore how meanings are made from visual histories of medicine, race and reproductive health. Arabindan-Kesson and Nelson focus on a mid-nineteenth-century image surrounding the life of Margaret Garner, an enslaved woman sensationally labelled 'the modern Medea' after she killed two of her children to protect them from enslavement. Garner's story asks us to consider racialized histories of reproductive health, and their implications for experiences of Black, Brown and Indigenous birthing people today.

Gabriella Nelson (GN): Margaret Garner's story resonates with me because it illustrates both the depth of a mother's love and the abhorrence of slavery in creating a situation where infanticide was the ultimate expression of maternal care. Garner wasn't the only person that did this, or attempted to do this.

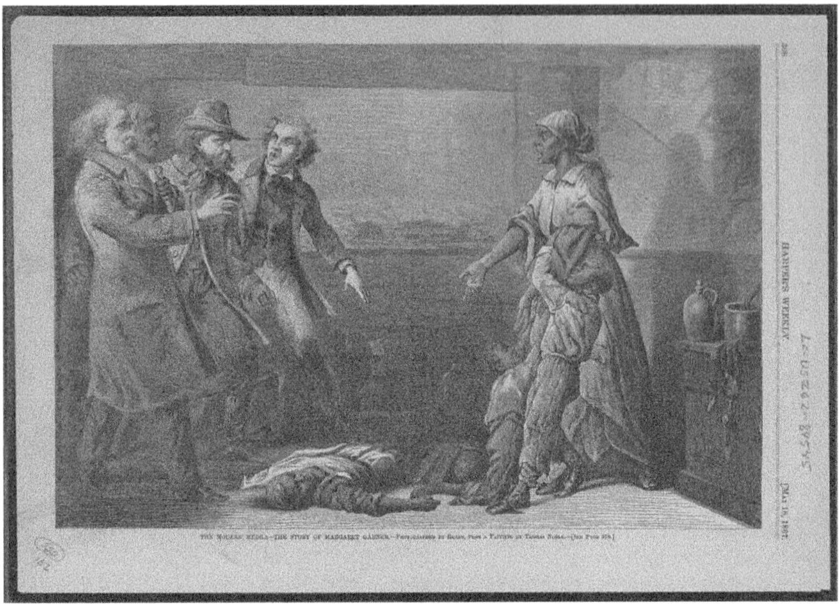

FIGURE 15.1 Thomas Satterwhite Noble. *The Modern Medea – the story of Margaret Garner, a slave who escaped from Kentucky to Ohio; her 4 children, 2 of which she killed so they would not have to endure slavery, lying dead on floor; and 4 men who pursued her*. 1867. Retrieved from the Library of Congress, www.loc.gov/item/99614263/.

The only known nineteenth-century depiction of Margaret Garner was created by Thomas Noble, a White artist from a slave holding family in Kentucky. This image, entitled *The Modern Medea*, is a wood engraving of the original painting that was reproduced in newspapers for public consumption. Noble's portrayal of the scene elides an important fact: Margaret Garner was mixed race, as were three of her four children. This makes me think deeply about inheritance. As a mixed-race woman, even though her father was white, Garner wasn't afforded freedom. The law *Partus sequitur ventrem* (or 'offspring follows belly') meant that children born into slavery assumed the status of their mother, not their father; it assumed the Black woman's womb to be the producer of inferior fruit, regardless of paternity. This built the conceptual and legal foundations for the devaluation of Black bodies – and specifically Black women's bodies and Black birthing people's bodies – today. The laws relating to reproductive rights are also connected to welfare and the criminal justice system. They all work to devalue Black women's bodies. The only time Black women's bodies are valued is when they are exploited to work, to produce something that is not a [Black] child, because our children are seen as inferior outside of profiteering. Garner's story is an excellent first introduction to the legal landscape around Black women's bodies.

Anna Arabindan-Kesson (AAK): Margaret Garner's story also inspired a profound piece of literature, the novel *Beloved* by Toni Morrison (1987). Is this one of the inheritances you were talking about?

GN: *Beloved* reminds us of how deeply Garner's story affected people, as well as the legacies of *Partus sequitur ventrem*. But we can also see how the inheritances of Garner's story continue in the ways that Black people are devalued today.

AAK: It's a powerful way to illustrate the bigger political and legal structures that frame histories of medicine and practices of social relation. The story's affective pull gives us the opportunity to deconstruct the pathologization of Black women's bodies and Black women's experiences as mothers. The image materializes the intersectionality of all these different components.

GN: The visual dynamic is important: the image was used in many different ways, both by abolitionists and also for arguments in support of slavery. For abolitionists it was a story and an image that could be reproduced in different ways to create empathy and support for the cause. But we know the limits of empathy to bring about change! To me, it's a way to reflect on the limitations of visual imagery for somehow 'validating' or 'proving' Black humanity.

AAK: These discourses continue today in the way images are used to mobilize support for certain causes and used to 'prove' that these people are 'human' too and encourage empathy based on this notion. But if you have to show this, that tells us we exist within a political framework whereby some people are not seen as human, or human enough, to begin with.

GN: That is clearly outlined in Garner's story. The authorities didn't know whether to charge her and her husband for murder: this would have been to acknowledge that her children were human beings deserving of fundamental rights. Garner and her husband were eventually charged for theft and destruction of property under the Fugitive Slave Law. When I look at this image, I am fascinated by how intentionally crazed her appearance is: the implication is mental instability and barbarism, but when interviewed she emphasized that she was in her right mind and had made a logical choice. The images of Margaret Garner also made me think about how we sensationalize Black bodies in relation to death, violence and trauma, to the point at which we're almost desensitized. This image frames Black suffering as entertainment, in a way that is still prevalent today. I don't think that I can bear to read another headline that says Black women are three to four times more likely to experience postnatal mortality, for example. I understand that images can convey information, but you cannot appeal to a society or an institution that does not value Black life. This made me think about Saidiya Hartman's book *Scenes of Subjection* (1997) where she explains how Black suffering is perceived or registered only in the most spectacular circumstances of violence. And I think this is one of those moments.

AAK: I'd like to introduce a provocation here, which is: can Black women be mothers?

GN: Garner's story is at odds with nineteenth-century discourses of middle-class respectability and gender politics, including the push for suffrage: Black women were kept out of all these conversations. But as Jennifer Morgan (2004) and Jennifer Nash (2021) have argued, Black womanhood is always doubly erased in its intersections with both racial and gendered norms. Garner's story asks us to see how these constructions of race and gender shape meanings of motherhood today, and consequently influence how you will be treated in a medical context, when you are not even seen as a woman, let alone a mother.

Another reason why I gravitated towards this image and story is because it's about choice. There have been so many occasions when choice and self-advocacy have not been possible for Black reproductive health: consider the histories of forced sterilization for example (Washington 2007; Roberts 1999). When I think about disparities in Black maternal health today and how to move forward in the future, it's about having the information to make autonomous decisions, which is a principle of reproductive justice.

AAK: Today, questions of reproductive choice remain connected to the spectacularization of Black women, and Black motherhood particularly.

GN: The choices of Black women, Black mothers, particularly working-class Black mothers, are scrutinized continuously.

AAK: In the media, in policy, Black women's choices are judged and used to denigrate their ability to mother, and also criminalized in some instances. We can think of other moments too, such as the publication of the Moynihan Report in the 1960s and the way government policies used and reinforced stereotypes about Black welfare and working Black women and mothers. This narrative completely disregarded the social structures that are available, or not, to Black mothers. And it has been used again and again as justification for ever more stringent policies: for example, the way Black women are prosecuted for their children's school attendance (Elliott and Reid 2019; Love 2023).

GN: In her book *Killing The Black Body* Dorothy Roberts emphasizes the way decisions around people's livelihood and freedom also hinged upon their ability or not to have children. And a lot of the discourse around the control of Black women's reproductive rights feeds into debates about the control and criminalization of Black children.

Our frameworks for understanding humanity are so deeply embedded in the structures through which we see. This story helps me see how different ways of knowing – medicine, visual culture, art – are imbricated in the framework of enslavement.

AAK: So again, Garner's story and its visual imagery helps us understand how the terms we have for acknowledging human-ness are embedded in ways of seeing that are both aesthetic and medical/scientific. And these frameworks emerge from the institution of slavery.

GN: The way we see, the way we think: histories of race are not just 'added' to these frameworks. No, the issue is that histories of race are a foundation for the emergence of all these other frameworks. This means we have to find a different way to see, even if that means acknowledging certain limits so as to move past them.

AAK: What can you do with a story like this? How do you use it to move beyond these limits and help people unravel these different strands? What interpretive practices do you want people to take up?

GN: Margaret Garner's story did something to me: I felt it in my body. That is where I started in my interaction with this artwork, by thinking about how the story and the images made me feel. Did it make me feel expansive or constricted? Where was I feeling these sensations in my body? From there I began to create a list of words. These are action words that can also be attributed to how the body works; I built on these words in formulating my response here, because I wanted other people who read her story to also sit with it, and think about how it made them feel.

AAK: What I love about the process that you're exploring here is that it's embodied. In traditional models of historical scholarship, we focus on observation and analysis, minimizing the significance of embodiment and affect. The practice that you've described here is important in moving us away from just looking, describing and connecting our observations to a set of ideas: you're actually asking the reader or the viewer to think about how the story and the image are working on them, and to then consider what that means. To me, this is the beginning of doing something very different in terms of historical analysis and art historical analysis, because it immediately requires self-reflexivity: it requires understanding how something works first on you, and then on the world. It's a pedagogical tool but it's also a different kind of methodology.

GN: It's a different way to interpret how something teaches us or brings us to knowledge or creates new knowledge. Here analysis is connected to feeling but is also about coming into action. To me, this is much more important, because how does something compel you to act?

AAK: How does this way of thinking or looking connect to your training and experience as an urban planner? I'm asking as someone trained in methods of art historical analysis. As a planner you're thinking about space, about positionality and embodied experience. These are important in Art History too, but I'd imagine that they are used in different ways. In particular, while Art History takes our relationship to the text or object into account, we're often looking for new ways to consider the broader environment of reception and the constellations of experiences that might create a particular experience of one's body or of the environment.

GN: I'm thinking about systems, the environment around an object, the people: about who did what and when. But I think, planning, or the way that I experienced planning, was often devoid of community. I'm supposed to be looking for the money, at the paid players involved, looking at the built environment where this building or green space might be placed. I wasn't trained to look at who will be displaced, or how displacement affects somebody's body. To feel, and find, feelings of community had to emerge from something outside of that discourse. It's connected more to the experiences I've had beyond professional training: feeling oneness was something that I had to do outside of that. We might be similar in our institutionalized learning!

AAK: In both discourses of knowledge, there is often a lack of engagement with embodied experiences. When you're working with Black histories or histories of oppressed people, the body becomes the archive so already you have to think very differently about how systems affect people, and how objects work.

GN: Thinking about people in these systems or histories can also be problematic or difficult: people become merely ciphers or spectacles, instrumentalized or demonized. There is a kind of alienation that is part of institutionalized learning.

AAK: This alienation mirrors the idea of the 'objective' researcher. The way you're thinking about these objects, as very visceral on a human level, is also a way to engage with people across communities.

GN: Because we all have to feel: I don't mean to say that we have go down the empathy path or that you have to feel what another person feels but I understand this affective response as a key part of [Black] revolutionary practices.

AAK: As someone who studies the nineteenth century, I've always been sceptical about empathy because of how it gets taken up in discourses of liberal humanism to reinforce ideas about who is human and who is not. Reframing empathy as a self-reflexive practice to understand your own embodied position and then stand alongside others, is really helpful and an important outcome that can be learnt from the kinds of analysis we do.

GN: It's just so important to work through that, because the disassociation that often happens then becomes a public one and then becomes a way to disassociate with what is happening in a political sense. We see that in the disparities so evident in Black maternal health, where there's no empathy for the Black body, and Black people's pain and suffering just becomes a part of everyday life. And so people die violently.

AAK: The form of analysis you're asking for draws on the language of therapy. It's a form of repair, right? It's not re-enactment, it's not asking you to imagine what it felt like.

GN: It's actually a kind of internal process. Like checking in.

AAK: A way of responding to these histories, that is not just about re-analyzing them but disassembling how they get put together in the first place. It is an active record of repair. These objects are difficult; what do you do with them? How do we deal with their violence?

GN: I don't want to seem like I'm exploiting stories like Margaret Garner's, but I want to find a way to incorporate them in our lives in ways that lead us towards joy. What really captivated me about Margaret Garner was her absolute love for her children.

AAK: This takes us back to the question of choice: her choice as a mother.

GN: I think finding joy means using your imagination. It's important that these histories don't dampen our ability to imagine, that we find ways to address them that actively expand what it is possible to imagine. To do this work of analysis is a different kind of intellectual work: it is a little more restful, it is collaborative – you can't do this work by yourself – and it's fundamentally about community building.

References

Elliott, S., and M. Reid (2019), 'Low-Income Black Mothers Parenting Adolescents in the Mass Incarceration Era: The Long Reach of Criminalization', *American Sociological Review*, 84 (2): 197–219.

Hartman, S. V. (1997), *Scenes of Subjection: Terror, Slavery, and Self-Making in Nineteenth-Century America*, Oxford: Oxford University Press.

Love, B. L. (2023), *Punished for Dreaming: How School Reform Harms Black Children and How We Heal*, New York: St. Martin's Press.

Morgan, J. L. (2004), *Laboring Women: Reproduction and Gender in New World Slavery*, Philadelphia: University of Pennsylvania Press.

Morrison, T. (1987), *Beloved*, New York: Knopf.

Nash, J. C. (2021), *Birthing Black Mothers*, Durham: Duke University Press.

Roberts, D. E. (1999), *Killing the Black Body: Race, Reproduction, and the Meaning of Liberty*, New York: Vintage Books.

Washington, H. A. (2007), *Medical Apartheid: The Dark History of Medical Experimentation on Black Americans from Colonial Times to the Present*, New York: Doubleday.

CHAPTER SIXTEEN

Reproductive resistance: Charmaine Watkiss's *Return of the Seed Keeper*

Jessica Womack

The daughter of Jamaican immigrants to England, artist Charmaine Watkiss (b. 1954, London) remembers her mother using plants to tend to her and her brother's ailments during her childhood in London:

> My earliest experiences of having a relationship with the natural world were of my mother treating my brother and myself with herbs. If we had a cough or a fever, my mother would boil herbs into a tea, or rub ointments on our chest to help shift the cold.... Her family lived off the land [in Jamaica], so when she came to live in Great Britain in 1962, she carried the knowledge of her mother and grandmother with her.
>
> (Watkiss 2023: 109)

Watkiss mobilizes this generational and embodied knowledge, passed down by the women in her family, to treat her own illnesses and inform her work, which presents what she calls a 'pantheon' of 'plant warrior women' who take on the qualities of a particular plant (Watkiss, 2023: 109–10). Additionally, she conducts extensive archival research, using historical books and documents to locate 'stories about the kinds of herbal knowledge and lifesaving treatments that would have crossed over during the transatlantic slave trade... the remedies that survived' (Bulley and Watkiss 2021). The artist intentionally invokes the drawings of seventeenth, eighteenth and nineteenth-century European botanists and naturalists like Maria Sibylla Merian (1647–1717) who learned of these remedies from their interactions with the enslaved. She also pays tribute to the labour, knowledge, and experiences of the enslaved themselves.

Watkiss's upbringing and research shape her 2021 series *The Seed Keepers*. Created using graphite, watercolour, ink and coloured pencil on paper, the works represent female figures who engage with, are adorned by, or are surrounded by depictions of various plants. An example is *The Warriors Way: Restructuring the Self*, in which the artist explores the tropical *cerasee* plant and its use in natural medicine to treat conditions such as hypertension, urinary tract infections, and diabetes (see 'Herbs For Life', 2018). Another such work is her *Return of the Seed Keeper*, which focuses especially on the reproductive experiences of the enslaved and offers a solemn meditation on the difficult decisions enslaved women made regarding pregnancy and childbearing during the colonial era.

Depicted on a flat, streaky goldish-brown watercolour background, Watkiss's protagonist in *Return of the Seed Keeper* wears a rich blue garment with a design of repeating, stacked semicircles on the collar and cuffs that recall the waves of the ocean. With a sombre expression, she gazes off to the work's left and tenderly cradles a terrarium with a single, large flower in her arms.

Watkiss's depiction of a singular figure from head to mid-thigh recall the conventions of traditional European portraiture. Additionally, the work is replete with moving symbolic meaning. Most significant is the central encased flower, a peacock flower (also known as a poinciana, the Pride of Barbados as it is Barbados's national flower, along with other names). A common variant has four or five brilliant orange and red petals, and each bloom has several long stamens. The flowers grow in clusters, or racemes, on shrubs or trees found throughout tropical climates.

The peacock flower was the subject of much study during the colonial period, with European physicians and botanists including Merian, Hans Sloane (1660–1753), and Michel Étienne Descourtilz (1775–*c.* 1835) discussing the plant and its properties in their writing (Schiebinger 2004: 107). For example, in her 1705 *Metamorphosis insectorum Surinamenstum*, Merian provided reports on and drawings of the flora and fauna of colonial Surinam. A section of the text chronicled the treatment enslaved Black and Indigenous women endured at the hands of the Dutch as well as their acts of rebellion.

> The Indians, who are not treated well by their Dutch masters, use the seeds [of the peacock flower] to abort their children, so that their children will not become slaves like they are. The black slaves from Guinea and Angola have demanded to be well treated, threatening to refuse to have children. In fact, they sometimes take their own lives because they are

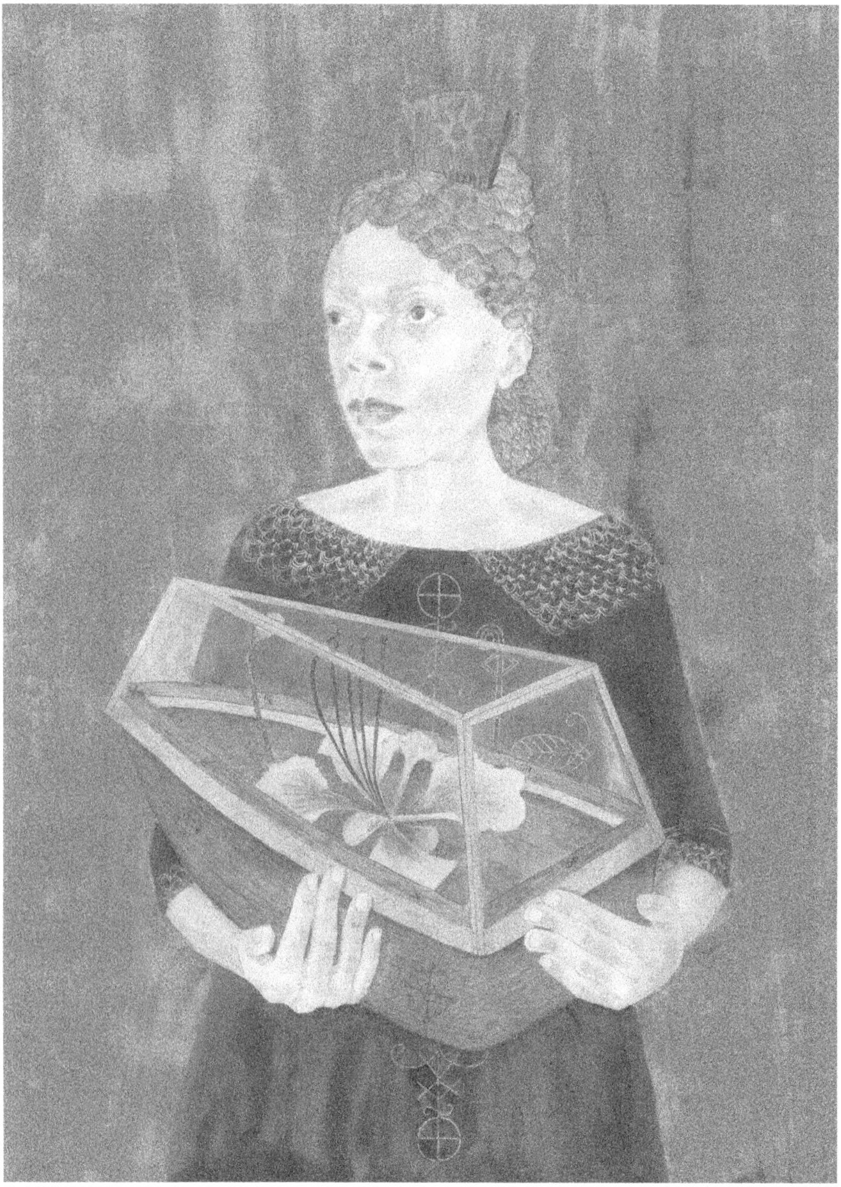

FIGURE 16.1 Charmaine Watkiss, *Return of the Seed Keeper*, 2021. @ 2024 Artists Rights Society (ARS), New York / DACS, London.

treated so badly, and because they believe they will be born again, free and living in their own land. They told me this themselves.

(Merian, as quoted in Schiebinger 2004: 1)

Several scholars, such as Jennifer Morgan (2004) and Deborah Gray White (1985), have discussed the experiences of enslaved Black women as they were forced to experience the double burden of 'production and reproduction'. In addition to being forced to plant and pick cash crops including cotton, sugar and tobacco – production – they were also expected by plantation owners to carry and give birth to the next generation of labour, individuals transformed in the womb from person to property by chattel slavery – reproduction.

As Londa Schiebinger writes in her book *Plants and Empire: Colonial Bioprospecting in the Atlantic World*, the fertility of enslaved women was of immense importance to colonial officials, planters, and physicians in the Americas, particularly as the eighteenth century wore on and conversation swirled about the end of the slave trade. Because trafficking and newly enslaving Africans from the continent was seen as unsustainable, the solution was to guarantee those already enslaved in the Americas successfully carried and delivered children (Schiebinger 2004: 128).

In the face of these expectations, enslaved women did what they could to undermine slavery's productive and reproductive mandates. Instead of planting and harvesting crops, they ran away, picked slowly, feigned illness and orchestrated work stoppages. Rather than birth children who would be taken from them, sold, and dehumanized, they refused to have children, committed infanticide, and induced abortions. To accomplish the latter, the peacock flower, ubiquitous in the region, was a crucial resource. 'By aborting, slave women were well aware that they saved their children from a life of servitude since, no matter who the father, the child inherited its mother's legal standing' (Schiebinger 2004: 132).

With this information, the terrarium in *Return of the Seed Keeper* is not simply a case for a beautiful, delicate flower. Its meaning expands: it is a coffin for someone whose mother chose death rather than despair, a ship returning a soul home.

Watkiss has emphasized in *Return of the Seed Keeper* that this death is not finite; there are several invocations of renewal and rebirth. An infinity sign on the ship's stern evokes eternity; and the Egyptian ankh at the bow is a well-recognized symbol for life. Finally, several circles separated into four sections in the work – on her dress at the chest and below the waist, and on the boat's stern and bow – suggest the Kongo cosmogram (*dikenga dia Kôngo*). A circular diagram used in the Bakongo religion, the cosmogram visualizes the relationship between the physical and spiritual worlds and how one passes through them during major life moments. In the *dikenga*, the arrows typically point counter-clockwise, indicating that one passes cyclically from conception to birth, then to adulthood and finally death (Fu-Kiau 2001: 26–35, 131).

However, in Watkiss's cosmogram – drawn subtly on the boat's hull near the figure's right hand – the arrows point clockwise, indicating her understanding that a different path was possible. By using the peacock flower, the cycle was reversed; after conception came death, a death which brought with it birth and a life outside of enslavement. This was the goal of the enslaved women who terminated their pregnancies: that their children would be free. The peacock flower facilitated Indigenous and African women's choice and resistance in a system predicated on depriving them of their agency and autonomy. Watkiss's *Return of the Seed Keeper* honours the power and complexity of that decision.

References

Bulley, V. A., and C. Watkiss (2021), 'Charmaine Watkiss on Reconstructing the Image of Black Womanhood', *Frieze*, 17 November, available online: https://www.frieze.com/article/charmaine-watkiss-interview-2021.

Fu-Kiau, K. (2001), *African Cosmology of the Bântu-Kôngo: Tying the Spiritual Knot: Principles of Life & Living*, 2nd edn, Brooklyn: Athelia Henrietta Press.

'Herbs For Life | Cerasee well worth enduring the bitter taste' (2018), *The Gleaner*, May 14. Available online: https://jamaica-gleaner.com/article/health/20180523/herbs-life-cerasee-well-worth-enduring-bitter-taste.

Morgan, J. (2004), *Laboring Women: Reproduction and Gender in New World Slavery*, Philadelphia: University of Pennsylvania Press.

Schiebinger, L. (2004), *Plants and Empire: Colonial Bioprospecting in the Atlantic World*, Cambridge: Harvard University Press.

Watkiss, C. (2023), 'Charmaine Watkiss', in T. Schoonmaker (ed.), *Spirit in the Land*, 108–11, Durham: Nasher Museum of Art.

White, D. G. (1985), *Ar'n't I a Woman?: Female Slaves in the Plantation South*, New York: Norton.

CHAPTER SEVENTEEN

Marian maternity and the medieval modern: engagements with contemporary un-reproductivity

Isabel Davis and Anna Burel

The *Madonna della Misericordia* (Madonna of Mercy) is an abiding subject in Catholic art, emerging from the religious communities – the fraternal and monastic orders and lay confraternities – of the late Middle Ages, where it articulated the shape and boundaries of pious community (Brown 2017: 131). In these images, Mary shelters kneeling figures beneath a cloak, imaging and spatializing the coverage of her maternal care, as she does, for example, in perhaps the most famous example by Piero della Francesca made for the church of the Misericordia in Sansepolcro, Italy (*c.* 1460). The emphases are on the sumptuous colours of rich draped fabric and sight lines – Mary looks down and her devotees look up. These were portraits of people in exclusive gated communities redescribed as humble devotees. Votive imagery of the Middle Ages worked like that, turning social and spiritual aspiration into pious humility with the kneeling pose. The separation of icon and devotee imagines status to be conferred by divine authority in response to unassuming prayer, rather than being self-warranting.

In her version, visual artist Anna Burel asks particularly about membership of community in reproductive experience. Whilst generations of feminist writers have sought to dispel the aura of piety which gathers

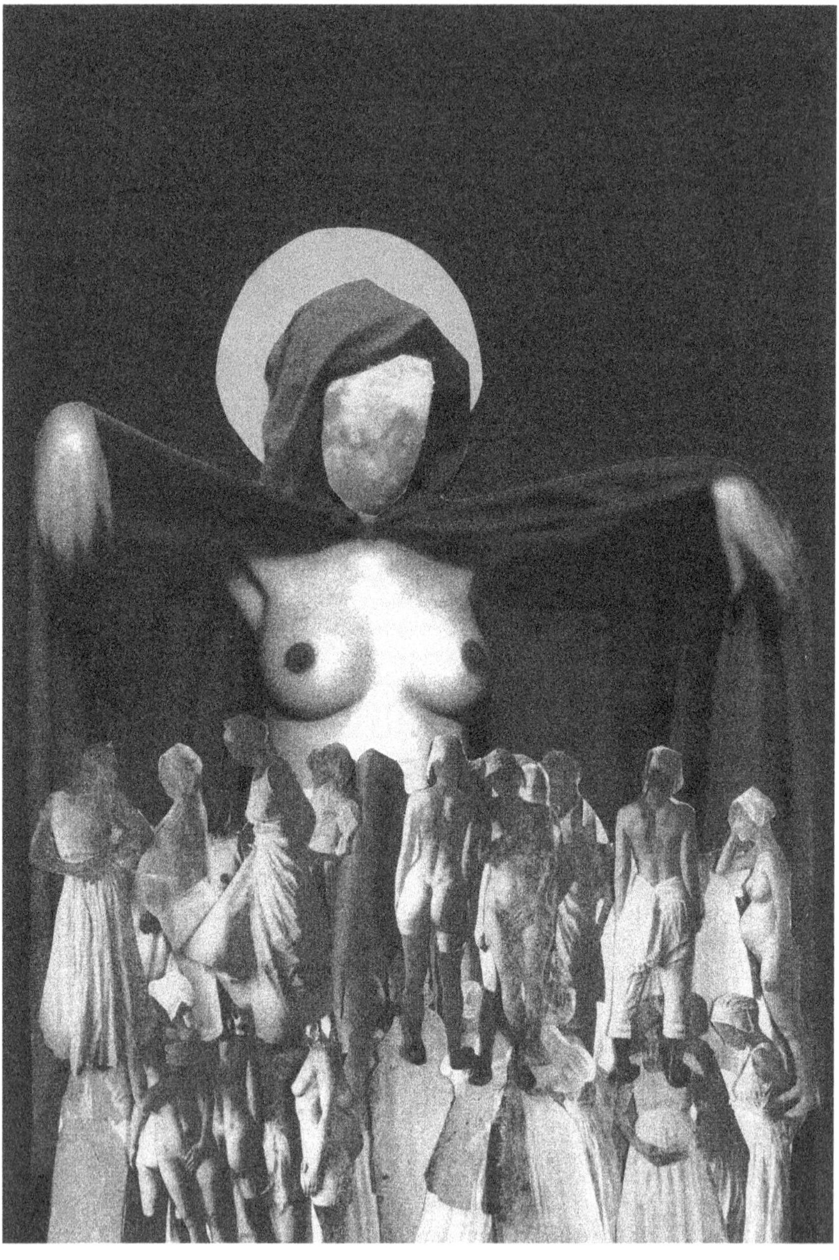

FIGURE 17.1 Anna Burel, *Madonna della Misericordia,* made for *Conceiving Histories: Trying for Pregnancy, Past and Present* (Cambridge, MA: MIT Press, 2025). Reproduced with the permission of the MIT Press.

around motherhood, and called for 'full-spectrum solidarity', regardless of reproductive desires or outcomes, those calls will always need iteration in the face of the perpetual formation and reformation of reproductive hierarchies (e.g., Rich 1976: chapter 2; quotation from Browne 2023: 124). Those hierarchies are differently drawn across diverse cultures and subcultures – whether geographical or in virtual spaces. What is in and what out, is framed differently in the medieval as in the modern, London as in Lagos, Mumsnet as on Instagram. Hierarchies rank and value reproductive loss and suffering as much as reproductive 'success'. Who is and isn't entitled to speak – particularly to complain – is determined by rules not always indexed to feminist demands for collective world-building. Burel's enfolded figures seem to stand in serried ranks, one on top of another. Ongoing feminist energy must perpetually challenge fantasies of perfection and purity, particularly as they are mythologized in relation to motherhood and pregnancy (Freidenfelds 2019: 9–10; Rose 2018: 28, 56).

Mary's perfection may represent a soothing refuge for those pictured inside the cloak but operates as a shaming technology for those beyond its protection, refused the typical desire of the shamed to hide (Lyons and Dolezal 2017: 209). In their considerations of the historical formations of Marian devotion, medievalists have asked about the dark shadows her impossible model cast over ordinary women (e.g., Monagle 2020). How divisive was her maternity for women who patently could not be virginal mothers, who experienced pain in childbirth or the stigma of infertility, and whose pregnancies were ambiguous, un-annunciated? And, given Mary's contemporary global reach, we must also think about how her model continues to structure reproductive expectations and senses of selfhood across Christian mission fields. Even figures included in the community beneath Mary's cloak offer a point of contrast to Mary in the *Madonna della Misericordia* images, being necessarily smaller than her to fit the composition. The smallness of the under-mantled people can communicate the security they are afforded, as if they were in a womb-like space, yet Mary also towers over those she protects (Castaldi 2011: 23). Ambivalence about Mary's exemplarity is already, then, lodged in this iconographic tradition, as seen in della Francesca's unsmiling and spectral Mary, whose maternal perfection is forbidding even as it covers those demonstrably under her care.

Burel's version of the Madonna of Mercy downplays the theme of sanctuary. Whether there is even a world beyond the cloak is unclear as there is less margin outside the tented space than is typical for the motif. The cloaked figures are not, here, protected children or kneeling worshippers, but rather adult women in varying states of nudity and postures of distress. Mary too is nude. The emphasis on Mary's breasts, carried from Madonna and Child iconography, makes an impossible and confrontational standard of her maternity for the women she dwarves. Nimbed by the sun and with a face like the surface of the moon, Burel's Mary gives full expression to the way that the Madonna of Mercy, like other giants, becomes 'a violator of boundary and rule' (Stewart 1993: 73). And Burel adds to Mary's giantism – the sense of her as a towering architectural column 'almost terrifying in her immensity and stillness' – the faceless face and drooping hands of the revenant, incorporating the uncanny elements of prior examples like della Francesca's (Brown 2017: 21; quotation from Warner 1976: 327). Monstrosity and saintliness converge, just as they are often liable to do in accounts of the holy body (Mills 2003: 28–54). And Mary specifically offers an *unheimlich* (uncanny) hesitation between maternal affection, which is at human scale, and divine power, which is not.

Burel's image emerges from a long standing artistic–academic collaboration on the history of fertility health; it is one of several illustrations in our book, part memoir and part history, about trying to conceive (Davis 2025). The histories we have written and imaged together refuse chronological ordering, telling not a long diachronic story about medical and scientific development. Instead, we consider how history becomes a repository for those things that modernity would like to cast out from its cloak: doubt, ignorance, delay, disappointment. The premodern, frequently aestheticized using gothic modes, continues to haunt modern cultural silences. On this we take a cue from art historian Alexander Nagel, whose phrase 'medieval-modern' describes how medieval forms have been so 'metabolized' in contemporary art, as to be in effect made of them (Nagel 2012: 278). Socially as well as aesthetically, premodern forms have operated as a 'construction site': for family models, and gendered and sexual ideals (McDonald 2013: 63). History is often understood as change, yet making points of historical continuity explicit through arresting images and ideas can question our sense of the now. The constancy and continuation of maternal and reproductive perfection myths, which give feminists their Sisyphean task, have been carried into modernity by Mary's iconographic force. Here we give that force form through image.

Funding statement

This work was supported by funding from an AHRC Research Development and Engagement Fellowship: (Mis)Conceptions: A Cultural History of Pregnancy Ambiguity 2023–2025. GRANT NUMBER: AH/X006530/1.

References

Brown, K. T. (2017), *Mary of Mercy in Medieval and Renaissance Italian Art: Devotional Image and Civic Emblem*, London: Routledge.

Browne, V. (2023), *Pregnancy without Birth: A Feminist Philosophy of Miscarriage*, London: Bloomsbury.

Castaldi, T. (2011), *La Madonna Della Misericordia: L'iconografia della Madonna della Misericordia e della Madonna delle frecce nell'arte di Bologna e della Romagna nel Tre e Quattrocento*, Imola: La mandragora editrice.
Davis, I., illustrated by A. Burel (2025), *Conceiving Histories: Trying for Pregnancy, Past and Present*, Cambridge, MA: MIT Press.
Freidenfelds, L. (2019), *The Myth of the Perfect Pregnancy: A History of Miscarriage in America*, Oxford: Oxford University Press.
Latour, B. (1993), *We Have Never Been Modern*, trans. C. Porter, Cambridge, MA: Harvard University Press.
Lyons, B. and L. Dolezal (2017), 'Shame, Stigma and Medicine', *Medical Humanities* 43: 208–10.
McDonald, N. (2013), 'Gender', in M. Turner (ed.), *A Handbook of Middle English Studies*, 54–63, Oxford: Wiley.
Mills, R. (2003), 'Jesus as Monster', in B. Bildhauer and R. Mills (eds), *The Monstrous Middle Ages*, 28–54, Cardiff: University of Wales Press.
Monagle, C. (2020), *Scholastic Affect: Gender, Maternity and the History of Emotions*, Cambridge: Cambridge University Press.
Nagel, A. (2012), *Medieval Modern: Art Out of Time*, London: Thames and Hudson.
Rich, A. ([1976] 1995), *Of Woman Born: Motherhood as Experience and Institution*, New York: Norton.
Rose, J. (2018), *Mothers: An Essay on Love and Cruelty*, New York, Farrar, Straus and Giroux.
Stewart, S. (1993), *On Longing: Narratives of the Miniature, the Gigantic, the Souvenir, the Collection*, Durham: Duke University Press.
Warner, Marina ([1976] 2000), *Alone of All Her Sex: The Myth and Cult of the Virgin Mary*, London: Vintage.

CHAPTER EIGHTEEN

Birth knowledge and institutional experiences: Lyndsay Mann's *As You Were*

Camilla Mørk Røstvik

A team of women are rowing through a canal. We watch them work through a tracking shot from a distant drone. Steady, focused, together. Painfully, dangerously, triumphantly.

In Lyndsay Mann's art film *As You Were* (2023; 47 minutes), complex stories about reproductive choices, birth, parenting and work are intercut with a reoccurring image of these rowers. Breathe and focus, breathe and focus, push, wait and go.

The calm and strength of the rowing team is necessary because *As You Were* deals with disturbing material throughout. The artist has spoken to and recorded the voices of maternity specialists from the NHS who have themselves given birth, inviting a conversation about entanglements between the professional and the personal. Mann is well placed to ask these questions, because she is entangled in them herself. Can an artist be a mother (Judah 2022)? Can a midwife not be? And what is the rule of structures like the hospital, the law, and the professional in all of this?

Institutions shape reproductive choices, pregnancy, and birth. *As You Were* documents how medical, legal, and political bodies all bring to bear on the person in labour, and those labouring to assist them. Birth and associated experiences are sites of politics, events flooded with cultural and social meaning (Björklund and Jülich 2024; Heffington 2023; Hopwood, Flemming and Kassell 2018; Olszynko-Gryn 2023). The

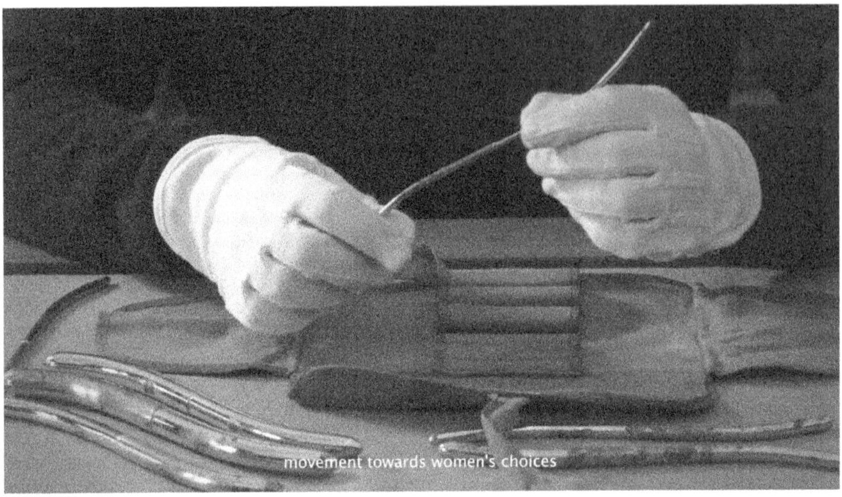

FIGURE 18.1 Lyndsay Mann, *As You Were*, 2024. Video still. Courtesy of the artist.

midwife, the obstetrician, the parent, the fetus, the baby are all produced by institutional norms: laws to follow, regulations to consider, advice to take, mistakes to make. Drowning in all of this, the only thing to do is keep going, keep rowing, keep pushing. Sometimes to exhaustion, then beyond.

Mann has been interested in the role of new parents for several years. In 2019 she initiated the New Mothers' Assembly at Surgeons' Hall Museum at the Royal College of Surgeons in Edinburgh. Over six weeks, the artist hosted weekly workshops with new mothers and their newborns. Inviting mothers and babies into the patriarchal space of surgery on their own terms is a radical act, and the resulting images and project documents how seldom people who have given birth can actually take up space in the institutions that have shaped birth as an increasingly medicalized event (Royal College of Physicians Museum 2018–19). Babies sitting in hundred-year-old mahogany chairs, strollers parked against lush red curtains, breastfeeding under ancient tools of horror. The visual contrast likely inspired *As You Were,* which skillfully and often surprisingly juxtaposes medical tools with the soft, strong, quick bodies of rowers, spiders spinning and snails strolling at a relaxed pace.

Mann first utilized the Museum's historic collection of obstetric tools to initiate conversations about the institutions and norms that shape experiences for pregnancy and birth for New Mothers' Assembly. In *As You Were*, we see these tools handled by white-gloved hands for several minutes at a time. Like the participants of New Mothers' Assembly, we are invited to think about how these objects might have been used (and misused). Rather than focus on the drama and gore of childbirth, however, these objects create space for wonder. What in the world is the pointy thing with a screw at the end? Who could the person using these objects have been? And what about their birth? How did it go? Did they survive? We fabulate about the history of birth in this way throughout the film, a history of the world itself (Hartman 2008).

We can see *As You Were* in the art historical legacy of important works on pregnancy, birth and motherhood. In recent years, several books have documented the importance of 'image-thinking' in this field, from cold clinical anatomy illustrations to the glamourized Hollywood vision, to feminist interventions exploring birth as ecstatic and beautiful, to shows including *One Born Every Minute* (Bal 2022; Fisher and Winick 2021). While different, all of these impactful visual representations focus on the birth event, whereas *As You Were* purposefully sidesteps the delivery room. Birth, as the film shows, is an event which is shaped by competing ideas that began a long time before and a long way outside the experience itself.

Mann's project was also entangled in a web of historic events, many of which have had a deep effect on medical institutions in Britain and elsewhere. Made before and during the COVID-19 pandemic, and released after, *As You Were* was documenting midwife and obstetric labour at a time of intense pressure on the health services. The effects of the pandemic were felt in the NHS, but also in the closure of museums like Surgeon's Hall, and in the interactions between Mann and her interviewees. Throughout the pandemic, midwives and obstetricians kept working because birth continued. I recall applauding this work for a while. When the applause stopped, the births continued. Life will out, but at a cost. The midwives which Mann spoke to were also caught in a moment in time before the mass exodus of the profession due to the pandemic and Brexit. Adding to this, the film was made immediately before the American supreme court's decision to overthrow *Roe v. Wade*, and in a period when reproductive choices in countries including Ireland, Poland and France restricted and loosened and restricted again. *As You Were* can already be seen in these historic contexts, documenting how key political events and institutional changes affect those who help in the birthing process. And therefore, the effects on birth itself. On life.

Mann does not want us to get stuck in these very real but very troubling realities. We keep moving. We return to the rowers. Working all the while, gently caring for their team and their vehicle, washing the boat together, ready to go again. While you watch *As You Were*, or read this text, people are birthing. Babies are disrupting work. Artists who are parents and who make work about parenthood are still seen as clichés in certain circles, especially mothers. Abortions are being carried out, legal and illegal. Midwives save lives and document death. Obstetricians carry on and on and on. Pushing, struggling. With a flood of new rules, restrictions, limitations, burdens, toil, struggle. And yet, with focus and strength, again and again, the world births itself.

References

Bal, M. (2022), *Image Thinking: Artmaking as Cultural Analysis*, Edinburgh: Edinburgh University Press.

Björklund, E., and S. Jülich, eds (2024), *Rethinking the Public Fetus: Historical Perspectives on the Visual Culture of Pregnancy*, Rochester: University of Rochester Press.

Fisher, M. M., and A. Winick, eds (2021), *Designing Motherhood: Things that Make or Break our Births*, Cambridge, MA: MIT Press.

Hartman, S. (2008), 'Venus in Two Acts', *Small Axe* 12 (2): 1–14.

Heffington, P. O. (2023), *Without Children: The Long History of Not Being a Mother*, New York: Seal.

Hopwood, N., R. Flemming and L. Kassell, eds. (2018), *Reproduction: Antiquity to the Present Day*, Cambridge: Cambridge University Press.

Judah, H. (2022), *How Not to Exclude Artist Mothers (and Other Parents)*, London: Lund Humphries.

Olszynko-Gryn, J. (2023), *A Woman's Right to Know: Pregnancy Testing in Twentieth-Century Britain*, Cambridge, MA: MIT.

Royal College of Physicians Museum (2018–2019), '*This vexed question': 500 years of women in medicine*, exhibition.

PART V

Rethinking art and therapy

CHAPTER NINETEEN

Perpetual custody

Suzanne Hudson

In 2018, I joined Loyola Marymount University's Art Therapy graduate programme to embark upon 'extra-disciplinary training', in the language of my fellowship. As an art historian with an interest in the relationship between modernism and art therapy, I started researching sites of art education outside of academies and museums in the United States and broaching questions about the justification for, and utility of, process-oriented practices therein. Moving beyond the clinical encounter, I was also curious about the exhibition of resulting works made by clients in session, and the framing that attended their display, when and if they survived, and when and if they were shown. What kinds of knowledge does this art produce and for whom? Beyond epistemology, I have also increasingly questioned the disciplinary competences undergirding professionalization, with the act of interpreting the art of others remaining chief among them for art therapists and art historians alike. This essay thus represents an examination of the professionalized assessor, reckoning with attempts at standardization and analysis within what I name perpetual custodial practices. In doing so, it argues that art history and medicine are in fact tandem disciplinary frameworks, shaped by diagnostic methods that take symptoms, broadly construed, as the basis for interpretation and classification.

So it was that I enrolled in a workshop teaching the Diagnostic Drawing Series (DDS). The DDS comprises drawings that a client produces in a choreographed sequence, or what creator Barry M. Cohen calls in DDS-sanctioned materials a 'three-picture assessment tool' (Cohen, Mills and Kwapien Kijak 1994: 105–10).[1] Intended for clinical application with

[1] I was trained in the DDS in March 2019, at the Expressive Therapies Summit: Los Angeles on 'Creativity & the Arts in Healing'.

identical directions, uniform materials, and a set rating scale, the series can be administered individually or in groups with the purpose of identifying pathology. Cohen, an artist and art therapist, developed the DDS at the inpatient psychiatric facilities of the Fairfax Hospital Association with Barbara Lesowitz in 1982, and extended the work with Anna Reyner and Shira Singer. Together they presented the pilot study the following year at the annual American Art Therapy Association (AATA) conference, where it won a Research Award. As recognized, it was novel in many regards, not least for being the first art therapy assessment for adults to correlate with the nomenclature of the Diagnostic and Statistical Manual of Mental Disorders (DSM). Since then, Cohen has spearheaded repeated tests for reliability and validity – a control commensurate with evidence-driven psycho-social research cultures but largely anathema to the field of art therapy as it was practised since the 1940s.

If art therapy long was based on the irreproducible specificity of one-on-one relationships, occupational therapy, by contrast, was from the very first concerned with codification.[2] Occupational therapy emerged as an allied health profession in the United States by World War I; inspired by the Arts and Crafts movement, adepts tending to the battle-wounded and infirm stressed the therapeutic value of handcrafts and nonalienated manual work. But important early occupational therapy curricula conceived by Susan Tracy, William Rush Dunton Jr., and others focused on training nurses for medical settings rather than teachers with knowledge of crafts (Quiroga, 1995: 71–89). When Tracy published *Studies in Invalid Occupations: A Manual For Nurses and Attendants* in 1910, she fronted her own course in occupations – a concept she nevertheless adapted from John Dewey's description of classroom 'activity… which reproduces or runs parallel to some form of work carried on in the social life' (Dewey 1906: 131–37) – with an endorsement by her collaborator, Daniel H. Fuller, MD (Fuller in Tracey 1910: 1–10).[3] The *Journal of the American Medical Association* (JAMA) reviewed it, noting: 'Although this book is not directly medical, it is of interest to physicians, and to all who have to do with invalids' (Review of *Studies in Invalid* … 1910: 722). While 'invalids' for Fuller exhibited 'physical, nervous, mental and moral characteristics' (Fuller in Tracey 1910: 2), physical ailments characterize a significant developmental axis of occupational therapy.

Stakeholders in the nascent field of occupational therapy seemed to understand the urgency of reproducing method, scaling the reach of their work, and naming the populations it served. In 1917, George Barton

[2]Occupational and art therapy share rehabilitative aims, but have differing institutional histories that are important to think together.

[3]In his introductory remarks, Fuller approved of occupations 'not as a panacea, but as an important adjunct to the other forms of treatment, and sometimes is quite all the treatment necessary.'

and colleagues gathered at his Consolation House at the Clifton Springs Sanitarium and formed the Society for the Promotion of Occupational Therapy; by 1922, *Archives of Occupational Therapy* became the official journal of the renamed American Occupational Therapy Association. A decade later, the association affiliated with the American Medical Association Council to encourage educational standards and to have a presence at American Hospital Association conferences (Quiroga 1995: 263). In contrast, art therapy, though similarly auxiliary to other forms of healthcare delivery, remained decentralized for decades. As art therapist and chronicler Maxine Junge characterizes, '[m]any art therapists working alone in different places thought they had invented the practice themselves' (2010: 11). Despite the naming of such art-based psychotherapeutic work by Margaret Naumburg in the early 1940s (alongside Adrian Hill), the first art therapy journal, *Bulletin of Art Therapy*, was established by Elinor Ulman only in 1961. (As Junge glosses further: 'Before the publication of the journal, art therapists had worked alone, often making it up as they went along' (2010, 12).)

To the point of Cohen's DDS, the analytical framework it centres to secure pertinence contravenes a legacy of wilfully particularized creative work. For Naumburg, art was useful *in therapy*, while for others including artist and educator-turned-therapist Edith Kramer, art *was therapy*. In neither case does art-making serve a solely diagnostic function, though debates around the founding of the American Art Therapy Association in the late 1960s do attest to a lack of consensus, and even antagonism, on this count. In 1968, a steering committee comprised of Myra Levick, Robert Ault, Don Jones, Elinor Ulman and Felice Cohen set about summoning a meeting for art therapists from the United States and Canada. The gathering, in 1969, had the purpose of making 'art therapy and its relationship to mental health and education more clearly defined and further developed' (Junge 1994: 175–79).[4] Perhaps unsurprisingly, delegates were conflicted regarding the ontology of art therapy and its presumptive nomination, with the assembly ultimately rejecting *art psychotherapy* in favour of the more catholic *art therapy*. The American Art Therapy Association later began awarding the A.T.R. (Art Therapist Registered) for those who met the then-developed standards, a precursor to state licensure for employment.

Levick – who began with a degree in painting, but ultimately received a PhD in psychology and served as the initial president of AATA – opened the first art therapy master's programme in the country with psychiatrists Paul Fink and Morris J. Goldman (at Hahnemann Medical College, subsequently absorbed by Drexel University College of Medicine, and later shuttered). Even before the events of 1968 and 1969, the three already had laid the

[4]The conflicts surrounding such developments were characterized by the concern that standardization would lead to a loss of independence for art therapists, who would be forced to work under, rather than alongside or separately from, psychiatrists.

groundwork for this venture. In 1967, they had published a manifesto, 'Art Therapy – A New Discipline' in *Pennsylvania Medicine*, the official publication of the Pennsylvania Medical Society. They call for organized self-determination within an undefined profession in the piece's first lines: 'Art therapy is a relatively new concept in the treatment of the mentally ill. One factor presently keeps it from reaching its full potential: art therapy is not organized and there are no particular standards of training' (Fink, Goldman and Levick 1967: 61).[5] They follow this by noting the lack of exchange among therapists that Junge later historicizes, and likewise lament the resultant dearth of unified and hence replicable knowledge. In short, they explicitly link formulating a programme to the mandate of redressing these problems.

Despite asserting the primary importance of an artist's approach to media, they acknowledge the need for the practitioner to have in-service training in 'psychiatric principles which would enable her to understand the patient and communicate with the psychiatrist' (Fink, Goldman and Levick 1967: 63).[6] If fluency across constituencies was requisite in the hospital, so was it brandished in such publications, albeit differently. This was, above all, an appeal to a medically affiliated readership in a paper lead-authored by two physicians for facilitating work within their own domains. They present evidence in the form of case studies. And they cite long-standing precedents: interestingly, of psychoanalytic interpretations of art based on Freud's model and the widespread use of the Rorschach and the Thematic Apperception Test (T.A.T.), projective tests 'constructed to utilize visual materials as a means of eliciting unconscious dynamics' (Fink, Goldman and Levick 1967: 62). Projective tests are otherwise key in their follow-up essay, 'Art Therapy: A Diagnostic and Therapeutic Tool', published in the *International Journal of Psychiatry* in 1973. Fink, Levick and Goldman make the distinction there between the reliance on readymade cards (whether abstract or figurative, as in Rorschach and T.A.T., respectively) to elicit verbal responses read against documented norms and art therapeutic methods that advance client art as '*a personal projection*' (1973: 109). This is the crux.

The authors prioritize the maker who 'has produced it, can speak about it, and can give his own ideas about it without the necessity of someone's interpreting his statements within a theoretical framework' (Fink, Goldman and Levick 1973: 111–12). Lest this tactic fall back on individuation,

[5]The heading above the text none too subtly broadcasts: 'This undefined profession, according to the authors, is a necessary ancillary service in an intensive, short-term treatment psychiatric unit.'

[6]Such gendered dynamics and resultant conflicts between male psychiatrists and women in the allied health professions are well-historicized in the realm of social work (Lunbeck 1994: 35–37) and here become relevant for both occupational and art therapies. Such professional relationships played out in a historical moment where psychoanalysis *writ large* was becoming feminized, as women entered the field in notable, if not majoritarian numbers (Zeavin 2022).

Fink, Levick and Goldman now take pains to disaggregate components of client art that have diagnostic significance: e.g., colour or the lack thereof, spatial relations, together with symbolism. At this pivotal moment of the discipline's consolidation – the 1973 text touts the new programme and further separates art therapy from occupational therapy, too (Fink, Goldman and Levick 1973: 17)[7] – the management of client art compels engagement with intractable questions, not least: who might adjudicate its meaning, and how, and with what interpretive techniques. In an eruption of rivalry over the point of diagnostic means and consequence, Fink, Levick and Goldman slam Margaret Naumburg for privileging her own 'fantasies rather than those of the patient' (Fink, Goldman and Levick 1973: 112). An irritated Naumburg challenged the trio's characterization of her work, assailing that they, not her, are at fault for imposing *their* understanding of art made in session (Naumburg 1973: 120).[8] Here is Naumburg's central argument, cited at some length, with emphasis preserved from the original:

> *Art therapy is primarily a therapeutic technique and not a diagnostic tool,* even though it may at times be adjunctive to diagnosis. In defining art therapy as a diagnostic instrument, the authors equate it directly with projective techniques, whose function is primarily diagnostic but not therapeutic. Art therapy should be recognized as an important and specialized form of psychotherapy in which the therapist encourages patients to associate verbally to the images they create, concerning their unconscious art projections. In this way, both patients and therapist may arrive at a better understanding of the nature of a patient's conflicts.
>
> (Naumburg 1973: 119)

More succinctly, this distinction is encapsulated in the opposing camps' two titles: 'Art Therapy: A Diagnostic and Therapeutic Tool' is at odds with Naumburg's 'Art Therapy: A Therapeutic Technique'.

A decade later the DDS fell on the side of the former, radicalizing the promise of the diagnostic impulse become 'tool' and seeking to instrumentalize it across various factions; in the words of Cohen, now together with Anne Mills and Adrienne Kwapien Kijak, in the piece for *Art Therapy*, they meant to effect a '*lingua franca*' (1994: 109). As introduced at the outset, Cohen and his collaborators worked with this goal to establish a system of three prescriptive, sequential drawings – 1) Free Picture, 2) Tree Picture and 3) Feeling Picture – that could be administered quickly and cheaply, and compared across locations of supervision. The test is intended for table-top application and must use a twelve-colour pack of chalk pastels

[7]They state this as a matter of fact in the conclusion, but do not offer any thoughts on the matter beyond declaring it so.

[8]Hanna Yaxa Kwiatkowska defends Naumburg, and importantly flags that artworks made in therapy 'are vulnerable to differences in interpretation' (1973: 121).

without paper wrapping on full-sized (18" × 24") white drawing paper with a slight tooth (Diagnostic Drawing Series 2021). Clients are told in advance that they will be asked to draw three pictures – each to be completed within fifteen minutes – and to talk about them afterwards. The instructions are brief: 1) 'Make a picture using these materials'; 2) 'Draw a picture of a tree'; 3) 'Make a picture of how you're feeling, using lines, shapes, and colours'. The second directive bears most directly on existing tests, including the H-T-P (House-Tree-Person) put forward by clinical psychologist John Buck in 1948 (though in use a decade before, and already based on the Draw-A-Man personality test created by Florence Goodenough in 1926, both of which were originally designed to assess children's intelligence).

Cohen's model insists on the multiple drawings, conceived of as 1) unstructured, 2) structured, and 3) semi-structured. Instead of a single effort, this heterogeneity abets tracking the presence of co-occurring aspects within or across them. In 1986, Cohen published the *DDS Rating Guide*, which provides twenty-three would-be empirical criteria. These include the presence or absence of blending, formal integration, line quality and line pressure, the use of space, and the incorporation of inanimate objects, symbols, or words; 'raters' also confirm whether something is abstract or representational. Summoning a long history of medical representations embodying knowledge, Cohen reached for an anatomical metaphor of skeleton, muscle and skin to describe the order of operations for incorporating the scoring. The skeleton refers to structural elements, the formal aspects of composition. As Cohen synopsizes the others:

> The muscle level consists of the latent content (including metaphors and symbols) that emerges from narrative, art historical and cultural contexts. These are the qualities that clinicians looked for in light of their personal associations, theoretical orientation, and professional experience. The skin level is the manifest content, the process of making the picture, including the artist's physical behaviour, verbalizations, associations, and the title given to the picture.
>
> (2016: 563)

While the scheme forges a language to describe clinical artwork, it admits not just the drawings but also the behavioural dimension of their instantiation as evidence: the *process* of art-making as well as the product. The client response to the directives' relative structuring and materials remains in the therapist's written evaluation – witnessing the subject into legibility – more explicitly than in the art.

Given how this circles back to interpretation exceeding the rating scale, it is unsurprising that the DDS remains contested for being both too mechanistic and not regular enough. (Note, as well, the language of 'artist' not 'client' in Cohen's explication, now assumed as the protagonist of a kind of contemporary art history in the making.) Defending it on its thirtieth anniversary, Cohen maintained that 'the most significant misperception about DDS research is that the art therapist administering it is responsible for making the diagnosis' (2016: 562). This distinction is extrapolated from clinical routine but made specifically in this sentence in relation to the DDS Archive of some 4,500 drawings he and colleagues have amassed for research. The collected series are each labelled on the back along the lower edge behind the left corner establishing the correct bearings; they are further sorted with the participants' demographic information and DSM diagnoses, with the latter 'established by two agreeing diagnoses, usually by psychiatrists' (2016).[9] The DDS remains a diagnostic method subordinate to the corroboration of doctors using a medical framework of DSM-regulated normalizations of health against which psychopathology registers. Predicated upon terms that it seeks neither to challenge nor repair, Cohen posits instead the efficiency and capacity of method to help a client find clarity of diagnosis – to convince them of their diagnosis – as a precondition to treatment.

In the training I attended, we practised rating drawings from the DDS Archive, made under the above conditions, collected and shared with client consent. To my art historian's mind, the exercises recalled Carlo Ginzburg's influential analysis of the modern medical-semiotic paradigm based upon clues, which emerged simultaneously among the detective, the psychoanalyst, the forensic scientist, and the art connoisseur; here, we almost comically play-acted the detective on the case, looking for pathologies (depression, dysthymic disorder, dissociative identity disorder) and observing the coincidence of items compared to controls (1979: 273–88). I found out that many tropes of modernist art are also flags of named disorders: monochromy, say, is not a badge of aesthetic-political avant-gardism but potentially a marker of schizophrenia. The course materials I received include a slide excerpting Anne Mills's 1995 work on binaries of 'healthy' versus 'unhealthy' qualities in these drawings: 4+ colours is healthy and monochrome is unhealthy; the use of blending is healthy and no blending is unhealthy; medium pressure is healthy and extreme light or heavy pressure is unhealthy; and so on.[10] There is inevitably more to say about this, not least regarding the medical model of fixed disability on which the DSM and hence the DDS relies; the DDS lexicon, inclusive of the slippage between *drawing* and *picture*; and the broader implications of clinical art-making in the service of diagnosis.

---

[9]This would seem to invalidate the 'efficiency' argument, specious because the diagnosis still requires a psychiatrist.

[10]Barry M. Cohen, Anne Mills, and Kathryn Johnson, 'The Diagnostic Drawing Series Two-Day Workshop Presentation Materials' (2006/2019), 39.

The dimension I want to press further here though regards that of the consensual gathering of so much client art, and more specifically, what happens to client work beyond the clinic. Cohen's is an unusual instance to be sure. In the absence of protocols aiming at standardization and dissemination, more commonly a client might hold onto their work, potentially reworking it across multiple sessions, or they might decide that its proximity is contraindicated; in that scenario, the therapist keeps the work, subject to state laws around preservation as part of a private medical record. In the United States, art made in session is the client's property unless it is not. Many artworks that stay in protected files do so until the destruction of such records, except when breached for forensic or other sanctioned reasons (Salomon and Levinger 2020).[11] In some cases, such as the instructive example of Edith Kramer, this might include the passage of the art therapist's archive (inclusive of clinical notes and other materials, together with art made by clients *and* the therapist) to a library or other repository where materials are still subject to restricted access as individual health records.

In 1951, Kramer was hired as an art therapist at the Wiltwyck School for Boys in New York's Hudson Valley. She kept art made by children and adolescents with whom she worked, and it ended up in the residential treatment facility's administrative files at Columbia University. The board gifted the records to Teachers College in 1983, and access to them remains limited, restricted for seventy years after their completion. Granting that those implicated in this material might wish to consult it, the finding aid further notes that former students may access their own files, if only after registering as a researcher. Kramer's personal papers are held elsewhere, at New York University, where she had joined the faculty in 1973 and worked to develop an art therapy graduate programme after the first was established at Hahnemann. However, the distinction between the two archives is not absolute. The guide to these papers summarizes the holdings as documenting:

> Kramer's work as a practicing art therapist, most notably her work at Wiltwyck School for Boys [....]. Kramer's notes about patients at Wilkwyck, artwork created by these patients in the course of art therapy, and example artworks created by Kramer are all included, as are documents related to and drafts of her 1958 book, *Art therapy in a children's community: a study of the function of art therapy in the treatment program of Wiltwyck School for Boys*. Slides and photographs also document patient artwork.
>
> (Schmeling 2011)

[11]See also the formal standards maintained by the AATA, which stipulate conditions for the release of patient artworks (Ethical Principles for Art Therapists: 5–6). Such standards exist in the United States as a response to privacy and records rules stipulated by state entities and federally by the Center for Medicare and Medicaid Services.

Her personal archive comprises, among many other things, five drawings and forty-two paintings on paper ranging from portraits, real and fantastical animals, to an urban scene.

That Kramer makes for an especially keen object of study owes to the endurance of the student materials and Kramer's role in prompting them. Kramer developed a technique known as the Third Hand. At decisive, often vulnerable moments in the art-making process she functioned like an art educator or even a studio assistant: mixing paint to the desired colour, demonstrating techniques, propping up a sculpture until the client could materially scaffold it, and so on. A Bauhaus-trained artist who studied with Friedl Dicker-Brandeis, Kramer worked in drawing, printmaking, painting and sculpture (Otto 2024). Considering the maintenance of one's own practice as requisite – 'that art therapists [should] be practicing artists first and foremost' (Thompson 2017: 85) as Geoffrey Thompson puts it – she likewise stressed the parallel use of one's 'artistic competence ... for the empathic service to others' (Kramer 2000: 48). She described needing a 'third eye' to 'perceive the multifaceted messages embodied in artwork produced in the course of art therapy – messages that may defy translation into words' together with a 'third hand' which helps 'the creative process along without being intrusive, without distorting meaning or imposing pictorial ideas or preferences alien to the client' (2000). The point was to engage in supportive work that met a client at their point of resistance and then facilitated but did not determine the activity beyond it, allowing for a mobility of response as work progressed.

From conservation research undertaken by Laura McCann and collaborators, we learn that in addition to Kramer's interventions in the framework of the session, she seems to have continued to modify the work thereafter, engaging in what they call 'post-custodial interventions' (McCann et al. 2021: 184–201). These interventions sometimes were strokes of conscientious protection, such as when she redacted a name or changed a date to obscure the identity of the maker. This proved especially common for works that circulated during the children's early lifetimes as part of a 1957 travelling exhibition, 'Art and the Trouble Child', dedicated to the school and Kramer's work, or that were published in her book the following year. In this show and its catalogue, Kramer used pseudonyms and changed the clients' ages and dates of the artworks, acting to protect the confidentiality of her charges, who were also minors. An act of benevolence, she nevertheless marginalizes the makers in determining the conditions of appearance for their work (in which some details of personal history would anyhow be preserved). One might note the ways this tactic is familiar from exhibitions of works made by psychiatric patients which became the hallmarks of 'outsider' art. It reproduces a version of medical paternalism that was baked into the American Medical Association's 1847 Code of Ethics and implicated in subsequent practice that has similarly obfuscated significant information for the ostensible good of the patient.

Still more interesting than the fact of Kramer's anonymizing efforts though is that the conservators found evidence of Kramer having overpainted and 'fixed' other sections of student compositions beyond those meant to veil their identities. They describe the varnish Kramer used to stabilize the inexpensive art materials for presentation in the exhibition, and distinct overpainting atop the surfaces, 'often crudely applied, which appears to be Kramer's continued use of the Third Hand approach when repairing the object' (McCann et al. 2021: 192). In one notable instance, a painting called *Young Man with Switchblade*, they show how such involvement did change the composition, with later retouching extending the figure's head above the background skyline, which previously had formed a higher horizon. In discussing available conservation treatment options, the authors explain their initial plan to restore the work to its prior, 'original' state, before revising this 'to include preserving all evidence of Kramer's interventions as insights into her art therapy methodology' (McCann et al. 2021: 197). They were guided in this choice by the siting of these papers in Kramer's archive, not that of the maker or the school. While they saved marks made upon the images, they also kept the redactions in place, acknowledging that they can later be removed when restrictions expire.

These intercessions reveal rather less about the child than the art therapist. One might acknowledge the role of the art therapist in setting up a directive or seeing the work through, as well as extending this custody after the paints are put away. In contrast to McCann, I would characterize these actions less as post-custodial than custodial in perpetuity. And it is this concept that I think bears directly on the work of modern art history as well, entangled as it has been with that of conservation. The period of art therapy's professionalization under consideration here also overlaps with that of art conservation in the United States, through Edward Waldo Forbes at the Fogg Museum, and others, including George L. Stout. (Stout believed the Fogg's technical laboratory should rest on the collaboration of art historians, scientists, and practising conservators as a 'three-legged stool') (Stoner 2005: 42–43). The physical alteration of the material as a form of stewardship distinguishes conservation, of course, but the framework of perpetual custody might help us to question the ethical limits of conceptual apprehension as a form of possession, too. It poses a heuristic for the limits of access and ownership; moreover, it begs what difference it makes to these operations whether the custodian watches (or has a literal hand in) the art being made.

Indeed, for the art therapist, observing a client making art is a cornerstone of practice, which yields critical behavioural information about the subject apart from whatever form the object might also assume. By contrast, while it is true that from the 1960s on plenty of non-clinical art (inclusive of happenings and performances) was made in situations of 'being watched' (Lambert-Beatty 2008) as Carrie Lambert-Beatty brands it, most modernist art was analyzed by someone other than the maker, sometime or somewhere other than where it was made. Interpretation of art happened – or happens in perpetuity – only when the maker leaves the work behind. This art historical response relies heavily on ideas of art's autonomy, the better to uphold the salience of the expert authorized to handle its meaning, to confirm, retroactively, its 'intention' and consequence. It obtains in the basic unit of instruction, the endless production of 'formal analysis' as a pedagogical paradigm of disciplinary competence prerequisite for professionalization. Yet the formal analysis is a means not an end. The larger goal is to connect the reading of a single work (or series) to an ordering system – boorishly: geography or period, culture or context, class or race, etc. – in an enterprise at knowing through classifying familiar from Foucauldian critiques of post-Linnean taxonomy. Art history wields interpretive dexterity with and jurisdiction over visual evidence; it rationalizes competences that accredit one to speak for others.

While art therapy remains internally divided on whether art made in its name is diagnostic, art history has never pretended to be therapeutic, much less reformist. In these terms, it is diagnostic, and not just by default, in extracting professional power out of the work of categorizing. In some instances, this work comes surprisingly close to a clinical assessment; the standard artist biography is the mirror image of a case report. Despite the fundamental difference of circumstance in its regard for objects not made in clinical conditions – by and large, though not exclusively (see again 'outsider' art) – I insist that art historians rely upon unacknowledged medical models. To return to Ginzburg's influential framing, the connoisseurship upon which modern art history is based seeks instances of deviance, clues that help one to determine if something is real or fake, and privileges skills associated with finding significant details that reveal deeper phenomena (1979: 273–88). In using medical models of assessment presumptively, in finding pictorial traces as clues over which the maker exerts no control precisely because they are involuntary, the discipline of art history manages art as though it were transparent to meaning for the one doctoring instead of producing it.

This shared approach has been confirmed somewhat paradoxically by art history's use value within medical training as an instrument in the service of science (Dolev, Friedlaender and Braverman 2001: 1020). In a recent review of art in medical education, Yoseph Dalia, Emily C. Milam, and Evan A. Rieder introduce the apposition of art history to medical education proper as follows:

> Physicians utilize pattern recognition and visual acuity skills to recognize physical examination findings and associate them with diagnoses. Examining and studying fine art could theoretically supplement a resident's training in this task. In the modern era of medical training,

> art has not been a curricular focus, despite having a role in the early days of medical training. Recently, however, there has been an effort to incorporate the use of fine art into medical training. Proponents purport that learning how to analyze fine art may improve not only clinicians' intellectual curiosity and critical thinking, but also their diagnostic skills and ability to empathize with patients.
>
> (2020: 686)

This is applied art history. Alongside but also exemplified by techniques for aesthetic development branded as Visual Thinking Strategies (VTS) (Housen 1983; Yenawine 1999, 2005, 2013), it is often lamented by those invested in the humanities as dislocating humanist skills of interpretation, ostensibly with no relation to medicine, into spaces of clinical training and care without recourse or remainder. But this passage runs so smoothly exactly because those skills were always already diagnostic tools, compatible because of a shared epistemic ground. These are similarly grounded in individualism, and accepted for self-governance which leaves the private subject, whether patient or artist, as the isolated bearer of otherwise social problems – an ameliorative therapeutic discourse for upholding productive neoliberal subjects, as Maria Walsh convincingly establishes (2021). As a necessarily provisional conclusion, we might find ways to think beyond this, and in so doing, to admit mutual disciplinary entanglement and shared responsibility.

References

American Art Therapy Association (2013), *Ethical Principles for Art Therapists.*

Cohen, B. M., Mills, A., and Kwapien Kijak, A. (1994), 'An Introduction to the Diagnostic Drawing Series: A Standardized Tool for Diagnostic and Clinical Use', *Art Therapy: Journal of the American Art Therapy Association*, 11 (2): 105.

Cohen, B. M., and Mills, A. (2016), 'The Diagnostic Drawing Series (DDS) at Thirty: Art Therapy Assessment and Research', *The Wiley Handbook of Art Therapy*, ed. David E. Gussak and Marcia L. Rosal, Chichester, England: John Wiley & Sons: 558–68.

Dalia, Y., Milam, E. C. and Rieder, E. A. (2020), 'Art in Medical Education: A Review', *Journal of Graduate Medical Education*, 12 (6): 686–95.

Dewey, J. (1906), 'Psychology of Occupations', in *The School and The Child*, ed. J. J. Findlay, London: Blackie and Son, 81–88.

Dolev, J. C., L. K. Friedlaender, and I. Braverman (2001), 'Use of Fine Art to Enhance Visual Diagnostic Skills', *Journal of the American Medical Association*, 286: 1020–21.

Diagnostic Drawing Series (2021), *About the Diagnostic Drawing Series*, available at https://diagnosticdrawingseries.info/About.html

Fink, P. J., Goldman, M. J. and Levick, M. F. (1967), 'Art Therapy – A New Discipline', *Pennsylvania Medicine*, 70 (11): 61–66.

Fink, P. J., Goldman, M. J. and Levick, M. F. (1973), 'Art Therapy: A Diagnostic and Therapeutic Tool', *International Journal of Psychiatry*, 11 (1): 104–18.
Foucault, M. (1970), *The Order of Things: An Archaeology of the Human Sciences*, New York: Pantheon Books.
Ginzburg, C. (1979), 'Clues: Roots of a Scientific Paradigm', *Theory and Society*, 7 (3): 273–88.
Housen, A. (1983), *The Eye of the Beholder: Measuring Aesthetic Development*, PhD diss., Harvard Graduate School of Education.
Junge, M. B. (1994). 'The Formation of the American Art Therapy Association', *Art Therapy*, 11 (3), 175–79.
Junge, M. B. (2010), *The Modern History of Art Therapy in the United States*, Springfield, IL: Charles C. Thomas Publisher.
Kramer, E. (2000), 'The Art Therapist's Third Hand: Reflections on Art, Art Therapy, and Society at Large', in *Art as Therapy: Collected Papers*, ed. Lani A. Gerity, Philadelphia and London: Jessica Kingsley: 47–72.
Kwiatkowska, H. Y. (1973), 'Discussion of "Art Therapy: A Diagnostic and Therapeutic Tool"', *International Journal of Psychiatry*, 11 (1): 121–25.
Lambert-Beatty, C. (2008), *Being Watched: Yvonne Rainer and the 1960s*, Cambridge: MIT Press.
Lunbeck, E. (1994), *The Psychiatric Persuasion: Knowledge, Gender, and Power in Modern America*, Princeton: Princeton University Press.
McCann, L., C. Stein, J. Pace, A. Wolf and K. Parks (2021), 'Legal and Ethical Considerations in the Conservation of Artwork Produced During Art Therapy', *Journal of the American Institute for Conservation*, 61 (3): 184–201.
Naumburg, M. (1973), 'Art Therapy: A Therapeutic Technique', *International Journal of Psychiatry*, 11 (1): 119–20.
National Academy of Sciences. 2005. *Scientific Examination of Art: Modern Techniques in Conservation and Analysis*. Washington, DC: The National Academies Press. https://doi.org/10.17226/11413.
Otto, E. (2024), 'Bauhaus for Children Care Work and Art Therapy with Friedl Dicker-Brandeis and Edith Kramer', in *Modernism, Art, Therapy*, Suzanne Hudson and Tanya Sheehan (eds), New Haven, CT: Yale University Press.
Quiroga, V. A. M. (1995), *Occupational Therapy: The First 30 Years*, Bethesda, MD: The American Occupational Therapy Association.
Salomon, M., and S. Levinger (2020), 'The experience of art therapists who work in private practice when retaining clients' artworks after therapy termination', *The Arts in Psychotherapy*, 70: 101684.
Schmeling, S. (2011): Edith Kramer Papers [Finding Aid]; MC 215; New York University Archives.
Stoner, J. H. (2005), 'Changing Approaches in Art Conservation: 1925 to the Present', in *Scientific Examination of Art: Modern Techniques in Conservation and Analysis*, 40–57. Washington, DC: The National Academies Press.
Studies in Invalid Occupation. A Manual for Nurses and Attendants. JAMA (1911), LVI(10):772. doi:10.1001/jama.1911.02560100064044
Thompson, G. A. (2017), 'Edith Kramer: Beyond the Studio', in *The Legacy of Edith Kramer: A Multifaceted View*, Lani Gerity and Susan Ainlay Anand (eds), New York: Routledge.
Tracey, S. (1910), *Studies in Invalid Occupation, a Manual for Nurses and Attendants*, Boston: Whitcomb and Barrows.

Walsh, M. (2021), *Therapeutic Aesthetics: Performative Encounters in Moving Image Artworks*, London and New York: Bloomsbury Academic.

Yenawine, P. (1999), 'Theory into Practice: The Visual Thinking Strategies', presented at the Aesthetic and Art Education: A Transdisciplinary Approach, Lisbon, 27 September 1999.

Yenawine, P. (2005), 'Thoughts on Visual Literacy', in *Handbook of Research on Teaching Literacy Through the Communicative and Visual Arts*, James Flood, Shirley Brice Heath and Diane Lapp (eds), International Reading Association, Mahwah, NJ: Lawrence Erlbaum, 845–46.

Yenawine, P. (2013), *Visual Thinking Strategies: Using Art to Deepen Learning Across School Disciplines*, Cambridge: Harvard Education Press.

Zeavin, H. (2022), 'Therapy With a Human Face', *Dissent* (Winter): https://www.dissentmagazine.org/article/therapy-with-a-human-face/ (accessed 20 November 2024).

CHAPTER TWENTY

Is there room for critical studies in art therapy?

Leah Gipson and Katharine Houpt

An essay about the Oscar-winning film *Parasite* (Bong Joon-ho, 2019) – published on the blog of the American Art Therapy Association (AATA) (Keane 2020) – provides a starting point to imagine how a wider cultural discourse might inform necessary dialogue on the politicized educational landscape of the profession of art therapy. In *Parasite,* the character Kim Ki-jung pretends to have studied art therapy in the United States as part of a complicated plot that eventually sees her entire family employed in a wealthy Korean household. Keane's text praised *Parasite* for 'breaking a historic cultural barrier, becoming the first non-English language film to win the best picture Oscar' (2020), while simultaneously criticizing the film for failing to offer a more didactic portrayal of art therapy as a regulated mental health profession. Our initial impulse to write about the reception of the film arose in response to global political events, including former US Second Lady Karen Pence's White House art therapy initiative and the rescinded US Immigration and Customs Enforcement (ICE) international student ban during the COVID-19 pandemic. We were interested in the potential for new critical ideas on art therapy, but more imperatively, we wished to advocate for a value-based inventory of professional actualizations of emergent social justice and decolonizing frameworks within US mainstream multicultural education and its emphasis on cultural competence and identity awareness.

Art therapy as a profession is growing and changing on an international scale. Seeing a tendency within the AATA to promote and embrace the growth of the field through a dominant and US-centric point of view, we believe that a critical approach to art therapy education is needed to question neoliberal values in the field as it accelerates an international agenda. Neoliberalism is both a set of economic policies and a social analysis: 'not only or even primarily focused on the economy; it involves *extending and disseminating market values to all institutions and social action*, even as the market itself remains a distinctive player' (Brown 2005: 39–40). In neoliberal academia, knowledge production is shaped through preferences in the format of publication, research methods, and the absence of axiology or value concerns (Gjorgjioska and Tomicic 2019). We view critical studies as a tool with which scholarship and pedagogy in art therapy might resist neoliberal modes of knowledge production. In this chapter, we question the potential consequences of defending the profession against critical cultural viewpoints such as those expressed by *Parasite*. We suggest that the defensive position articulated by Keane (2020) on the AATA blog favours a presumed body of authority – an 'insider' professional community dominated by white, US-centric, non-disabled, cis-heteronormative perspectives. Our analysis interrogates the cultural influences of US art therapy education, while situating the field within an international landscape of contemporary political concerns impacting students, professionals, and consumers of art therapy services (Gipson 2017). Klein suggests that studying Korean cinema challenges American studies scholars to abandon thinking that situates 'foreign' cultural production as a 'material and representational field upon which American agents act' (2008: 872). We propose that the study of transnational cultural works such as *Parasite* can encourage critical thinking in art therapy and destabilize societal norms in the global North that assimilate, co-opt, exclude and disappear Black, Indigenous, and all people of colour. Rather than reject Bong's satirical art therapist, we purposefully view the character Ki-jung as a resource to explore issues of power in US notions of professional identity. Bong's art therapist character is a reminder of the specificity of place, culture and positionality that are embedded in the critical praxis of teaching art therapy students.

Toward art and critical cultural studies in art therapy education

In the summer of 2020 during the first wave of COVID-19, many academic institutions and professional organizations began to publicly acknowledge the insidiousness of US racism in response to a reinvigorated Black Lives Matter movement. Ongoing protests in the US resonate with a growing number of art therapy students seeking more critical perspectives in the field (Johnson et al. 2021). Critical perspectives are often thought to be in competition with other presumably more practical skills deemed of greater use value for art therapy students entering the job market. Yet it is dangerous to limit the study of culture in art therapy to the exchange value (commodity) of cultural competence in professional terms. George et al. (2021) surveyed art therapists from the United States to explore the values that informed positive or negative associations with the AATA partnership with Karen Pence in 2017. Survey participants who supported the initiative articulated the following values: visibility at all costs; blanket-inclusivity; the personal is not political; and educating Karen Pence. Despite many art therapists' general alignment with promoting the visibility of the profession, visuality is not an equal sighted field. Marginalizing critical discourse in art therapy relates to a logic of control that concerns the academic production of knowledge.

The tendency within art therapy to readily adopt dominant ideas in mental health has been raised as an ethical and pedagogical issue representative of white supremacy culture within the field (Hamrick and Byma 2017). The role of US-centrism and nationalist discourse should be more closely examined in art therapy research, practice and education. For example, US students might inform their research and professional practices of helping through a cultural contextual lens that often erases patriarchal and racialized settler-colonial histories. A political analysis of neoliberal globalization and the dominance of US education in the field of art therapy has been notably absent from art therapy scholarship. Publications in English about art therapy on an international scale have not thoroughly examined the influence of art therapy education in the United States and other countries of the global North. Bordonaro described international art therapy as having two distinct constructs, 'the growing global practice of art therapy and the formalization of the field in countries around the world, including educational criteria and standards of practice... [and] the cross-cultural application or introduction of art therapy in international and cross-cultural contexts by international practitioners' (2015: 675). Although educational criteria and standards of practice are mentioned, no substantial attention is given to the role of education in international art therapy, or to the racial/ethnic and national contexts where people studied art therapy. Potash et al. (2017) have acknowledged the need for art therapists to individually examine their positionality when establishing art therapy in a country outside of their own national context:

> Beyond project stakeholders, art therapists working internationally are accountable to the profession of art therapy, to represent it accurately and uphold its ethical principles. Further, there is a responsibility to represent one's country well, as every international encounter is an opportunity for cross-cultural exchange.
>
> (2017: 80)

What are the international politics and invisible processes that metamorphose US art therapists' international encounters into 'positive' representations of their country? In viewing *Parasite,* art therapists might ask how race and trauma are related to militarized interventions and policies between the United States and places where Indigenous American, African, and Asian peoples are the majority. Art therapy educators must begin to evaluate modes of professionalization that reflect existing political concerns in the field.

Graphic medicine: An example of critical awareness of audience

Art therapy is a field that is challenged by its own multidisciplinary conceptualization. Answering the question of what art therapy *is* has proven far more elusive than asserting who art therapists are; as Phillips describes, 'Art therapy is what art therapists do' (2016). It is remarkable that art therapy, as a blended discipline, has existed without a significant and sustained dialogue with other fields. A prominent place for critical cultural studies at the core of understanding both disciplines of art and psychotherapy has not yet taken root in art therapy education and research (Leigh 2020). Additional approaches to art from critical theoretical positions are needed in art therapy. We find it then necessary to ask, what are the connections between seeing and treatment? Marxen addressed distinctions between challenging hegemony and reifying social control through uses of art (2018). What types of images and narratives are disseminated about what happens in art therapy?

Graphic medicine is a broad interdisciplinary field which inhabits the intersection of the comics medium and healthcare discourse. Emerging in the 2010s, graphic medicine is described as a 'movement for change that challenges the dominant methods of scholarship in healthcare, offering a more inclusive perspective of medicine, illness, disability, caregiving, and being cared for' (Czerwiec at al. 2015: 2). Graphic medicine recognizes people with lived experience hold important knowledge about mental and physical health and trauma, and have communicated it through art, specifically through the low-cost, largely DIY medium of comics. In contrast to perspectives in art therapy that strive to establish disciplinary authority, graphic medicine openly embraces its interdisciplinary origins and looks to subvert notions of medical expertise through art.

Graphic medicine takes art reception seriously, elevating a multiplicity of subjective experiences through the graphic medicine platform. Donovan and Ustundag note that autobiographical comics allow for de-pathologized self-representation of trauma without expert mediation (2017), and analyze the form's ability to portray individual embodied experiences as part of a collective experience of trauma within a sociopolitical context, 'beyond the limits of biomedical and institutional frameworks' (2017: 234). Other critical perspectives in graphic medicine challenge professional knowledge about madness, contesting dominant medical and psychiatric narratives of normalcy, treatment and systems (Spandler 2020). Graphic medicine positions art as decentralizing knowledge from commodity-driven, biomedical, paternalistic constructs of care. Wegner further complicated the application of these ideals by asking who the implied readers of graphic pathographies are (2020).

Art therapy is situated within a wider medical industry where empathy and creativity can become forms of human capital. The Organization for Economic Co-operation and Development (OECD) defines human capital as the 'knowledge, skills, competencies and attributes embodied in individuals that facilitate the creation of personal, social and economic well-being' (2001: 18). In higher education, the concept of human capital reduces learning to the development of skills linked to an economy.

Bong's satirical image of the art therapist in *Parasite* competes with a capitalist representation of the art therapist as 'trauma expert'. These contrasting images – expert and impersonator – unmask a difficult and messy reality of neoliberalism. Art therapy is a profession made up of skilled and empathic individuals, but the field still exists within a promotionally driven, capitalist economy made for a global elite whose objective must be to specialize in trauma and never dismantle violence that contributes to it. Keane's observations on the AATA blog about the character Ki-jung's forged art therapy degree (2020) interestingly relate to class conflict in the history of art therapy professionalization in the US. In 1975, the chair of the AATA Ad Hoc Committee of Third World People, Lucille Venture, wrote to the AATA president, Felice Cohen:

> Another stumbling block that our committee has come up against that acts as adeterrent to minority folks in college is the requirement (of art therapist) for graduate level study. By the time Black folkes (sic) and other minorities have managed to complete their undergraduate education a job is a 'MUST.' ....Thus $$$$$$$$$$$$ keeps the minority groups out of the field of art therapy as well as the graduate degree requirements... AATA is not only "NOT HELPING us" but our association, in tightening the reigns (sic), is strangling minority groups out of the art therapy field of action.
>
> (1975: 2)

Keane's response to *Parasite* is indicative of unexamined issues of social class within the field (2020). Empathy from a normative gaze empowers professionals who can mobilize emotional narratives more freely than individuals whose 'othered' subjectivities are routinely co-opted or used to define them. Professional advocacy in art therapy seldom questions issues of power which shape empathy and its relationship to therapeutic discourse.

The role of advocacy in establishing the recognition of art therapy in mental healthcare has taken multiple forms. Keane's insistence that Bong 'fully flesh out' the usefulness of art therapy is an attempt to advance the profession in alignment with an exchange-value education, one in which the field's relevance is determined by its fragile and contingent legitimacies under US imperialism. Keane's essay invites film audiences to ignore the fact that Ki-jung lives in a dingy basement apartment where an elevated toilet is the only place she can get a WiFi signal. It is certain that an art therapy master's degree from Chicago would be nearly impossible for her to obtain. Art therapists in the United States have more in common with Ki-Jung than Keane suggests. Both happen upon the kind of low- to mid-salary range jobs reserved for a middle class of service professionals. While Ki-jung manages to con her way out of the exorbitant cost of a graduate art therapy degree in the United States, her fate reveals that she cannot get away with being an imposter. If art therapists wish to see the inherent goodness of art and art therapy in *Parasite*, they will not find it. To do so, they would need to overlook the entire plot – a mythical norm collapses for a moment, just long enough to laugh at its horrors.

Conclusion

We wish to offer an alternative to narrowly defensive responses to any form of critical representation of art therapy. Professional ideas about educational training, licensure and credentials draw upon cultural notions of subjectivity. Issues like these reveal political processes that give certain groups authority to intervene on behalf of society – to raise children, educate citizens, and treat sick and disabled people. What types of knowledge are centred by assertions that art therapy must only be professionally defined or even represented? Art therapy's limited critical engagement with outside perspectives, as exemplified by Keane, is a form of neoliberal knowledge production that closes possibilities for the field. Interacting with cultural works like Bong's *Parasite*, a work of Korean cinema, opens the possibilities for decolonial values to finally take root in the profession.

References

Bordonaro, G.W. (2015), 'International Art Therapy', in D. Gussak and M. Rosal (eds), *The Wiley Handbook of Art Therapy*, 675–82, West Sussex, UK: Wiley.

Brown, W. (2005), *Edgework: Critical Essays on Knowledge and Politics*, Princeton: Princeton University Press.

Czerwiec, M. K., I. Williams, S. Merill Squier, M. J. Green, K. R. Myers and S. T. Smith (2015), 'Introduction', in Czerwiec et al. (eds), *Graphic Medicine Manifesto*, 1–20, University Park: Pennsylvania State University Press.

Donovan, C., and E. Ustundag (2017), 'Graphic Narratives, Trauma and Social Justice', *Studies in Social Justice* 11 (2): 221–37.
George, J., G. B. Yancey, D. A. Sharpe and A. K. Moore. (2021), 'Taking a pulse of the American Art Therapy Association's values: A study of a nonprofit organization in conflict', *The Psychologist-Manager Journal*, 24 (1): 48–83.
Gipson, L. (2017), 'Challenging neoliberalism and multicultural love in art therapy', *Art Therapy*, 34 (3): 112–17.
Gjorgjioska, M. A., and A. Tomicic (2019), 'The crisis in social psychology under neoliberalism: Reflections from social representations theory', *Journal of Social Issues*, 75 (1): 169–88.
Hamrick, C., and C. Byma (2017), 'Know History, Know Self: Art Therapists' Responsibility to Dismantle White Supremacy', *Art Therapy*, 34 (3): 106–11.
Ho, Bong Joon (dir.). 2019. *Parasite*. United States: Neon.
Johnson, T., S. P. Deaver and C. Doby-Copeland (2021), 'Art Therapy Students of Color: The Experience of Seven Graduate Students', *Art Therapy*, 38 (1): 50–56.
Keane, C. (2020), 'Unpacking the so-called art therapist character in "Parasite"', American Art Therapy Association Blog, https://arttherapy.org/blog-unpacking-the-so-called-art-therapist-character-in-parasite/ (accessed 28 November 2024).
Klein, C. (2008), 'Why American Studies Needs to Think about Korean Cinema, or, Transnational Genres in the Films of Bong Joon-ho', *American Quarterly*, 60 (4): 871–98.
Leigh, H. (2020), 'Signature Pedagogies for Art Therapy Education: A Delphi Study', *Art Therapy*, 38 (1): 5–12.
Marxen (2018), 'Artistic Practices and the Artistic Dispositif – A Critical Review', *Antípoda. Revista de Antropología y Arqueología*, 33: 37–60.
Organization for Economic Co-Operation and Development (2001), 'The Well-being of Nations: The Role of Human and Social Capital', https://www.oecd-ilibrary.org/education/the-well-being-of-nations_9789264189515-en (accessed 13 December 2024).
Phillips, J. (2016), 'Identity of the Art Therapist' in D. Gussak and M. Rosal (eds), *The Wiley Handbook of Art Therapy*, 777–86, West Sussex: Wiley.
Potash, J. S., H. Bardot, C. H. Moon, M. Napoli, A. Lyonsmith and M. Hamilton (2017), 'Ethical implications of cross-cultural international art therapy', *The Arts in Psychotherapy*, 56 (1): 74–82.
Spandler, H. (2020), 'Crafting psychiatric contention through single-panel cartoons', in S. M. Squier and I. M. Krüger-Fürhoff (eds), *PathoGraphics: Narrative, Aesthetics, Contention, Community*, University Park: Pennsylvania State University Press.
Venture, L. (1975), Letter 'Re. Committee Report', AATA. The Association's Archived Records. Historic Figures: Lucille Venture, https://www.arttherapy.org/ARCHIVES/Historic%20Figures/Lucille%20Venture/Correspondence%201973-74.pdf (accessed 13 December 2024).
Wegner, G. (2020). 'Reflections on the boom of graphic pathography: The effects and affects of narrating disability and illness in comics', *Journal of Literary & Cultural Disability Studies*, 14 (1), 57–74.

CHAPTER TWENTY-ONE

Beyond therapy: Lula and Rogério's *estrutura viva*

Kaira M. Cabañas

An *estrutura viva*, or living structure, is a simple object: it is made of interlaced rubber bands that form a flexible geometry or net. Brazilian artist Lygia Clark first developed her *estruturas vivas* in the late 1960s in Paris as part of her larger corpus of sensorial propositions. When in use, the bands' elastic materiality acts as a 'dynamic index of sensorial mediation between the various participants pulling and stretching it' (Martins 2019). To the best of my knowledge, Clark introduced the (feminine) adjective *viva* (living) into her texts in 1960, when referring to art as a '*coisa viva*' or living object or thing (Clark 1998: 113, 140). Perhaps unsurprisingly, Clark continued in the course of her career to describe the art object as a living entity, blurring the distinction between the organic and inorganic, subject and object: the object is 'lived' as a force rather than a form. This distinction, as well as Clark's emphasis on the immanence of the encounter, is brought up again and again by her disciple, artist and psychiatrist Lula Wanderley. He explains, the 'relationship established between [sensorial and relational] objects and body is not attained through meaning or shape… but through its sensorial image: Something vague "lived" by the body' (Wanderley 1998: 29).

In 1988, in the context of ongoing psychiatric reform in Brazil, Wanderley created the Espaço Aberto ao Tempo (Space Open to Time; EAT), one of the first clinical spaces in Brazil to use artistic-cultural practices, including Clark's *estruturas vivas*, within contemporary psychiatry. EAT is located on the grounds of the Instituto Municipal Nise da Silveira (formerly the

Centro Psiquiátrico Nacional Pedro II) in the Rio de Janeiro neighborhood of Engenho de Dentro. As an institution, EAT emerged in collaboration with hospital staff and clients (*client* is the preferred term for patients in this context) and from Wanderley's search for a new ethics, aesthetics, and politics of working with individuals who experience acute psychic suffering. EAT embraces multiple activities – for example, painting, collage, silk screen, movement workshops, drawing, and music – and Wanderley also maintains a consulting room to treat clients with Clark's *Estruturação do self* (Structuration of the self) therapy sessions, using, at times, an unorthodox combination of her objects in his highly individualized engagement with clients. Beyond the space of the individual consultation room, Wanderley also activates Clark's sensorial propositions in public.

*

Rogério, Wanderley explains, was 'adrift, immersed in an intense hallucinatory image, everything about Rogério was surprising and terrifying.... The family (the brother) filed a complaint with the Health Department for the lack of solution to Rogério's suffering and, guided by other professionals, demanded electroshock be used on him' (Wanderley 2021: 33). Called upon to intervene in 2002, Wanderley established a small team that would accompany Rogério through his daily activities at the hospital. Leandro Freixo, a professional musician, explored a chaotic sound universe with him, while Ana Mittelback produced affective maps based on his wanderings on the hospital grounds. Wanderley in turn devised ludic experiences to help Rogério find, 'through sensoriality, the completeness (of body and world) lost in psychotic fragmentation' (Wanderley 2021: 34). In the course of this therapeutic companionship – embracing treatment modalities as varied as engaging with sound and playful behaviour – Rogério slowly showed signs of improvement. Wanderley also noticed that his client began mimicking his (Wanderley's) gestures as a way of bringing 'awareness to his own' (Wanderley 2021: 34).

Around this time that same year, Rio-based dancer and choreographer Angel Vianna (aka Maria Ângela Abras Vianna) was organizing a festival on dance and physical rehabilitation with participants from Brazil and Italy; she asked EAT to participate too. In turn, Wanderley invited Rogério to publicly present with him a version of Clark's *estrutura viva*. Rogério accepted the invitation. To recreate Clark's proposition, Wanderley formed two Y's made of rubber bands. He and Rogério faced one another and crossed the structures at the point where the tail of the Y meets its two arms. When attaching the rubber band Y to their bodies, each connected the longest end of their Y to a foot and the smaller ends to their hands; thus, one foot on each participant remained independent of the structure. In this way, the bands crossed and intertwined at the junctures of the Y's upper and lower

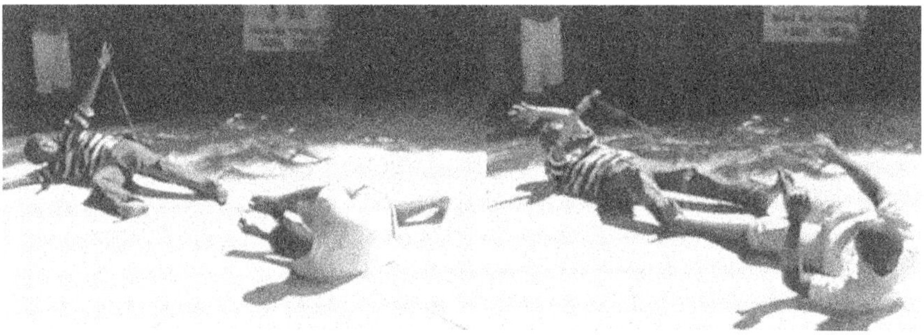

FIGURE 21.1 Lula Wanderley e Rogério with an *estrutura viva* (living structure) as part of their public presentation titled *O prazer é todo meu com Lula e Rogério* (The pleasure is all mine with Lula and Rogério). Two screen captures from the film that captures their actions, *Sutis Laços que nos unem* (Subtle ties that unite us), 2002. Filmmaker unknown.

parts. Wanderley and Rogério did not follow a script. Instead, enabled by the variable and elastic structure, they responded to each other's movements in the form of an improvised dance, which was captured and preserved on film.

Wanderley recalls how the *estrutura viva* created

> a continuum between my body and his, but the structure is absorbed in an interior [immanent] time and, simultaneously, returned to space by action in the form of a dialogue, which yielded in each of us the consciousness of the gesture – an awareness of difference. Rogério reaches me (and vice versa) through the rubber bands, we communicate and recognize each other from the other.
>
> (Wanderley 2021: 35)

As with Clark's use of an *estrutura viva*, Wanderley's 'dance' with Rogério was not primarily about a performance in front of an audience (though, in the context of the festival, one was present in the makeshift theatre on the hospital grounds). The living structure and how it came to life in the co-movement of the participants' gestures are not only constitutive of the immanence insisted upon in Wanderley's practice; the immanence of the encounters – that is, between him and Rogério, between them and the *estrutura viva*, and between their actions and the viewing audience – is also key to the ethics and politics at the heart of Wanderley's art of psychiatric reform. Rather than represent inner visions or speak for others, Wanderley's mobilization of Clark's *estrutura viva* reveals different modes of being and subjectivation, uniting art, body, and psychology so that stable subjectivities are never assumed or uncritically reproduced.

Wanderley's practice diverges from that of many professionals in the psychiatric reform movement (as well as from practising art therapists), who often seek to 'augment' the quality of a patient's creative production so that it will be legible outside the asylum as art; that is, they attempt to discover 'talent' so as to transform clients into art professionals (Wanderley 2021: 16). Accordingly, rather than go in search of 'talent' à la Prinzhorn or Jean Dubuffet, or as in the recent market and museum craze for 'outsider' art (evinced by the Pompidou's acquisition of Bruno Decharme's collection of Art Brut in 2021), Wanderley's primary task is to engage his clients' creativity to build relations to the world, thereby also promoting their social integration. It follows that one 'object story' of the *estrutura viva* is to cast in relief how Wanderley's practice displaces the power relations that often subtend therapeutic care.

With Wanderley and Rogério's public engagement of an *estrutura viva*, they bypassed representation and the representational codes of illness and psychic suffering to foreground the immanence of the aesthetic experience, an immanence that paradoxically enabled Rogério's communication with and participation in a socially recognized form of cultural production (in his case, a dance festival). Psychiatric clients contribute to culture through their artistic production (independent of whether its aesthetic quality is deemed 'good'), whereby their 'cultural citizenship' is an acknowledgment of the cultural resiliency and rights-claiming agency of marginalized groups.[1] Together with the *estrutura viva*, Wanderley and Rogério affirmed their time-based collaboration as a form of cultural citizenship capable of existing beyond a therapeutic frame.

References

Clark, L. (1998), 'The Full-Emptiness' (1960) and 'Untitled' (1960), in *Lygia Clark*, Barcelona: Fundació Antoni Tàpies.

Martins, B. (2019), '14th Bienal de Cuenca', *Artforum* 57 (7), March, available online: https://www.artforum.com/events/14th-bienal-de-cuenca-243830/.

Rosaldo, R. (1994), 'Cultural Citizenship and Educational Democracy', in 'Further Inflections: Toward Ethnographies of the Future', special issue, *Cultural Anthropology* 9 (3): 402–11.

[1]Here I expand the use of *cultural citizenship* to respond to the context of psychiatry and psychiatric reform. The term seems to have been first used by anthropologist Renato Rosaldo, who in the 1980s argued for the democratization of higher education with an eye to Latino civic participation. In this way, the term also calls attention to debates between cultural pluralism and universal citizenship in the nation-state. See, for example, Rosaldo 1994.

Wanderley, L. (1998), cited in Guy Brett, 'Lygia Clark: Six Cells', in *Lygia Clark*, Barcelona: Fundació Antoni Tàpies.
Wanderley, L. (2021), *No silêncio que as palavras guardam: O sofrimento psíquico, o Objeto Relacional de Lygia Clark e as paixões do corpo* [The silence that words hold: Psychic suffering, Lygia Clark's Relational Object and corporeal passions], ed. Kaira M. Cabañas, São Paulo: n-1 edições.

PART VI

Caring, collaborating, curating

CHAPTER TWENTY-TWO

Healthcare intimacies: Vanessa Bell and Dr Marie Moralt

Alison Syme

In December 1918, the painter Vanessa Bell was pregnant with her third child at Charleston in Sussex. She had been living there since 1916 with the two sons she had with her husband Clive Bell; the artist Duncan Grant, father of the baby she was expecting; and David Garnett, Grant's lover and fellow conscientious objector, in a typically unconventional Bloomsbury ménage. The baby, called Angelica, was born on 25 December but, alarmingly, did not put on weight in the weeks after her birth. Bell's milk was suspected to be inadequate. A local doctor prescribed a mixture of orange juice and carbolic acid, a cocktail which gave the baby 'green motions', and under this regimen 'she shrank to skin and bone' (Garnett 1955: 195). When things became desperate, Garnett contacted his childhood friend Noël Olivier, a former neo-pagan known to the Bloomsbury circle who had recently qualified as a doctor, and she sent her friend Dr Marie Moralt to Charleston. After an intervention with the local doctor described by Garnett as 'awkward' and more dramatically by Bell's sister Virginia Woolf as 'scenes, explosion, dismissal' (Garnett 1955: 195; Woolf 1976: 326), Moralt stopped the carbolic mixture, put the baby on Glaxo (a form of powdered milk), and prescribed a couple of doses of grey powder, after which the baby began to recover and gain weight.[1] Moralt stayed on for two or three weeks to look after both mother and child.

[1]Grey powder was the common name for a mixture of chalk and mercury given to children as a laxative, to treat diarrhea, or while teething. A 'favourite in the nursery', it was used in Britain into the 1940s (Chavasse 1878: 67). For a detailed account of the medical crisis at Charleston as well as concurrent and compounding drama with the servants, see Spalding 1983: 176–78.

Angelica did recover, but over the next months, Bell's letters recurred to the traumatic situation. In February, she described the experience to Roger Fry as one of 'absolute horror and chaos', noting that while the baby was recuperating, at six weeks she still weighed 'less than when she was born' and was 'fearfully small and thin' (Bell 1998b: 229, 230). Nearly eighty years later, Bell's son Quentin recalled that when he and his brother, who had been sent away for the birth, returned, there was 'no coal, little wood, no butter, no meat, and no hope in the house' (1997: 17). Subjection and submission to the male doctor's authority had been injurious to mother and baby alike. Both Bell and a nurse had suggested alternatives to the carbolic and orange juice, but, as Bell put it, 'out of sheer obstinacy… (and fear of its being *our* remedies and not his that cured her) he wouldn't give them' (1998b: 230). Letters and Woolf's diary attest that the ordeal and 'the idiocy and obstinacy of that old man' haunted Bell for years (Bell 1998b: 230; Bell 1995: 40). When Moralt arrived, Bell pretended the two had known each other for ages (Spalding 1983: 178), presumably to minimize confrontation over the male doctor's replacement and to allow him to save a little face. Bell's ill feelings towards him were tenacious, but his dismissal also occasioned the first of multiple salutary acts of collaboration between Bell and Moralt in the fiction of their long acquaintance.

Indeed, the acute tension with male medical authority, coupled with the women's shared concern with health and recuperation in Bell's domestic sphere in 1919, precipitated an intriguingly entangled, creative, therapeutic and collaborative relationship between female artist and lady doctor – a relationship which elicited the artist's care and the doctor's artistry as much as the other way around, and frayed disciplinary distinctions and other phantasms of autonomy from the start. In what follows, I propose that the artworks and reciprocal care springing from their mutual involvement articulate a kind of semi-autonomy, through the semi-autonomous brushstroke and other signifiers of in- and interdependence. While this lens might seem to cement a historical refusal to accord women artists and professionals the same autonomy, agency, self-sufficiency and mastery which their male counterparts have been presumed to possess, I see Bell and Moralt's collaborative endeavours as embodying alternatives to those paradigms and attesting to the messy complexities of modern art, life, and medicine. I take seriously James Herbert's critique of the way art history has tended to assume male artists' agency and his reminder that agency is 'an emergent tactic – always partial and never certain; a maneuver, not an essence' (2015: 95). Bell's and Moralt's histories demonstrate that medical authority, too, is a matter of ongoing negotiation.

The pair's experience at Charleston in 1919 was emblematic of women's more protracted struggles for authority and some degree of autonomy in the period. Such contestations were intimately familiar to both of them. Bell was, as she mockingly described herself, 'that terrible low creature, a female painter' (1997: 118) in a male-dominated art world. And despite Bloomsbury's generally progressive politics, the demands of her roles as wife, mother, lover, manager of a household and professional artist entailed compromise (Elliott and Wallace 1994: 79). Moralt, a graduate of the London Royal Free Hospital School of Medicine for Women, had held posts at various London hospitals during the war but almost certainly suffered from the postwar backlash against women doctors and medical students, which reduced admissions and barred them from many positions, leading her to set up in private practice (Taylor 1932; Dyhouse 1998b). It is perhaps unsurprising, given the circumstances, that Bell and Moralt developed a relationship which lasted over a decade. Bell considered her 'sensible and quite easy to say anything to, which is more than most doctors are' (1998b: 230). Moralt's interest in modern art undoubtedly helped; she patronized the Omega Workshops, the Post-Impressionist home furnishings firm founded by Fry, Bell, and Grant in 1913 (Bell 1998b: 230; Taylor 1932: 67).

In May 1919, Moralt returned to Charleston for a check-up on mother and child, and on that occasion, she sat for a half-length portrait by Bell, one of several material manifestations of their inventive and attentive solidarity I examine here. The portrait was not commissioned by and never belonged to Moralt, but she was a willing and cooperative sitter; Bell described her as 'simply wonderful to paint' (Shone 1976: 193).[2] In the painting, which exhibits Bell's 'austerely simple and direct' manner (Fry 1922: 237) and muted postwar palette, Moralt is depicted frontally, seated in a wooden chair before a grey wall (Figure 22.1). The bulk of the canvas is dedicated to her torso, a substantial, ovoid form built up through layers of clothing beneath a small, serious-looking face with a somewhat abstracted expression. Moralt wears a dark hat with a black ribbon, a thick fur collar over a black jacket or cardigan and no jewellery. Although her attire is not recognizably medical garb, it reflects the professionalization of women in the period. Her shirtwaist, typical of white-collar female workers, is conspicuous in its lack of feminizing lace or frills, and her hat is similarly plain. Historian Carol Dyhouse's research into medical education for women in Britain has shown that female medical students and doctors generally dressed in a way which downplayed signifiers of femininity to signal their seriousness

[2]She sat for Grant at the same time, who often painted side by side with Bell. A letter of 23 May 1919 shows that she also sat for Fry later the same month (Fry 1972: 452). She posed again for Bell and Grant in December, as drawings by Grant attest (Shone 1999: 188). It is beyond the scope of this essay to analyse the portrait by Grant, which is less finished than Bell's and was considered unsatisfactory, as portions of the painted surface were folded back to obscure the sitter's hands and part of the background, but, as will become evident below, Moralt's collaborations with Bell extended to Grant as well. Nevertheless, her relationship with the Bloomsbury group was anchored in Bell.

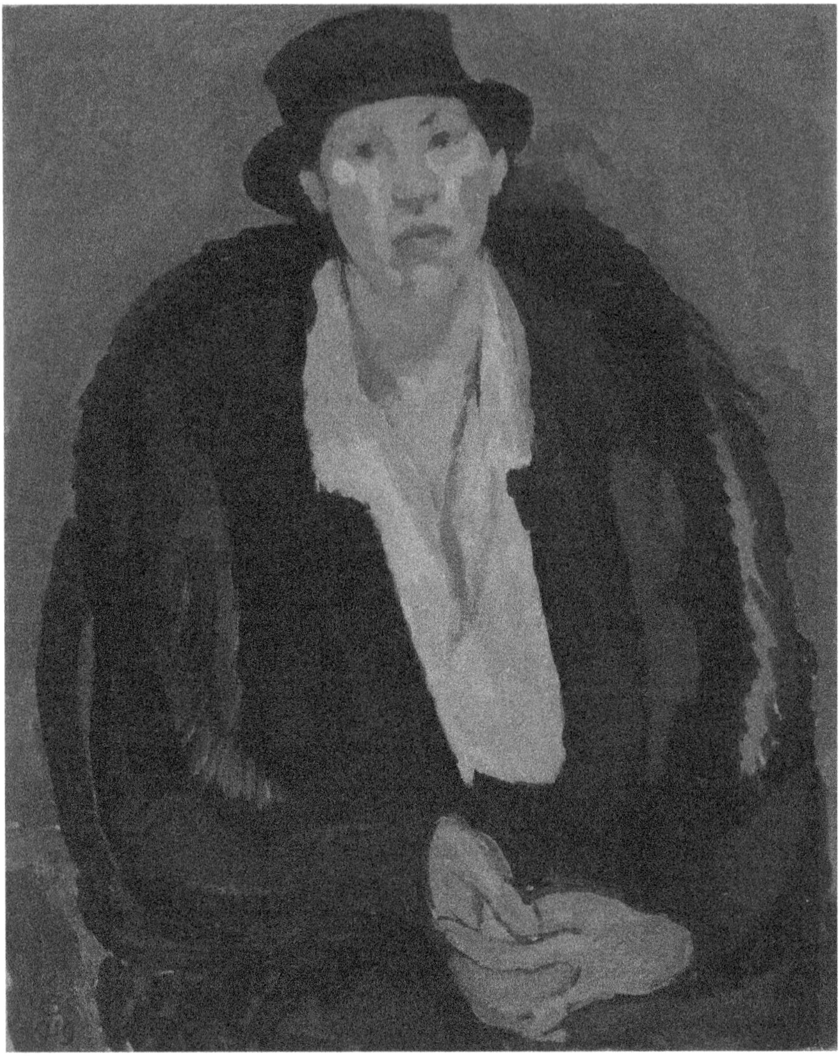

FIGURE 22.1 Vanessa Bell, *Dr Marie Moralt*, 1919. Oil on canvas, 68.2 × 56.8 cm, Fitzwilliam Museum. © Vanessa Bell / DACS, London / CARCC Ottawa 2024.

(Dyhouse 1998a). For many women, navigating the medical profession entailed wearing 'a severe style of dress and the plainest of hats' (Malleson 1919: 24–25).[3]

[3]Bell's painting gives Moralt's dress considerable pictorial weight, perhaps because of her own professional engagement with clothing. While Bell, in her artistic milieu, dressed rather differently than Moralt, she had, during the 19-teens, taken up designing dresses for the Omega Workshops, and as Wendy Hitchmough has argued, her Omega dresses 'rejected conventional ideals of prettiness' and cultivated an air of 'intellectual gravitas' as well as Bohemianism, partially in response to Gertrude Stein's example (2020: 101, 98). Both Bell and Moralt, in other words, cultivated simplified forms of dress that helped them navigate their professional milieux.

The task of portraiture is to capture something of the inner character as well as the outer appearance of the sitter, and if Bell's portrait subtly intimates Moralt's professionalism via external trappings, it also suggests the painter's probing beneath the surface. Various critics have observed that Bell's portrait is inward-focused, one writing that this is a painting of a 'real', 'grown-up' woman who has 'suffered and adjusted and made allowances', and that she is portrayed with 'knowing, affectionate solidarity' (MacCarthy 1999). Bell had painted professional women before, and Bridget Elliott and Jo-Ann Wallace argue that such portraits, made between 1912 and 1919, including paintings of Woolf, often have 'curiously featureless and dissolving faces', which they link to the tensions attached to women's professionalization during this period (1994: 61). Grace Brockington points out that if features in these works are obfuscated to some degree, they are never entirely absent, and contends the paintings place a double emphasis on 'the formal and the psychological' (2013: 148). Bell's portrait of Moralt is not as featureless as those of Woolf; the face is not dissolving, exactly, or not only. But the portrait does similarly conflate formal, psychological and even anatomical layering.

When Bell exhibited the painting in her solo show at the Independent Gallery in 1922, Fry singled it out in his review, calling it 'the most brilliant thing in the whole exhibition', which showcased what he considered Bell's quality of 'allow[ing] the motive to unfold itself gradually to the apprehension' (Fry 1922: 238, 237). The face's painterly construction is fully on display, in the flush Bell renders on Moralt's cheeks, which is framed by conspicuous brushstrokes of a pale flesh colour which simultaneously model bone structure and hover as patches of paint on the surface of the canvas; in the accretion of flesh-coloured facets alongside and over blue and green ones in the chin; and in the furry strokes shaping upper lip and nose. If this painterly composition of feature and face allows the motif to unfold, it also gestures to some of the tensions in Moralt's, and, implicitly, Bell's, inhabiting of their embodied identities. While there is likeness here, there is also slippage and blur. The face is caught between being put on or coming into being and threatening to dissolve. The brushwork, which in places hints at the écorché tradition with its glimpses beneath the flesh-paint even as it foregrounds Bell's modernist credentials, suggests that substance, flesh, and face can be lost as well as gained, literally and figuratively – our capacity to be discomposed, anatomized in diverse settings and, eventually, decomposed. The sitter's patient and painter looked at Moralt with a gaze both diagnostic and empathetic of the psychological and physical effort that living and selving, professional and otherwise, entailed.

I write physical advisedly, for one of the most striking features of Bell's rendering of Moralt's face is the hectic flush of her cheeks. An ambiguous sign, flushing may be an index of pleasure, embarrassment, health, or illness. Here the rose-coloured marks can read both as surface and depth, vitality and ailment. However ambiguous the painterly mark is, in reality, Moralt was ill, as Bell knew. She had suffered from chronic bronchitis, a type of obstructive pulmonary disease that in her case was a 'serious physical disability', from childhood (B. 1931: 9). One of her obituaries mentions that 'the periodic acute attacks, which interrupted her work as a student, made it seem unlikely that she would ever be able to practice medicine' (Taylor 1932: 66). She did qualify, though, and practised for a decade before her last few years were spent travelling for lung treatments and to stay in more congenial climates, including at Bell's house in Cassis in 1930 (Shone 1999: 188), until she died of tuberculosis in 1931. Moralt's ill health was apparent during her first stay at Charleston, Bell writing at the time that her chronic bronchitis 'threatens to become acute at any moment!' (1998: 229), Garnett observing that Charleston was 'doing her good' (1955: 196). In July 1919, when Moralt returned to vaccinate Angelica, she walked the three miles from the station at Glynde and 'almost collapsed en route & wouldn't eat anything' (Bell 1919b). The doctor's health and substance were fragile; the care went both ways. The country air and Bell's ministrations – which her mother's example and the 1883 book *Notes from Sick Rooms* would have taught her were a form of 'art' (Stephen 1883: 2) – doubtless helped Moralt.[4] But the portrait, with its ambiguous indices of both frailty and solid vitality, may also be seen as a form of care: a means of lavishing attention on Moralt's embodiment and professional identity, one that gave the subject breathing room, as it were, through a pose that offered repose, and sittings that created space and stillness for her to compose herself.

Bell's female figures tend to be depicted with reddened cheeks, but they signify differently in each instance. An artistic epiphany in 1912 paved the way for her portrait of Moralt. While suffering from measles in Italy that year, she played with paper mosaics, gluing pieces of cut, coloured paper onto board – an activity that led to a formal shift in her painting. After returning to England, she wrote on 5 June 1912 that she was 'trying to paint as if I were mosaicking, not by painting in spots, but by considering the picture as patches, each one of which has to be filled by one definite space of colour, as one has to do with mosaic or woolwork, not allowing myself to brush the patches into each other' (Bell 1998a: 119). The painting *Byzantine Lady* from the same year depicts a model, in strict profile, in Byzantine-inspired attire. A bright red circular spot on the figure's whitened cheek emblematizes a form of face painting both theatrical and feminine, while the static pose and larger blocks of colour evoke Byzantine icons. According to Christopher Reed, Byzantine mosaics offered Bell 'a model for a modern idiom of power and permanence' (2004: 84). The construction, performance, and possibilities of feminine identity and agency are raised in the painting not only by the conspicuous make-up but also by the symbolic

---

[4]Julia Stephen's writing anticipates medical humanities scholar James Thompson's work and its attention to forms of 'artful care' and 'careful art' (Thompson 2023).

role of this elaborately dressed figure inspired by the mosaic of the Empress Theodora at Ravenna. Theodora was 'a paradigm in Bloomsbury's vision of a Byzantine-inflected modernism' (Reed 2004: 84), and the mosaics at Ravenna, which Bell visited in 1913 and again in 1926, became a touchstone for the group.

In 1919, long after Bloomsbury's romance with Byzantium had begun, Bell still drew on its precedent (and would continue to do so into the 1930s). Fiona McCarthy has described the portrait of Moralt as having a hieratic quality (1999), conjuring up the sacred and archaic in keeping with the Ravenna mosaics' precedent. The painting also exhibits a similar construction of visage: lighter flesh tones cup the eye on the right in both works, for instance, and although Bell's rectangular brushstrokes are larger than the mosaic's tesserae, both works juxtapose different-coloured patches of paint or stone; this mode of fabrication is particularly visible on Moralt's cheeks and chin. The Bloomsbury artists' familiarity with the mosaics was based on both first-hand experience and photographs. The Omega Workshops decorated its walls with framed photographic enlargements of details of mosaics from Ravenna ('Post Impressionist Flat' 1913: 3), and while the lighter eye-cup is particularly distinctive in situ, it is also evident in photographs such as the one of Theodora in Clive Bell's 1913 book *Art*. Frances Spalding regards the construction of the faces in Bell's portraits of Woolf, which veer away from naturalism, as a refusal to depict likeness at a particular date, thus opening up 'the formation of identity to both past and future' as well as 'the obscurities of the self' (2017: 69, 71). The 'mosaicking' brushwork of Moralt's portrait ties this formation of identity, in all its complexity, to a longer historical past and associative lineages than Spalding perhaps envisaged with her remark.

Bell's portrait of Moralt, then, makes use of semi-autonomous brushstrokes, signifiers of in- and interdependence that slip between painterly surface, representational duty and psychological depth as well as between face, with all its connotations, and physiology. They evoke 'power and permanence' along with infirmity and gesture to continuities between the tribulations of modern women and historical precursors. Just as importantly, they are a site of connection and differentiation between the painter and the doctor. Fry considered 'every touch' of Bell's brushwork an index of her 'complete absorption in the general theme' (Fry 1922: 237), an immersion which blurred boundaries between painter and subject. The very existence of the portrait, even before its attributes, embodies the affective entanglement between the two. But the portrait's intimations of warmth, respect, gratitude and solidarity are balanced by a certain reserve and graveness of the sort regularly attributed to Bell herself, whose 'lapidification of character' Leonard Woolf remarked upon (1964: 27). Bell, in other words, presents Moralt's, and implicitly her own, emergent autonomy through painterly allusion to mosaic precedent while acknowledging, through blur and flurry, the haptic quality of her strokes, the ineluctable partiality of the process. If Moralt's torso conveys 'the strength of a boulder', as one commentator has it (Go 2006: 138), the portrayal of her face betrays her corporeal vulnerability: lapidification of character can never be complete. Virginia Woolf succinctly articulated the nature of our only-ever-semi-autonomy in her diary on 15 September 1924: 'we're splinters and mosaics; not, as they used to hold, immaculate, monolithic, consistent wholes' (1977: 313–14).

The year 1919 was a time of change for both Bell and Moralt, who showed themselves open to new possibilities. The Omega closed, and Bell took on more decorative commissions in partnership with Grant. Moving out of hospitals into private practice, Moralt cultivated other passions – including politics and art – and connections. The most conspicuously unfinished part of her portrait is her clasped hands, and their unfixed, partially obfuscated forms suggest their multiple valences: they could examine and help care for infant and mother yet could also be put to other uses. For in addition to the injections and suturing of her medical practice, the doctor performed other sorts of needlework for, with, and outside of the Bloomsbury set. Two extant examples of Moralt's needlework are based on designs by Grant, one of them part of an interior co-designed by Bell and Grant. Moralt was almost certainly working on the first of these when the portrait was painted, for Bell wrote to Grant, 'Moralt has almost finished your embroidery... – it's certainly lovely quality' (1919b), referring to a fire screen based on a painted collage (Figure 22.2).

The act of translation from Grant's assemblage of cut, painted papers to the finished woolwork involved considerable sensitivity and decision-making on the part of the embroiderer. In the collage, a simplified orange fish (or duck) floats in a central pool in the shape of an irregular pentagon, which is framed by layers of coloured rectangles. Most of the papers are painted in a single, if modulated, hue, though several show chromatic layering and one at the bottom centre has noticeable divided red brushstrokes over a yellow ground. In the fire screen, Moralt's stitches follow the direction of Grant's brushwork in some places, for example in the long stitches of a bright orangey-pink vertical at the left. In others, she has chosen not to sew in the direction of the paint but selected stitches that create a comparable effect. In the greenish rectangle at the far right and the one that slopes upward from its top, she has used vertical chain stitch running perpendicular to Grant's semi-transparent brushwork. The parallel links of the vertical chains create their own horizontal striations, and the slight openings in the stitches create a subtle chromatic modulation that complements that of the multiple colours of wool. In the central horizontal rectangle along the bottom, Moralt has similarly managed to find a woolly language, of angled long stitches in different hues, to emulate Grant's conspicuous coloured brushstrokes. And although there has been significant fading of some of the dyed wools, a number of the rectangular sections of the embroidery incorporate multiple colours to suggest the differing intensities, contrasts,

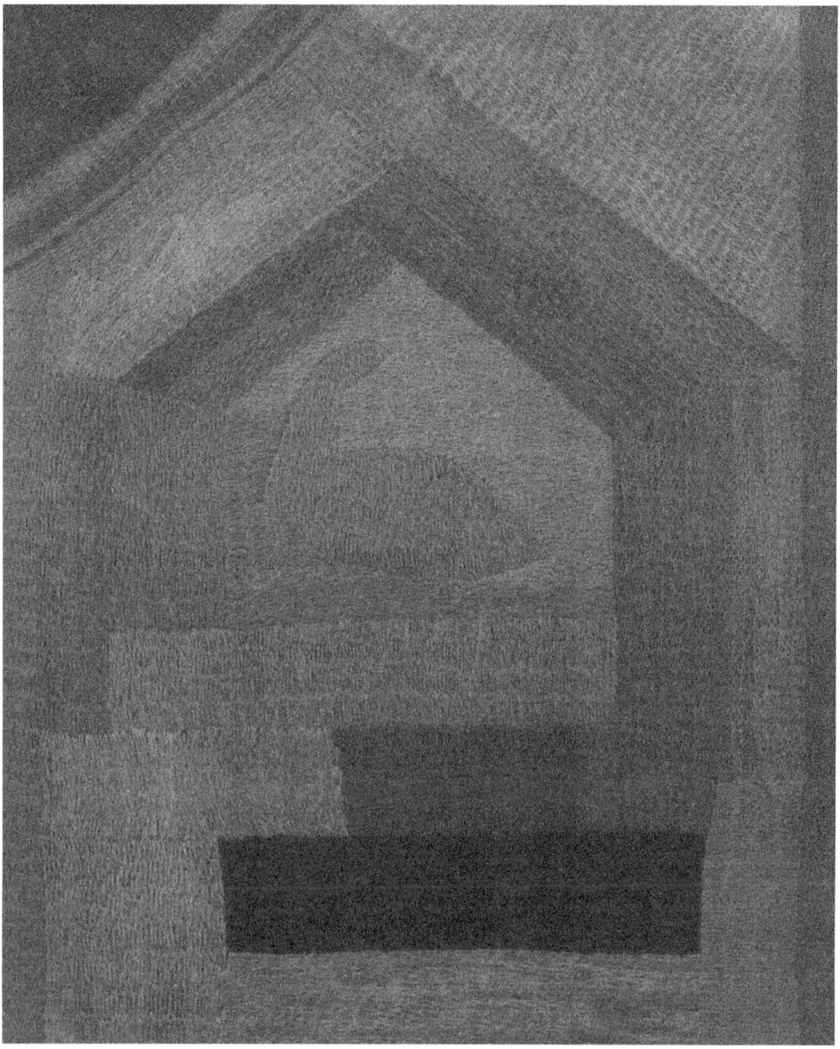

FIGURE 22.2 Firescreen designed by Duncan Grant and embroidered by Dr Marie Moralt, *c.* 1919. Polychrome wools stitched on linen canvas, 75 × 61 cm, Charleston Trust. © Duncan Grant / DACS, London / CARCC Ottawa 2024.

and flows evident in Grant's collage. Moralt would have worked most of the screen out of Grant and Bell's presence and made her own aesthetic decisions, including larger departures in the translation process than those described above. The goldfish or waterfowl at the heart of the composition is surrounded by a modulated blue in Grant's collage but a two-tone field in the fire screen, which works differently to signify a sense of light-filled, reflective space. Unsurprisingly, Bell lauded Moralt's ability to 'embroider[]

intelligently' (1919c). Like Bell's brushstrokes, Moralt's stitches were semi-autonomous.

The fire screen belonged to Maynard Keynes. Moralt also undertook woolwork, dated to 1920, that formed part of the redesign of his King's College rooms by Bell and Grant. The theme for the decoration was the muses of the Arts and Sciences, represented in eight painted panels by the two artists as four draped female figures and four male nudes (Reed 2004: 220–22). It is unclear which arts or sciences most of the figures represent, and the pair embraced this interchangeability: Bell wrote to Fry in August 1920 that 'they are supposed to represent law, science, history, etc. though you mightn't think it – in fact we're always changing their arts and their sciences' (Shone 1976: 234). For this fluid milieu, Moralt worked covers for the upholstered seat and back of an eighteenth-century chair in cross-stitch (Figure 22.3). Grant's design for the back consists of a still life of a ewer and a pear on a table in front of a window. Curtains framing the view at either side connect the chair to its architectural setting, for which Bell designed and made appliquéd curtains. The range of chromatic nuances Moralt would have had to effect are less visible today due to fading of some of the dyed wools, though the tabletop gives a sense of them. While Moralt's creativity and skill in needlework were required for the creation of the panel, the resonance of its iconography is of particular interest here. Reed has argued that 'the jug-and-fruit motif' became a kind of 'signature for Grant in this period', and that its inclusion on the chair was a way for Grant to mark the décor as partly his own (2004: 222). Partly is right, for in addition to the rooms being a Bell-Grant rather than a solo commission, the figure of the vase or jug was also historically a symbol of Mary. Moralt's first name (which appears as Mary in some documents) links her to that mother, and Bell frequently associated herself with the Madonna pictorially (Humm 2001: 123).[5] This indeterminate signature was sewn by Moralt into a collaborative project that celebrated and conflated doctors and artists of different kinds, and both imaged and materialized interdependencies, its very manufacture attesting to the interoperability of the arts and sciences.

Beyond its role as signature, though, the ewer as stitched by Moralt evokes and calls into question fantasies of plenitude and self-sufficiency. If Bell's portrait of Moralt builds up a sense of her solidity (and, implicitly, autonomy) through paint and material allusion, without definitively securing them, the vessel in the chairback functions similarly. Its upright form ostensibly holds wine, its swelling form suggesting abundance. Yet the coloured interior of the ewer also reads as sand running through its hour-glass shape. The liquid or solid identity of its contents forever suspended in the woolly medium, the vessel simultaneously signals amplitude and presence, on the one hand, and

[5]Bell's mother had modelled for Mary in Burne-Jones's 1879 *Annunciation* while pregnant with her. In the finished painting, she stands next to an elegant amphora.

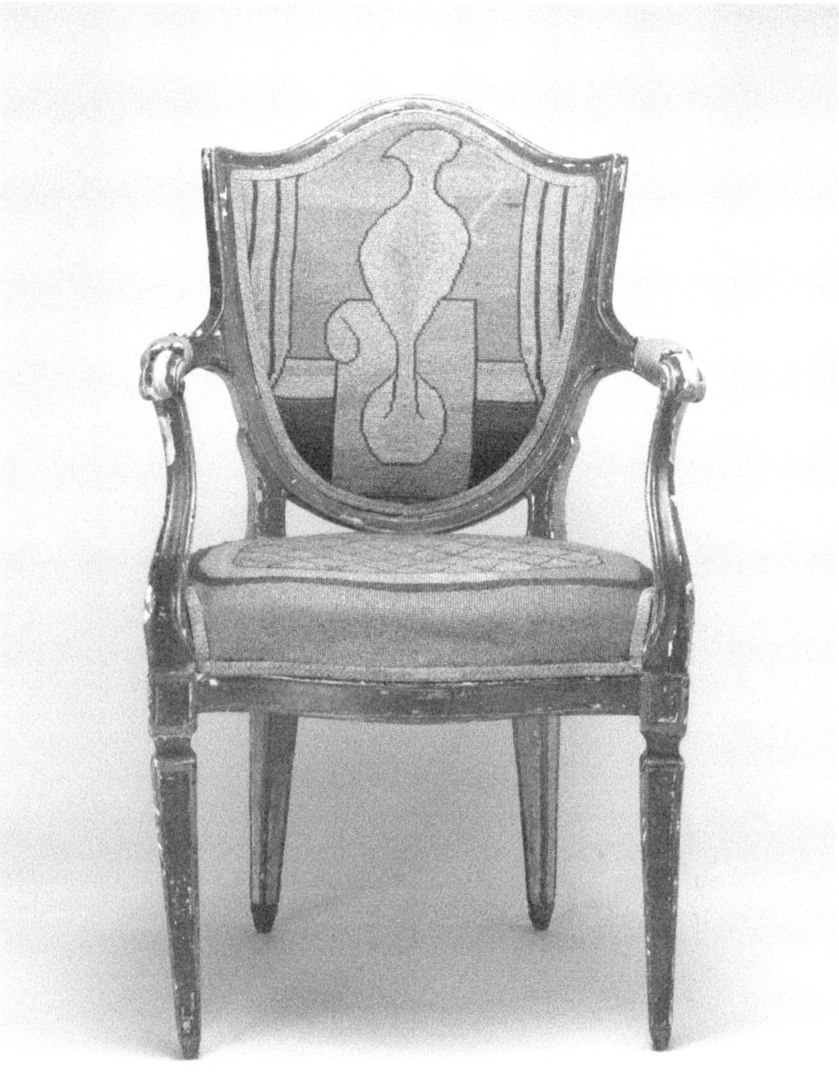

FIGURE 22.3 Needlework panels stitched by Dr Marie Moralt after a design by Duncan Grant, 1920. Polychrome wools, Fitzwilliam Museum. © Duncan Grant / DACS, London / CARCC Ottawa 2024.

ephemerality on the other, a still life conjuring thoughts of our mortality, our perishable substance. For Bell, the reality and connotations of substance – milk, flesh, paint, stone, wool – were tied to both artistic style and matters of care. Calibrating the right degree of substance was central to the case of the baby in what has been dubbed the 'nutritional drama' of January 1919 (Gill 2019: 318) that revolved around nursing and nourishing. Substance was also a criterion by which Fry evaluated Bell's paintings: he owned numerous works by her and in an April 1919 exchange of letters concerning Angelica's health, among other things, he described an early abstract work by Bell that had 'gone thin' on his hands and thus didn't mean anything to him anymore (Fry 1972: 449). And the vulnerability of women's substance – of their mattering and sufficiency in various senses – is registered in Bell's portrait of Moralt as well as the pair's other collaborations, as here.

Needlework in this period still carried connotations of feminine subservience, but it was also open to other associations. Fry liked it 'because it is so durable and strong' (B. 1913: 10). And as various historians including Joseph McBrinn have observed, it was prescribed to wounded soldiers in World War I 'as a form of rehabilitative therapy' for mind and body (2020: 73). McBrinn takes Woolf's well-known comment that 'knitting is the saving of life' as his starting point for a discussion of Bloomsbury needlework of all kinds as therapeutic, linking them not only to the textilic metaphors that are rife in Woolf's writing but also to Bell and Grant's woolwork designs. In addition to its somewhat contradictory associations of strength and recuperation, woolwork, particularly in projects like the ones just described, represented both communal and solitary, contemplative activity. In the quietude and solidarity of her needlework, Moralt stitched together her salubrious relationship with Bell, which offered friendship, care, artistic employment, and professional validation.[6] And through this needlework as well as her portrait of Moralt, Bell consolidated her understanding of her own practice as growing out of a particular medial matrix, or an intermedial dialogue that can itself be seen as embodying the collaboration between fine and applied arts that characterizes her oeuvre. The material and medial interchangeability implied in her description of her aim to treat 'the picture as patches, each one of which has to be filled by one definite space of colour, as one has to do with mosaic or woolwork', is evident in Moralt's portrait. Even in the most mosaic-evoking places in her complexion, Bell has used a series of parallel brushstrokes to create planes that can also appear furry or woolly. Her paint gestures toward stony autonomy, woolly warmth, and fleshly interdependence.

When Bell made her painting-in-patches analogy with needlework, she concluded, 'I think this ought to give something of the life one seems to get with mosaic' (1998a: 119). And it is life that Walter Sickert found in Bell's portrait of Moralt in his review of Bell's 1922 exhibition. In his meditation on painting in general as well as Bell's in particular, he describes

[6]Bell and Moralt's careful acts of attentiveness and their material manifestations suggest, as Des Fitzgerald and Felicity Callard have it, that 'holistic understandings of the body, as well as its illnesses, require much richer conceptions of both doctoring and healing' (2016: 38).

the phenomenon that can occur 'under accomplished fingers', wherein the painter becomes 'a conduit for strange insights greater than, and outside himself'. While a female painter could hardly ignore the default 'he' in this formulation and the art world at large, the idea of the painter as conduit for that which is not exclusively self surely resonated. Sickert sums up his, or Bell's, insight as follows: 'The subject of painting is, perhaps, that it is not death. It is, perhaps, nothing more' (1922: 34). That the portrait of Moralt is not death, or rather, is life in its ongoing dance with death, was true for Bell: it represented the life of her daughter, of Moralt herself, and of Bell's own return to a life of art, all of which had to be nurtured collaboratively. Woolf noted in her diary on 5 March 1919 that Grant was painting but not her sister, who had to wash bottles and nappies, prepare meals, and manage the servants (1977: 249), attesting to the gendered distribution of labour in Bloomsbury as well as more normative households. The month of May and this portrait marked Bell's return to art.

In his review, Sickert also posited that 'It is love alone that clings to what is unique and unusual in its object, and makes, of what are called defects, a *desiderium*' (1922: 34), and we can read the brushwork of Moralt's flushed cheeks in this relatively unidealized depiction as traces of affection as much as a dissecting gaze, as recognition of the mutable body. A decade later, when she was very ill and receiving treatment for her worsening lungs at Bad Reichenhall, Moralt wrote a letter to her friend Noël Olivier, 'My life creeps wretchedly along. I wish I had a husband and two children. I wish I hadn't got emphysema. I wish I had a job. I wish I could see you all' (1929). In her letter, Moralt describes a life and an 'I' whose meaning comes from a vocation and affective connection. She expresses a simultaneous desire for independence and dependents, for an ongoing, generative semi-autonomy. Her letter also speaks to the coexistence of life and the ever-present fact of death that Bell's painting of its black-clad figure, and Moralt's stitched ewer so eloquently embody: the fact that, at the end of the day, artistic and professional autonomy are tactics, sometimes tangents, and often phantasms and only ever part of the picture of our vulnerable mattering. The unexpected manifestations of Bell and Moralt's healthcare intimacies – what the lady doctor and the female painter created together – allowed these fragile threads to show.

Note: I am grateful to dress historian Alison Matthews David for discussing Moralt's attire with me and to Tamsin Majerus for permission to quote Moralt's letter, along with Sarah Watling for the connection. I also thank Emily Doucet, Miranda Purves, and Allison Morehead for their generous and insightful comments and suggestions.

References

B., A. (1931), 'Obituary. Dr. Moralt', *The New Age*, 5 November: 9–10.

B., M. M. (1913), 'Post-Impressionist Furniture', *Daily News and Leader*, 7 August: 10.

Bell, Q. (1997), 'A Vanished World', in Q. Bell and V. Nicholson (eds), *Charleston: A Bloomsbury House and Garden*, London: Frances Lincoln.

Bell, V. (1919a), letter to Duncan Grant, *c.* 6 July, Tate Gallery Archives 20078/1/44/94, London.

Bell, V. (1919b), letter to Duncan Grant, 11 July, Tate Gallery Archives 20078/1/44/96, London.

Bell, V. (1919c), letter to Duncan Grant, *c.* July, Tate Gallery Archives 20078/1/44/102, London.

Bell, V. (1995), letter to Margery Snowden, Christmas 1923, in A. Garnett, *Deceived with Kindness: A Bloomsbury Childhood*, London: Pimlico.

Bell, V. (1997), 'Memories of Roger Fry', in *Sketches in Pen and Ink: A Bloomsbury Notebook*, L. Giachero (ed.), 117–47, London: Hogarth Press/Chatto & Windus.

Bell, V. (1998a), letter to Roger Fry of 5 June 1912, in R. Marler (ed.), *Selected Letters of Vanessa Bell*, 118–20, Wakefield, RI: Moyer Bell.

Bell, V. (1998b), letter to Roger Fry of 6 February 1919, in R. Marler (ed.), *Selected Letters of Vanessa Bell*, 229–31, Wakefield, RI: Moyer Bell.

Brockington, G. (2013), 'A "Lavender Talent" or "The Most Important Woman Painter in Europe"? Reassessing Vanessa Bell', *Art History*, 36 (1): 128–53.

Chavasse, P. H. (1878), *Advice to a Mother on the Management of her Children and on the Treatment on the Moment of Some of their more Pressing Illnesses and Accidents*, London: J. and A. Churchill.

Dyhouse, C. (1998a), 'Driving Ambitions: Women in Pursuit of a Medical Education, 1890–1939', *Women's History Review*, 7 (3): 321–43.

Dyhouse, C. (1998b), 'Women Students and the London Medical Schools, 1914–1939: The Anatomy of a Masculine Culture', *Gender & History*, 10 (1): 110–32.

Elliott, B., and J. Wallace (1994), 'Professionalism, Genre, and the Sister(s') Arts: Virginia Woolf and Vanessa Bell', in *Women Artists and Writers: Modernist (Im)Positionings*, 56–89, London: Routledge.

Fitzgerald, D., and F. Callard (2016), 'Entangling the Medical Humanities', in A. Whitehead et al. (eds), *The Edinburgh Companion to the Medical Humanities*, 35–49, Edinburgh: Edinburgh University Press.

Fry, R. (1922), 'Vanessa Bell and Othon Friesz', *The New Statesman*, 3 June: 237–38.

Fry, R. (1972), *The Letters of Roger Fry*, vol. 2, Denys Sutton (ed.), London: Chatto & Windus.

Garnett, D. (1955), *The Flowers of the Forest, Being Volume Two of The Golden Echo*, London: Chatto & Windus.

Gill, G. (2019), *Virginia Woolf and the Women Who Shaped Her World*, Boston, MA: Houghton Mifflin Harcourt.

Go, K. (2006), 'Artistic Expression, Domestic Desires: Vanessa Bell's Vision of Modern Life and Modern Art', PhD diss., Cambridge University.

Herbert, J. (2015), *Brushstroke and Emergence: Courbet, Impressionism, Picasso*, Chicago: University of Chicago Press.
Hitchmough, W. (2020), *The Bloomsbury Look*, New Haven: Yale University Press.
Humm, M. (2001), 'The Domestic Photography of Virginia Woolf and Vanessa Bell: Modernism, the Erotic and the Maternal', in M. Barbeito (ed.), *Feminism, Aesthetics and Subjectivity: Essays on Women and Culture in Early Twentieth Century British Literature*, 99–130, Santiago de Compostela: Universidade de Santiago de Compostela.
MacCarthy, F. (1999), 'A radical regained', *The Guardian*, 23 October: https://www.theguardian.com/theguardian/1999/oct/23/weekend7.weekend3?CMP=share_btn_link
Malleson, H. (1919), *A Woman Doctor*, London: Sidgwick & Jackson.
McBrinn, J. (2020), '"Knitting is the saving of life; Adrian has taken it up too": Needlework, Gender, and the Bloomsbury Group', in J. Amos and L. Binkley (eds), *Stitching the Self: Identity and the Needle Arts*, 67–79, London: Bloomsbury.
Moralt, M. (1929), letter to Noël Olivier, collection of Tamsin Majerus, London.
'A Post Impressionist Flat: What Would the Landlord Say?' (1913), *The Daily Mirror*, 8 November: 3.
Reed, C. (2004), *Bloomsbury Rooms: Modernism, Subculture, and Domesticity*, New Haven: Published for the Bard Graduate Center for Studies in the Decorative Arts, Design, and Culture by Yale University Press.
Shone, R. (1999), *The Art of Bloomsbury: Roger Fry, Vanessa Bell and Duncan Grant*, New Jersey: Princeton University Press.
Shone, R. (1976), *Bloomsbury Portraits: Vanessa Bell, Duncan Grant, and Their Circle*, London: Phaidon.
Sickert, W. (1922), 'Vanessa Bell', *Burlington Magazine for Connoisseurs* 41 (232): 33–4.
Spalding, F. (1983), *Vanessa Bell*, San Diego: Harcourt Brace Jovanovich.
Spalding, F. (2017), 'Among Friends: Vanessa, Virginia, and the Modern Portrait', in S. Milroy and I.A.C. Dejardin (eds), *Vanessa Bell*, London: Philip Wilson Publishers for the Dulwich Picture Gallery.
Stephen, Mrs L. (1883), *Notes from Sick Rooms*, London: Smith, Elder, and Co.
Taylor, L. D. (1932), 'Marie Moralt, M.B., B.S.', *The Medical Women's Federation News-letter*, January: 66–7.
Thompson, J. (2023), *Care Aesthetics: For Artful Care and Careful Art*, Abingdon: Routledge.
Watling, S. (2019), *The Olivier Sisters: A Biography*, Oxford: Oxford University Press.
Woolf, L. (1964), *Beginning Again: An Autobiography of the Years 1911–1918*, London: Hogarth Press.
Woolf, V. (1976), letter to Katherine Arnold-Foster of 5 February 1919 in N. Nicholson and J. Trautmann (eds), *The Question of Things Happening: The Letters of Virginia Woolf, Volume* 2: *1912–1922*, London: Hogarth Press.
Woolf, V. (1977), *The Diary of Virginia Woolf*, A. O. Bell (ed.), New York: Harcourt Brace Jovanovich.

CHAPTER TWENTY-THREE

Flight as method: a *Sick Women* exchange in material encounters, and the time it takes to care

Gemma Blackshaw and Alice Butler

'It's kind of spectral', writes the poet Eileen Myles in their foreword to the book of visual correspondence enacted by Moyra Davey (b. 1958) with Peter Hujar (1934–1987): 'But in the enormity of time in this graveyard (or in the work of these two photographers) you can do anything you want' (Davey and Hujar 2021: n.p.). Davey described her staging of this dialogue-beyond-death as 'a risky act' (ibid.). Lingering in Hujar's archive, placing works in new proximities, responding with images of her own, this photographic 'conversation' comprises transmissions across time, space, sickness and care: the grey foam of a wave at Jones Beach Island that is a Hujar waterscape that is also life and death.

Myles is writing for the book that commemorated the Berlin-based exhibition *Moyra Davey Peter Hujar*, which they could not fly to see after its closure during the COVID-19 pandemic. Myles describes printing 'the pictures out' and restaging 'some parts of the show right there on that empty wall at the end of the bed' (ibid.). The intense nowness of this practice is distorted by the poet's looking at the artists' pictures within a domestic space not dissimilar to Davey's own citational illness narratives on film, conjuring not only the grief of the photographic image itself, but also the loss of Hujar, who died of an AIDS-related illness in 1987: engulfed by an epidemic which would take out so many more of his artist-friends.

Davey's 'cross-generational (cross-dimensional?)' (Wilkie 2021) correspondence with Hujar – and Myles's situated gaze at it – across Downtown apartments, an ocean, an archive, a letter, two essays and blank pages, inspires the '*Sick Women*' exchange that follows: a series of 'flights' which have been formed by more than one correspondent. It is an epistolary essay that expands our collaborative letter writing project – 'Sick Women: correspondences and performances' (2020–ongoing) – which develops a multiform, multidisciplinary approach to its embodied, critical and theoretical investigation of sickness, gender and cross-historical correspondence and care. Throughout we have been indebted to Johanna Hedva's 'Sick Woman Theory' (2016/2022) – a manifesto-essay for a subject of 'many guises', representing all of the 'un-cared for, the secondary, the oppressed, the non-, the un-, the less than'; it is a text that in its embodied materiality, citational form and affective register has also inspired the intimate politics of how we address our '*Sick Women*' historical subjects – artists and muses from across the twentieth century.

In this exchange we also attend to the neglected, uncared-for properties and textures of our archival materials, summoning a practice of the *shabby* which echoes the title of Davey and Hujar's correspondence book, *The Shabbiness of Beauty*. Through this material-epistolary lens, we circle and theorize affective, alternative forms of knowing and historicizing that register and revitalize the potentials of temporally deviant care. Our flights are visioning, haptic thought experiments; they are projections through the air and not; they are temporal, spatial, material movements *in writing*, however suspended, distracted or belated. In non-linear murmurations that mix tenses and timelines, swirling above the physical and digital locations of our research, these flights spend time with the 'archives of feeling' (Carland and Cvetkovich 2013: 70–77), which are attached to the sticky, shabby lives and works of the sickened subjects we seek across methodological encounters of looking, waiting and writing.

We write to each other about our flights to, from and between a further two addressees: Cookie Mueller (writer, actress, portrait sitter, 1949–1989) and Liliana Amon (writer, actress, portrait sitter, 1892–1939), 'sick women' whom we bring together across time in letter-like visual and textual flights of synchronicity, serendipity and resonance. Specifically, in our letters to each other (around which we have also meditated on the ecological meets maternal anxieties of air travel; remembrances of reading Davey's *Mother Reader* on a flight while seven months pregnant), we dare *to look* at them as the mother and not-quite mother; to wait with them and the pressure-points for thought that they pose; and to do so in the endurance, remembrance, belatedness and ongoing goodbyes of our writing-as-flight, which in turn revitalizes the complexities of our sick women subjects' sickened lives, works, bodies and minds, their creativities and cares.

A note to our readers: neither of the images we write about are illustrated here; they are held in the collections of the Morgan Library and Museum (Peter Hujar Collection) and the Leopold Museum. We encourage your own flights of imagination and visioning from our descriptions of our encounters with them, focusing attention instead on Cookie and Liliana's writing, and our own writing-as-method.

Flight 1

May 2023

It's my last day in New York before I fly home. It could be my last archive trip of the year.

Despite being in the US to research the archives of others, I can't stop communing with Cookie. She surfaced in a black leather journal embossed with '1990 Appointments'. It belonged to her friend, the artist who made Schiele-inspired stuffed nylon dolls using surgical stitches, Greer Lankton. I found a lined back page strung with a sketched list in black and blue inks. The list begins 'Dead from AIDS'; it ends in a comma, hanging expectant and waiting in the hardening time of sickness and care, its negative space. Just one horizontal line apart: Peter Hujar and Cookie Mueller.

I recall the appointments they shared. I dream of appointments made possible *in the beyond death of writing* as I arrive for another kind of appointment: with a student-turned-curatorial-fellow at the Morgan Museum and Library. It is our first encounter meeting in person after the pandemic. I've come to the side entrance of the library to meet with her because she's working with the contact sheets of Hujar's archive, its sideways, slantwise pieces.

Previously, we'd talked about Nan Goldin's *The Cookie Portfolio* over Zoom – its handwritten accompaniments to fifteen colour images documenting the maternal holdings, queer kinships, pleasures, pains, and sickened precarities of the writer-actress's life and death.

It was a surprise and a gift when a snapshot arrived in my inbox months later: a never-before-seen contact sheet comprising Hujar's greyscale, interior, intimate portraits of Cookie. Receiving this surreptitious letter felt contagious: a spectral transmission of Cookie's illegitimate acts of librarianship, which the eternal-adolescent re-enacted in retrospective, piecemeal writing. In 'My Bio – Notes on an American Childhood', Cookie describes smuggling her handmade historical novel – which narrativized the world of care-worker Clara Barton ('the American version of Florence Nightingale') and was finished 'the day before [her]

11th birthday' – onto the local library's 'shelves in the correct alphabetical order' (Mueller 1990: 141).

I think of this story as a 'resource of survival' for Cookie in the precarious, then sickening, present of her writing, its own relation of radical care, to cite Eve Sedgwick's return to the queer excesses, mysteries and pleasures of high and low cultural attachments in childhood, found in the 1993 essay 'Queer and Now', which was published in the 'omnipresence of somatic fear and wrenching loss' that was the continuing AIDS emergency at this time (3), only four years on from Cookie's death from AIDS-related causes in November 1989. In chronic, then terminal, *sick time*: Cookie returned to the story of her adolescent novel belatedly, composing and re-composing it in a collection of multiple parts, amounting to an unfinished novel.

I gasped when I opened the contact sheet. First, I turned away. I struggled to look at Cookie naked, resplendent, erotic, side by side with the rawness of her mothering. Was this withdrawal of my gaze an act of care? Or shame? Or *both*? I did not download the unsanctioned image to my files that day.

But now I'm in the archive, I stay with the trouble of her: seven pages of three columns and four rows (likely two film rolls in one dragged-out sitting), documenting the trials, experiments, encounters, surprises and interruptions of a day-long session in a studio, which appears like a salon, at times just a living room, its bodies strewn across a bed covered in black-and-white fabrics: striped pillows, polka dot throw, undone sheets. I feel unsure of how to read these photographic things, how to 'fit' them into my research, how to neaten them up by making them legible to a concept, these episodic images of a white woman reclining – '*nude*' – performing the horizontal dance of an eroticized figure, and more banally of a dressed mother at work, juggling the needs of her young son, Max, who is seeking the attention of the lens. I sense all kinds of embodied labour in these shifting acts, the tangled mess of art and life: an experimental film.

It unravels in slow frames a version of Cookie stripped back, unclothed, partially submerged in her close friend and creative partner's sheets. He photographed her inside and outside (clothed and naked); from the salon stuffed with cotton sheets to the Manhattan rooftop that backdropped her sky-high wedding in lace. She would write beside Hujar too, in loving correspondence, affinity and with the affirmation of a mother; as she propositioned in *Details* magazine: 'What else do I have to say? He's one of the best artists in the world' (Mueller 1986). It was a gesture of political resistance and community formation – a reply to the contact and light in his tender, *mothering* images of her – in the stigmatizing absence of medical funding, research and treatment for people living with AIDS.

In devotion to this devotional practice, I pluck up the courage to look again at her illumined naked body (save for the gold rings on her right hand, the bangles stacked on her left wrist), her penetrating stare, her loose, matted blonde hair (the same locks I've long copied) – captured in the quiet hum of black-and-white, not the fireworks of Goldin's colour (the hues in which I've long placed her, and loved her in letters). Somehow, it's different with the contact sheets: these minor, intimate, private, expectant, scrappy, shabby (but also careful and full-of-care) *preliminary* things, which denote rectangular pieces of paper (for printing, for writing) and which etymology suggests is rooted in the verb 'to project'. A contact sheet is a projection of light writing, an imaginative surface, an image-to-come. Not quite. Not yet. It is close to the intimacy of a cloth covering at home, or in the hospital, or more likely spaces in-between. And like the letters-in-letters of our archive, the contact sheet is multiple, shifting; comprising images-in-images, like the enchantment of being born with eggs which might make a child-to-come, bound by cellular connectivity. With her son nearby and her friend beside her, Cookie is communing in the commons of this photographic apprenticeship.

From 45 degrees to full frontal.
She's holding me here.
Dead on.
Exposing all my letters addressed to her.

Flight 2

June 2024, January 2018, November 2019; all the yearly returns

I had flown to Vienna in the third trimester of my second pregnancy, to work in the archive of the Josephinum museum for the history of medicine. I had left my three-year-old at home with my mother. The work I was doing had started soon after their birth, ebbing and flowing through those first years of parenting – ebbing and flowing still, submitted to as tidal, such are the changing/unchanging labours of care. The work concerned a set of drawings of 1910 by Egon Schiele (1890–1918), completed in one of the two new Women's Clinics for gynaecology and obstetrics at the University of Vienna General Hospital, which had opened two years previously. Schiele's girlfriend, Liliana, was receiving antenatal care there. While visiting, Schiele drew the pregnant and labouring women on the ward: bodies divided by hospital gowns and raised on hospital beds; undulating, pulsing, full-term bellies circumnavigated with a line so swift and sure it never fails to unnerve me – artist's charcoal as surgeon's scalpel, in all its irreparable potential. Though it may not be Liliana, there is one sheet that summons Liliana; a sheet which instrumentalizes Schiele's immense ability to convey through alternately soft and hard charcoal, the individual – vividly drawn, irrefutably known, *her*, surely, channelling her lived experience through his materials, methods and marks.

Looking at this sheet unframed in the conservation room of the Leopold Museum in November 2019 (nearly two years after the Josephinum visit – the research swells, recedes), I found myself incapable of engaging in the art historical analysis I had returned to Vienna to do: how did this drawing replicate the paper, charcoal and watercolour, the composition, line and form of others I had seen from Schiele's time in the clinic, contributing to a technically and aesthetically coherent whole; how, then, could it be deployed to think about what I was proposing in academic papers of the time as Schiele's 'clinical modernism'?[1] I faltered, made self-conscious by the model's absolute sense of herself, a subjectivity produced by the most inconspicuous of details: the ring that rests between knuckle and nail, being too small now to slide down her swollen finger; a ring I could imagine her twisting, tapping, *testing*; returning to as a circular window on to an interiorized view, as something to look at whenever it became necessary to look away. The ring was the punctum, as Lauren Berlant and Kathleen Stewart describe it, meaning 'whatever grabs you into an elsewhere of form' (2019: 5), but I pushed it away. In doing so, I also refused the directness of her stare (which is not the same as her gaze through that window of my flight) at me, the viewer-artist-doctor between her knees. To lock eyes with this subject – to wonder about her worrying of this ring – was to submit to the risky, critically speculative work that would become so much a part of our sick feminist art history of attention, affect and care. I wasn't ready to do it. I/she/we had to wait.

You write of your confrontation with Cookie, her 'penetrating stare', ringed in (char)kohl, at you and your letters. It has taken time to look back, and this has been my experience too. I could not meet the eyes of the model who may or may not have been Liliana, observing my observation, as she had observed Schiele's, and the doctors', which Schiele's position while drawing invokes. Shame-faced, I looked instead to the side of her, focusing on everything Schiele had left out; on nothing, then, but the blank paper ground upon which I projected the unpublished photographs I had discovered the previous year in the Josephinum, of the clinical environment and apparatus in use through Liliana's care that Schiele, in his modernism, had erased.

I reasoned that to turn to the negative space which surrounds the model was to devote my time and attention to the regulatory powers at work in her blind spot. It was to think about new clinical instruments for viewing the outside and inside of her body; about new clinical protocols on the concealing of her view of her body, and those of other bodies – of medical staff and patients – through the sheet and screen; about new clinical hierarchies which asserted the authority of the doctor over that of

[1]See Gemma Blackshaw, 'Egon Schiele's Clinical Modernism', *Artistry in the Spaces of Medicine*, convened by Mary Hunter and Natasha Ruiz-Gómez, Association of Art History, Annual Conference, University of Sussex, 2019.

the midwife; and about new clinical modes of representation including the drawn, fragmented illustrations of the surgical experiments in obstetrics and gynaecology that were conducted on those who could not afford to pay for treatment. But it was not to think with any newness about Schiele's model – 'Liliana' – as a subject; a process which would entail a meeting of her eyes, a fantasized projection through looking and writing, a *flight through affect* to imagine the drawing as an encounter in time – in that clinic, Schiele and Liliana – and across time – Liliana and me, in the conservation room, my books, my phone; wherever I saw the drawing reproduced.

Berlant and Stewart's thoughts on the punctum are contained in one of their 'exercises in following out the impact of things (words, thoughts, people, objects, ideas, worlds)', which is titled 'Dilations'; in the same piece, they argue that encounters 'are not events of knowing' (2019: ix; 5). Sometimes, they say, encounters 'stage a high-intensity tableau of the way things are or could become', performative work which 'pushes and follows histories out' (5). I struggled to engage in this work of dilating, pushing, following out. Ultimately, without such 'dead on' encountering, as you describe of Cookie, my work felt like a re-inscription of what I was attempting to critique: the clinic's scopic regime which screened, which partitioned, dividing the body into pieces.

I didn't write the article on Schiele's hospital drawings that the editor of *Art History* had invited me to submit. Was I stopping or was I waiting? Schiele's drawing is a scene of waiting. Liliana waits, too. For what? For whom?

Flight 3

Valentine's Day, 2024

It's February now, and I'm getting ready to pass the manuscript onto the publisher. It's what I've been waiting for.[2] I've grown up with and alongside the delayed birth of its writing, as I've grown into my desire with and alongside Cookie. For so long it was the wild glow of her writing, her life, her image, which led me to the light of things. Now, before I say goodbye to her, as I know I must, in an act of therapeutic closure which feels something like care, I can't shake the need – although it is difficult, although it is vulnerable – to stay with the mess and love and contradictions of her mothering; a part of her embodied, creative life, including the 'adolescent' productions she assembled and re-assembled in her sick time, so often erased, or neglected, 'partitioned' as you say (including by me). She asked me to on that day in

[2]See Alice Butler's forthcoming monograph on Kathy Acker and Cookie Mueller, Duke University Press.

the archive when she also recognized the mess and love and contradictions of my love letters to her. It was, I have come to realize, a necessary exposure.

How might I try to look back at her *in reply*, to stay with her – the most intimate version of Cookie I'd ever seen – with the kind of attentive tenderness David Wojnarowicz emitted in his reciprocal encounter with Peter Hujar's hospitalized deathbed? In images and words, Wojnarowicz devotedly, determinedly, directly 'looked' at his friend's 'body… completely still' with an intensity of proximity and accompaniment that 'his death is as if it's printed on celluloid on the backs of my eyes' (1991: 102). In this gesture of grieving care and 'form' (100), Wojnarowicz closes the door on medicalized knowledges, apparatuses and scopic regimes: 'the sounds of nurses and hospital gurneys far away in the halls' (86). Hardly an 'event of knowing' – instead, like Berlant and Stewart's strange and speculative absorptions, he holds the 'flight' (and 'light') of 'spirituality', as the eyes of the dead and living meet; and 'the water comes from my eyes' (103).

Is Cookie a sexual body in the sheets? A sensual body? A maternal body? A contagious body? Somehow, the images become less 'explicit' the more time I look at them and stay with her and Peter and Max. She emerges as a woman opening herself up to the dance of embodied life, in all its desiring, distracted and indeterminate choreographies, dreamlike wanderings, erotic folds and temporal surges: as a mother, as a writer, as a companion to her queer kin. I guess I am opening too. But not quite; not yet. The contact sheets course and current like this; they rip, ebb, drift, drag, flow (but not in a straight or 'well' line; the contact sheet is 'all side effects') (Berlant and Stewart 2019: 18). I sense the charged but tender atmosphere of rooms opening into more rooms, trying out its textures and shadows and dimensions naked, then dressed, then topless (recalling her go-go dancing era). Her pre-adolescent child (aged nine or ten; almost the age of her novel-smuggling) interrupts the experiment but is also part of it, slowing the shoot down, in eyes-closed reverie, making room for laziness, boredom and play, in this doll's house of mothering, art-making and affective labour, as the child curls into the mother, and the mother folds back into the child. Her published words from not long after return in the sheets: 'I have a twelve-year-old son, who I believe has taught me the most' (Mueller 2022: 330).

It is unlikely that in 1981 (the time of the photographs) Cookie knew she was ill, but it's possible she was already infected. It was only a year later that her friend Gordon Stevenson died of AIDS; the last letter he sent to her from hospital is transcribed by Cookie in the dead-on, proximate, posthumous, bedside stare of the epistolary piece 'A Last Letter'. All I can say is that the difficulty I have had in confronting dead-on the slantwise contact sheets is connected to the irresolvable, unknowable pain of imagining conversations or utterances or estimations that may have taken place between mother and son at various stages of Cookie's illness through to her need for palliative, accompanied care.

I think of Sedgwick's reading of Melanie Klein and AIDS activism in her essay on paranoid and reparative reading; its moving away from the 'dogged, defensive narrative stiffness of a paranoid temporality' shaped by the Oedipal vertical generational line to an affective embodied reparative sense of horizontal, transhistorical relations, which offers something like hope amidst 'the brutal foreshortening of so many queer life spans' during this time (2003: 147–48). In this devastating abbreviation of life and deroutinization of time (148), Cookie crafted communality, kinship and care, beside those closest to her; it was a reparative 'project in survival' (Sedgwick 2003: 150), of queer and sick mothering care, 'in spite of' the stigmatized absences of medicalized treatment and research that got legitimized in the dominant biomedical 'queer paradigm' of 'risk-taking behaviours' causing AIDS (Patton 1985: 3–6). The first utterance of the disease only came from the president in 1985, but this was not the only 'silence'; and it is within silence that 'people find others looking for connection' (Juhasz and Kerr 2022). I think Cookie found it in the resourcefulness of words, stories, images, writings: the letter, the photoshoot, the autobiographical manuscript of adolescent returns, in which the misbehaving, malfunctioning, reclining female body *delayed* in its social norms due to infected fallopian tubes, returns. Cookie remembers this childlike, not-quite-mother in 'Female Trouble', which I thought of when I received the clinical data on my egg reserves, and which I think of now as offering hope in the horizontality of a capacious care network, if only in the imagination.

I return, too, to the otherworldly perceptions and hallucinations of her metaphorical visionings in youthful childbirth (in the Provincetown hospital, again): where the moon 'had turned to blood'; the cries of women 'in the next rooms were as earsplitting as the wrong songs of distressed humpback whales'; the baby she had been growing 'slipped out… like a bloated mackerel' (Mueller 1990: 63–64, 68). How gigantic, planetary, interspecies, strange, and aquatic it all is, this feverish but tender exploration of mothering, occupying it as a continuing state, in the to-and-fro flux of her remembrance writing.

I am staying with her there. In grey: the blur of the in-between.
And just knitwear.
Or naked.
Possibly ill.

Flight 4

April 2024; my son's sixth birthday

I write about Liliana. The writing is stark and spare. It can only seem to describe. It makes an attempt at the *elsewhere* and then retreats. One of the sentences risks nothing more than a single word:

> Schiele depicts a woman on a chair, naked apart from a gown about her shoulders, one hand resting on top of her pregnant belly. Her eyes are swollen with exhaustion and yet, she looks back. Though seated, she lists to one side, to stretch, to open out, to make room, somehow, for the baby inside, turning, pressing, pushing against the womb that is closing in. Confinement.
>
> (Blackshaw 2021)

I return to Berlant and Stewart's 'Dilations'. 'Amplified description', they say, 'gets at some quality that sticks....' (2019: 5). The metaphors they use for this sticking are that of the primary object, usually the mother or the mother's breast, and the floater, the loose particle suspended within the eyeball which causes small dark shapes to appear across one's field of vision – in the eye's flight, it cannot alight.

Again, I try to write about Liliana. Again, the writing is stark and spare. I cannot seem to amplify description, to get at that which sticks, by which I mean at vision, gestation, lactation. I retreat. I recount:

> Liliana Amon, aged 18, model, was admitted to the clinic on 17 May 1910 and gave birth there three months later. According to the autobiographical novel she published later in life, she was already pregnant when she met Schiele. She gave birth to a girl who was noted as being handed over to the foundling home, but does not appear in its records.
>
> (Blackshaw 2021: 23)

I am forty-seven-years-old. The same age as Liliana when she published her first and only literary work, her own life story yet written as one 'Anna Lisser', a name which reversed the first letters of her own, abbreviating 'Liliana' to 'Anna'. Liliana wrote in German, but her book was published in French. Its discovery was announced in 2019, some time into my own research; the original manuscript has yet to be found.[3] Prior to this date, no one knew the name of the model identified in correspondence between Schiele and a doctor at the clinic with the initials 'L.A.'.[4] No one could have imagined her as the author of a novel that rushes onwards through nearly four hundred pages. The novel's title is *Barrières*.

Barriers is a breathless text: reams of pages on a lifetime of abuse which begins in Liliana's infancy. Somehow, incredibly, the uncared-for baby

[3]Walter Schübler announced his discovery of the novel in 'Geniale Sprüche im Literatencafé', *Frankfurter Allgemeine Zeitung*, 23 March 2019, p. 16.

[4]Letter from Erwin Graff to Egon Schiele, 18 May 1910, Albertina, Vienna, Inv. ESA 169; Egon Schiele Autograph Database, ID: 239. Available online at: http://www.egonschiele.at/.

pushes through to adulthood, through prostitution, sickness, addiction, abandonment, despair. Pleasure is longed for, is fleeting, is lost. A life of nearly fifty years is described in unremitting, unmodulated detail and in the third person because 'Anna' is a character. But 'Anna' is also the author, Liliana, who switches to the first-person pronoun for similarly long, stylistically undifferentiated interior monologues, which she surrounds with speech marks, taking refuge in punctuation which imposes if only at the level of grammar something of a distance between lived and narrated experience, such as this: '"I can't live, I'm being chased, I can't see anything, I have to see something, I'm crazy. That's it, I'm crazy. And everyone knows it and won't do anything for me… My future is in my hands… but my past is on my back…"' (Amon 1939: 124). In these sentences, which ebb in the much-repeated ellipsis before flowing back, Liliana seeks to make sense of the hostilities, fragilities and intensities of her situation. She waits for care which never comes. While waiting, she describes, in paragraph after paragraph, a life so unrelenting the text itself cannot draw breath.

When will I write not about but *with* Liliana, with the methods she seems, in the stare from Schiele's drawing of the patient who may or may not be her, to be asking of me. When will I write with my experience, and Liliana's experience, of waiting for writing (there are nearly thirty years between her time in the clinic and her time of writing); with states of expectancy which refer to my own as well as those of my sick women subjects, waiting for so many forms of care, including the care of different research questions, methods, modes and forms of writing, before revealing something more of themselves (a *novel*, no less). When will I gather the ephemera of forgotten work on Liliana, amassed through many years, along with the shabby records against the forgetting that is mothering that is waiting for writing that returns me to my son's first, joyful steps, his cheeks scarlet from teething, his suck, his cough, his cry. When will I reflect on the writing already done for the writing yet to come, considering it as an archive itself, which takes me not only to forgetting, recording, ebbing and flowing but also to entangling, mothering, embodying and surviving, as the chronically criss-crossing verbs which activate *waiting as writing*.

As I give up, move on, then return to find not only what was left but also what she or a historical me has chosen to offer since, it transpires I am always writing with Liliana. The waiting *is* the writing. And in this state of waiting-as-writing which provides both space and time, which is open to the 'unexpected intuitions and fortuitous insights' that philosopher Harold Schweizer defines as waiting's welcome, experiential effects (2008: 2), which does not ask if it is process or production, which exists as part of everything else – children, sickness, seasons, love – I realize I am practising the cross-historical care that is so much a part of *Sick Women*, which works both ways, with affinity and serendipity, likeness and resonance, to truly attend to the deeply traumatized Liliana – the writer who describes everything except the birth of her child, who recounts everything except the days she spent with her child – and to the writer of 2024 who waited to become a mother, who endured numerous clinical procedures to become pregnant and to maintain the pregnancy, who submitted to the 'cascade of medical interventions', as it is termed, that follow the inducement of birth, who can hardly bear to read such flattened, deadened, dissociated sentences as: 'He came to the clinic several times, made some drawings of the new-born child in red and blue, wished her luck, and left' (Amon 1939: 63–64).

Flight 5

I'm thinking of the verbs in our flights: *staying*, *waiting*, *writing*; these suspended states as mothering. To mother: as verb. What might it mean to mother, which also means to write, in the sickness and care of a time suspended: for me, for you, for Liliana, for Cookie? While not as excessive and strange as Cookie's childbirth remembrance writing, I wonder if Liliana's bare, attentive sentences and sentence-withdrawals summon their own kind of directional gaze, as if she's swallowing Schiele's clinical gaze with her writerly eyes, decades after.

Cookie's clinical visioning following from natal encounters was *cosmic*; in the belated, *collected* sick time of her autobiographical manuscript, she situated her son's birth in gigantic time and space: 'From my antiseptic bed with the stiff flash-pasteurized sheets in a severely blank hospital room I could see, through the window... galactic nebuli and meteor dust' (Mueller 1990: 64). Her son was born in Hyannis Hospital, an umbilical cord of a drive down the skinny peninsula from Provincetown, also known as 'the end of the world': the wild, hazardous, undisciplined, tempestuous, otherworldly edge between land and sea. I've only visited the tip of the Cape in stories and pictures. Cookie's worldings of mothering care make that possible. Here she crafted families of new shapes – with experimentation, love and play. Here she apprenticed herself to girlish motherhood, to writing, the page and the stage.

And it was where she came back to in the summer of 1989. The return, a *retreat*. A space to remember and rest. I can't stop thinking about this, that, close to dying – struggling to speak in linear sentences after a stroke, to stand on sand without needing a cane – she not only escaped to the restorative climes at the extremity of the country's edge, a palliative abyss 'away from' the violences of the city, but she also retreated to the hook of endless beaches where she birthed her child into this precarious world. And all the while restlessly seeking to birth the manuscript she'd long been writing. Was the not-too-late life writing itself – as well as her son, her many-gendered friends, her ex-girlfriend-turned-carer, Sharon – the companions of care, the midwives, the birth doulas and death doulas, she needed: as reparative resistances to the structural injustices of medicalized care? As Sophie Lewis has drawn out, the etymology of 'midwife' is 'with-woman', so that to be 'a midwife is to be a woman *with*, a companion to another, especially during the more slippery, amniotechnical moments of social reproduction: partum, miscarriage, departure'. Such forms of accompaniment, as Lewis writes, denote a commitment to 'being-with' the birthing, sick and dying as a labour of 'holding; staying; witnessing; facilitating the crossing of liminal thresholds; lubricating the beginnings and ends of human life-forms' (2020).

'To mother' and 'doula' as interlinking verbs; for Cookie, it was happening in the embodied, sickened, palliative space of writing both at once.

I stay with one of the last of her photographic remains. She's submerged in dark grey water (the kind loved by Hujar), a pool painted black (to borrow her posthumous book title), and one of the peninsula's 890 freshwater 'kettle' ponds, which got etched into the earth by disappearing glaciers, 18,000 years ago. Like a baby, Cookie loved to swim underwater, but this is a moment – captured in a photograph likely rinsed in water – of her bursting forth from the surface, out from the amniotic sac of the pool. Her arms are outstretched like a starfish. She's still wearing the same bangles. It is a picture of ecstasy, joy, elemental enchantment, a meeting of sky and lake. Her hair is drenched through. She's smiling. It is a gesture that says loudly: I'm here on this earth.

Not quite, not yet.
Still here.
Suspended.
In the pool of her mothering writing.

References

Amon, M. (1939), *Barrières*, trans. A. Paraz, Paris: Les Éditions Denoël.

Berlant, L. and K. Stewart (2019), *The Hundreds*, Durham and London: Duke University Press.

Blackshaw, G. (2021), 'On Constellations or Seeing Stars: *Constellations* by Esther Teichmann and Christopher Stewart'. Available online: https://constellations.world/essay/on-constellations-or-seeing-stars (accessed 2 June 2024).

Carland, T. R. and A. Cvetkovich (2013), 'Sharing an Archive of Feelings: A Conversation', *Art Journal*, 72 (2): 70–77.

Davey, M. and P. Hujar (2021), 'Fierce Friends: Moyra Davey is inspired by Peter Hujar's archive – in pictures', *The Guardian*, 13 May. Available online: https://www.theguardian.com/artanddesign/gallery/2021/may/13/fierce-friends-moyra-davey-inspired-by-peter-hujar-archive-in-pictures (accessed 22 July 2025).

Davey, M. and P. Hujar (2021), *The Shabbiness of Beauty*, n.p. London: MACK.

Hedva, J (2022), 'Sick Woman Theory', *Topical Cream*, 12 March. Available online: https://topicalcream.org/features/sick-woman-theory/ (accessed 10 June 2024).

Juhasz, A. and T. Kerr (2022), 'An AIDS Conversation Script to be Read Aloud Timeline 2', in A. Juhasz and T. Kerr (eds), *We Are Having this Conversation Now: The Times of AIDS Cultural Production*, 95–98, Durham, NC, and London: Duke University Press.

Lewis, S. (2020), 'With-Women: Grieving in Capitalist Time', e-Flux Journal, Issue 111, September. Available online: https://www.e-flux.com/journal/111/343916/with-women-grieving-in-capitalist-time/ (10 June 2024).

Mueller, C. (1986), 'Art and About', *Details*, March, Serpent's Tail and High Risk Archive, BVII.1, F20, Fales Library and Special Collections, New York University Libraries.

Mueller, C. (1990), *Walking Through Clear Water in a Pool Painted Black*, New York: Semiotext(e).

Mueller, C. (2022), *Walking Through Clear Water in a Pool Painted Black: Collected Stories*, ed. H. El Kholti, C. Kraus and A. Scholder, Edinburgh: Canongate.

Patton, C. (1985), 'Heterosexual AIDS Panic: A Queer Paradigm', *Gay Community News*, 9 February.

Schweizer, H. (2008), *On Waiting*, London and New York: Routledge.

Sedgwick, E. K. (1993), 'Queer and Now', in *Tendencies*, 1–20, Durham: Duke University Press.

Sedgwick, E. K. (2003), 'Paranoid Reading and Reparative Reading, or, You're So Paranoid, You Probably Think This Essay Is About You', in *Touching Feeling: Affect, Pedagogy, Performativity*, 123–51, Durham, NC and London: Duke University Press.

Wilkie, L. (2021), 'Moyra Davey and Peter Hujar: The Shabbiness of Beauty', 7 September. Available online: https://c4journal.com/moyra-davey-peter-hujar-the-shabbiness-of-beauty/ (accessed 2 June 2024).

Wojnarowicz, David (1991), *Close to the Knives: A Memoir of Disintegration*, New York: Vintage Books.

CHAPTER TWENTY-FOUR

Manual: broken bodies for broken landscapes

cripxcess (Lorenzo Galgó and Maria Morata)

Take a moment to breathe.
Become aware of the space you are in.
Choose a landscape after reading this sentence.
This could be any object, body, agent or ecosystem that you can imagine as a landscape.
What is the relationship between your body-mind and your affects with this place?
What is the relation of this landscape to those who inhabit it?
Does this landscape fit in your hand?
Does the unwanted fit into this landscape?
Become aware of these dissonant elements,
In what ways can you generate kinship with them?
Take them with you when you think of this landscape again.
Come back here as often as you like.

How might crip experience and ecological thinking support each other? Working together as cripxcess, we – Lorenzo Galgó (LG) and Maria Morata (MM) – mobilize illness and disability as tools for a critical reading of the Anthropocene and ecological politics, establishing a relationship between sick bodies and sick landscapes. The conventional version of ecology is built on the sick/healthy binomial that refers to a romantic vision of nature and perpetuates the enabling structures of neoliberal societies. Resisting this,

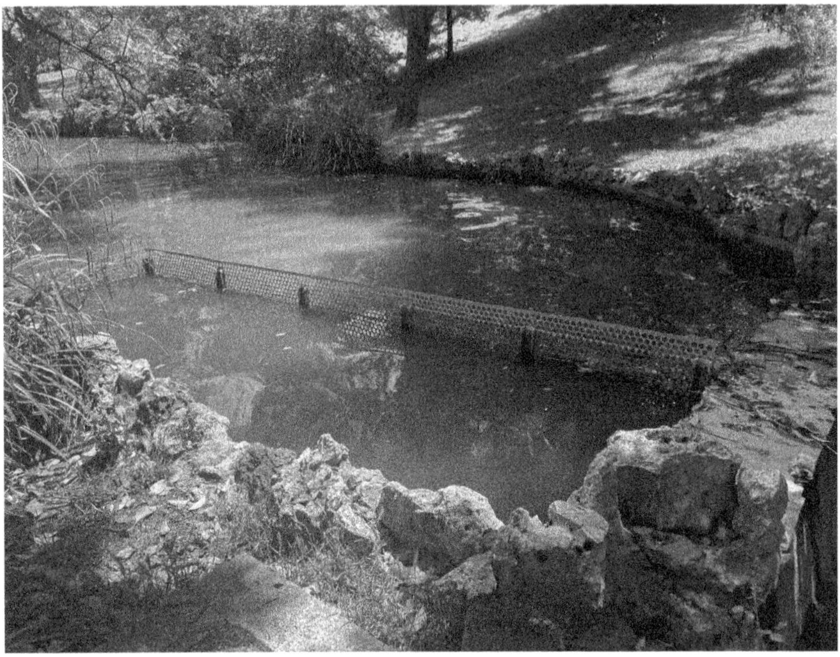

FIGURE 24.1 *End of La Ria de la Salud (River of Health) in the Parque del Oeste (West Park), Madrid.* Photo credit: cripxcess, 2023.

our research asks how working from our embodied positions of illness and disability might be used to rethink hyperproduction, extractivism, and the aesthetic, cultural and identity values of a given territory.

Our methodology is based on translating and expanding the practice of the access rider, a document used to help people with disabilities to communicate their needs with art institutions (Lazard 2019; Walden, 2020). Applying the access rider to diseased landscapes, we practise listening to, attending to and caring for landscapes from the limits of our inevitable human condition. Permeating text-body-landscape, we understand illness and disability as fundamentally relational: as aching bodies sharing vulnerability, as a crutch that supports another crutch, it is in this interdependent state that we generate our research.

Maria Morata (MM): In January 2023 we realized our project *Pain in the West: Access Rider for a Landscape* at the Parque del Oeste (West Park) in Madrid. The aim was to collaboratively develop an *access rider* for the park through somatic practices of listening to, and being with, the site. We began with research sessions on historical, political, cultural and biological aspects of the park, practising different forms of resonance and identification with real or imagined landscapes, either by ourselves or with other members of our research group (formed by Fernando Vílchez Rodriguez, Ana Jarosz, Lucía Bravo and Patricia Villanueva). Through this speculative exercise, which positioned our bodies as factors in the research, we were able to unearth a number of questions and tensions. The day we went to visit the park together was a sunny, magnificent day. The park was a gift, green, lush, shining in the light.

Lorenzo Galgó (LG): It was not a place sacrificed to economic interests through exploitation and extractivism, actions which correspond to an imaginary of illness (see Clare 2017).Within a landscape or ecosystem, relationships between assorted agents are diversely configured: atmospheric agents, animals, the relationships of trees with other trees, the soil with insects, with detritus... everything is connected; there is interdependence, with different layers operating simultaneously across different scales and times. Within these relations there is also the human factor, its material interventions and its ideological readings of the territory. We rethink the exclusionary binomial health/illness by working on a crip reading of the landscape, making visible the complex relations between ecological thought and crip theory, which reclaims the derogatory term crip as an expression of resistance and emancipation.

MM: To develop our crip vision of the West Park, we conceived of the park as a *dispositif* (Foucault 1977); that is, as an apparatus with its own functions and rules. Artificially created from natural features linked with technical, cultural and social elements, the park was designed and built at the beginning of the twentieth century for the production of pleasure according to an anthropocentric ideal of nature. Inspired by Marie-Luise Angerer's use of the term *intensive milieus* to articulate complex networked relations between human and nonhuman or para-human others (Angerer 2017), we identified what we call *zones of vulnerability*; that is, the places in the park where the *dispositif* breaks down and becomes fragile, either because what should remain hidden (to maintain the illusion of the natural) becomes visible, or because elements appear that were not planned in the original design, thereby altering the relationships that keep the system stable.

LG: These alterations can introduce changes that overwhelm the *dispositif* and turn it into something different, something outside of the control of the cleaning and maintenance services and the narratives officially attributed to that space. We are talking about an anthropocentric balance, about relationships between the elements of the park that have been created and maintained from a human perspective, and within which the imaginary of the 'healthy' to which the park must respond is implicit. Starting from this premise, we can think of illness and disability as something disruptive, uncontrollable and undesirable. It is this aspect that interests us for addressing three *zones of vulnerability* within the park: the River of Health

(*La ría de la Salud*), the so-called plague of the Argentinian parrots, and the monument to La Veneno, a trans woman and icon of the LGBTIQA+ collective in Spain.

MM: The first *zone of vulnerability* that we related to was the artificial river that crosses the park, called The River of Health because it originally started from a fountain that was attributed healing properties but was later sealed off for containing toxic elements. We think of this body of water as an aesthetic prosthesis which is in turn organic and produces life. The river ends abruptly when it reaches the spatial limit of the park and disappears into the ground. It is engulfed by the underground structure of the machinery that artificially moves it into a 'natureculture' (Haraway 2003) or 'postnatural' encounter zone.[1]

But not only. The park was a battlefront during the Spanish Civil War: the river was created by taking advantage of an existing indentation in the earth made by a line of trenches. No signage, no plaque or memorial gives any account of this re-appropriation of the landscape despite the fact that the park abounds in commemorative monuments of all kinds. We can speak here of a process of erasure, a concealing of the park's history. The trench received a 'cure' when it became a river, 'optimizing' its state under the logic of pleasure: this cure obscures, erasing the wounds of the war within the riverbed, which, although artificial, carries water, a symbol of purification.

LG: This line of water that proclaims the 'healthy' aesthetics of the park drags into its flow particles of cement detached from the walls of the artificial river; this greyish sludge ends in a sewage treatment plant which keeps the river circulating and clean. We are interested in including pain as part of the dynamics of a physical, social or cultural space: not to cover it up, not to purify it, or correct it, but to give pain a place in the complexities that constitute a landscape.

MM: There is no single optimal state for a landscape; landscape is dynamic. This brings us to another of the *zones of vulnerability* that we identified in the West Park: the Argentinian parrots. This bright green-plumaged species was introduced into Spain as an exotic pet in the 1980s from South America; their presence in the park is an echo of a neo-colonial mindset of species displacement. The institutional authorities considered the parrots to be a plague that endangers native flora and fauna and even the safety of park visitors (the parrots' nests can weigh up to 200 kilos and break tree branches). The alleged noise pollution from their song is also the cause

[1]On the 'postnatural' see the Institute for Postnatural Studies: https://www.instituteforpostnaturalstudies.org, accessed 18 November 2024.

of repeated complaints. The West Park was 'chosen' by the Argentinian parrots, yet it is a site where violent methods of population control have been practised on them.

LG: We are faced with an interventionist 'cure' to return the park to an imagined aseptic original state. This justifies the extermination that took place in this space: the large scale of mortality of the so-called invasive species as well as the cruelty of the methods used. The head of the environment department at the time made the following statement: 'We have to understand that in the environment there are good and bad ones, and that those who come from outside aggressively do not have the same ecological right to life that we all have.'[2] The resonances with xenophobic discourses and conservative immigration policies are evident.

When we walk down any street in Madrid, we hear the parrots blabbering. They awaken love and empathy in me, I feel them as fellow queer subjects, shouting and agitated.

MM: Perhaps we can push this metaphor further. Public discourse in Madrid is hostile to the Argentine parrots: the 'diversity' that they bring to the park's ecosystem is framed as harmful to a supposedly original (and therefore more valuable) ecology. Similarly, when body-minds diverge from normative standards, this diversity is often perceived as a challenge or a threat to existing structures of power.

LG: How would a *crip ecology* accompany these landscapes in their new precarious balances?

MM: Returning to the diversity of bodies and territories, this thought leads us to another *zone of vulnerability* that we locate in the West Park: the monument to La Veneno, aka Cristina Ortiz Rodríguez, a trans woman with a significant TV media presence in the 1990s. La Veneno was 'discovered' in 1996 while working as a sex worker in the West Park; she died in 2016, in a situation of poverty, aggravated by addiction and mental health issues.

LG: This monument consists of a memorial plaque affixed to a brick column; it is regularly visited by followers and admirers who demonstrate their affection through graffiti, photographs, objects, flowers, candles, honouring

[2]Cited in 'Madrid eliminará a 12.000 cotorras invasoras por amenazar la biodiversidad', *El Confidencial*, 7 October 2024: https://www.elconfidencial.com/espana/madrid/2019-10-07/ayuntamiento-madrid-eliminara-cotorras-invasoras-120_2272524/#:~:text=%22Tenemos%20que%20entender%20que%20el,la%20vida%20que%20tenemos%20todos%22. Translation provided by the authors.

the visibility that La Veneno gave to the LGBTIQA+ community. The plaque has been repeatedly stolen and vandalized, but nonetheless endures; a point of renewal and resistance in the official narratives of the park, it recalls less idyllic aspects of the park's history, such as its use as a prostitution zone during a period when sex workers were criminalized. Making visible activities that usually remain more or less hidden – the park also houses cruising areas and places for street drinking – the monument to La Veneno draws attention to unregulated social practices that expand the normative functions for which the park was designed.

MM: After traversing these crip moments in the West Park, we had to rethink our initial objective of creating an access rider for the landscape. We wanted to move away from the idea of issuing a set of instructions or recommendations, instead focusing on developing exercises for identifying and *being with* the crip elements of an environment.

LG: The idea of creating an access rider for a landscape foregrounds the limitations of our human condition; we can only relate to landscapes from our own embodied states as humans.

MM: Every access rider is dynamic; it has to be constantly modified. It is neither universal, nor unique. If the access rider represents the vulnerabilities of diverse bodies that exceed a normative ableist model, in the same way we want to acknowledge and respond to the vulnerabilities of diverse landscapes that escape normative standards of beauty or productivity created for human benefit.

LG: An access rider should be based on a process of empathy and affection towards the space. Creating a somatic relationship with the landscape, and imagining different ways of inhabiting that, allows us to rewrite and re-signify human-landscape relations from a *crip* perspective.

MM: We knew that ours was an exercise in overflowing the *access rider*; through this we intended to introduce ourselves into the continuum of bodies and lives that make up a landscape, fleeing from compartmentalization and questioning the classifications of the natural and the artificial, the healthy and the sick. Our crip vision of territories does not pretend to be the only or optimal possibility for responding to a landscape; it is simply based on making visible complex processes of destabilization.

LG: This is where we are, let's keep thinking together.

References

Angerer, M. L. (2017), *Ecology of Affect: Intensive Milieus and Contingent Encounters*, trans. Gerrit Jackson, Lüneburg: Meson Press.

Clare, E. (2017), *Brilliant Imperfection: Grappling with Cure*, Durham, NC: Duke University Press.

Foucault, M. (1977; 1980), 'The Confession of the Flesh', in *Power/Knowledge Selected Interviews and Other Writings 1972–1977*, ed. Colin Gordon, trans. Colin Gordon, 194–228, New York: Pantheon Books.

Haraway, D. (2003), *The Companion Species Manifesto: Dogs, People, and Significant Otherness*, Chicago: University of Chicago Press.

Lazard, C. (undated; first edition 2019), 'Accessibility in the Arts: A Promise and a Practice'. https://promiseandpractice.art/, accessed 21 July 2024.

Walden, R. (2020), 'Access Rider. What is an access document?', Diversity Arts Culture Berlin, https://diversity-arts-culture.berlin/en/magazin/access-rider, accessed 21 July 2024.

CHAPTER TWENTY-FIVE

Lying in: a conversation from the bedside

Angela Alves, Monika Ankele and Céline Kaiser

The starting point for this conversation is the performance and sound installation REST *(2019) by dancer and choreographer Angela Alves (AA). To develop this work, Alves invited three women to lie alongside her in bed to embody and explore resting as an act of care, surrender and rebellion. In response to the work, Monika Ankele (MA) examines practices of bed rest in the history of psychiatry, while Céline Kaiser (CK) traces literary and medical responses to Ivan Gončarov's 1859 novel* Oblomov, *in which the reclining hero has been variously read as a symbol of feudal decadence, a case study of a clinical pathology, and a refusal of the neoliberal idea of self-improvement. Together they reflect on the complex social, moral, political, and physical implications of lying in or being put to bed from the late nineteenth century to the present day.*

Angela Alves (AA): In 2019, I invited three women to spend time with me in my bed, talking about their relationship to rest; recordings of our conversations became the centrepiece of the sound installation *REST*, which explores resting as an act of care, surrender, and rebellion.[1] REST liberates an archive of voices usually silenced by a culture that equates resting with laziness: these women's experiences challenge the norms of constant activity

[1]The work was developed for the project 'The Space In-Between' and was shown for the first time at the Sophiensaele Berlin on 16 November 2019. 'The Space In-Between' is a co-production of the No Limits-Festival (GER) and Metal (UK).

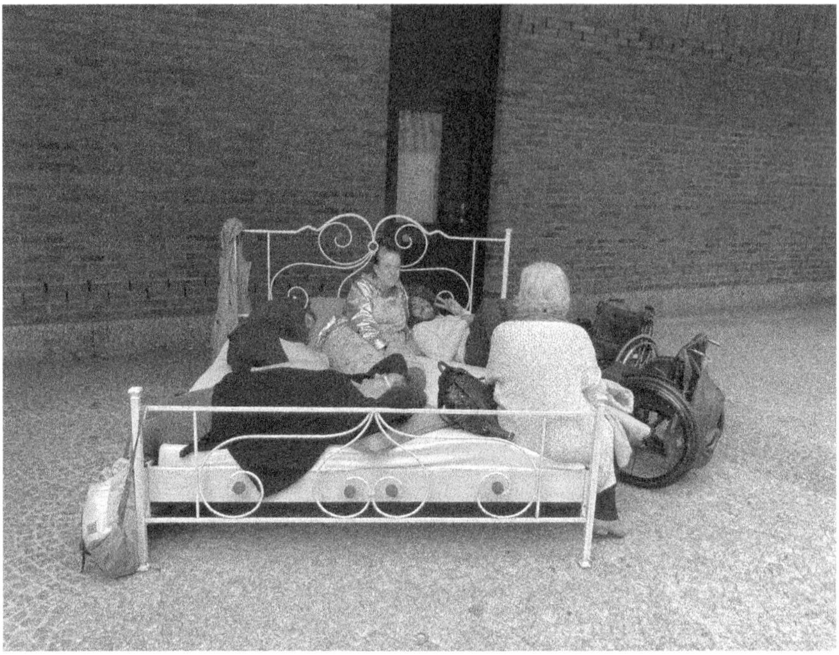

FIGURE 25.1 Angela Alves, *REST*, at Grenzgänger Festival, Munich, 2022. © Angela Alves.

considered healthy by a capitalist, neoliberal society. These personal stories – of coping and resisting, celebrating, loving and creating – become political formulations as soon as they leave the private sphere and become public.

I remember when my first conversation partner laid down on the bed with me and exhaled deeply. There was no shyness or awkwardness. We knew what connected us and that we had nothing to fear from each other.

> 'Would you like a smaller cushion for your lower back?' I asked.
>
> *'No, thanks, I'm fine, I like lying flat on my back'.*

After we had laid in pleasurable silence for a few minutes, I asked her:

> 'Is it different for you to rest in bed than on the sofa, for example?'
>
> *'Of course, you can also rest on the sofa, but that's not the same. Resting in bed goes deeper'.*

Céline Kaiser (CK): For the speaker, bed and sofa are not only associated with different bodily positions, but also with different qualities and temporalities of resting.

Monika Ankele (MA): Angela's dialogue with her conversation partner appeals to my interests in the hospital bed as it relates to the history of psychiatry. Bed rest was introduced in psychiatric hospitals around 1900, at the same time as Sigmund Freud adopted the couch for 'cathartic psychotherapy'. Bed rest was supposed to calm the patient as a result of the 'brain rest' ('Gehirnruhe') brought about through bodily posture and the reduction of sensual stimuli. Doctors complained that psychiatric patients often lacked an acknowledgment of their illness (in German they used the term *Krankheitseinsicht* to describe this phenomenon); lying in bed during the day was intended to bring the patient to an awareness of his or her condition (see Ankele 2022b; 2019). For Freud, lying on the couch was intended to help analysands block out their surroundings and concentrate on their thoughts. However, when psychiatrists realized that patients on bed-rest were more likely to occupy themselves with fantasies, dreams and imaginaries, this treatment came under increasing criticism. Psychiatrists attempted to overcome the negative effects of bed rest by intensifying work therapy, where a patient's attention was no longer directed inwards, but outwards towards an external object that they were supposed to care for, create or handle (see Ankele 2016). But Céline, I interrupted you. What points of relation do you see to your research?

CK: I have brought Ivan Gončarov's 1859 novel *Oblomov* to our discussion (see Kaiser 2021). A piece of furniture plays a central role in this text: a divan on which the eponymous hero, Ilya Ilyich Oblomov, spends most of the novel. Oblomov is a thirtysomething landowner who, after attending university and failing to hold down an official position, moves to Petersburg to live with his old servant. Throughout the 200-page-long first section of the text, Oblomov repeatedly raises his upper body to act, before sinking back down into his previous position and returning to his thoughts and dreams. The divan offers a permanent state of liminality between verticality and horizontality, waking and sleeping, socializing and retreating.

MA: Here, too, the (semi-)reclining posture facilitates a turning away from reality towards one's inner worlds, which are arguably not less 'real' – as one psychiatric patient on bed-rest put it: 'The life of thoughts is real' (see patient file of Else Blankenhorn from the Curanstalt Bellevue, Binswanger Archive Tübingen, Nr. 441/1696).

AA: Horizontality provokes a radical readjustment of the whole body-mind-system. Your eye-level turns to the sky. Your breath deepens and slows down. Your perception starts to dance.

> *'I'm not allowed to have a mattress in my study because my colleagues want to keep the room accessible'.*

Rest as resistance is about harnessing the power of horizontal perception as a space for liberation, resistance, ownership and connection.

MA: The Black Power Nap collective takes this a step further by linking lying down to sleeping and dreaming, to which they attribute emancipatory and empowering qualities. They ask: 'How can we dream if we don't sleep?' In the context of slavery, systematic sleep deprivation was a means of breaking the will of enslaved women, men and children, making it impossible to dream of a free life (see Acosta et al. 2021).

AA: Resting and daydreaming are deeply rooted in Black history. Performance artist, writer and activist Tricia Hersey explores rest as a practice of Black resistance and liberation (Hersey 2016; 2022). Other practices of rest as resistance include the Tangping movement (*tangping*: literally, *lay flat*, Koetse 2022), practised by the younger generation in China in order to visibly refuse the pressure to perform. Or 'Quiet Quitting', a protest trend practised by employees who draw boundaries with their employer, responding with a friendly but firm 'no' to exploitation, overtime, and grind culture in general (Green and Baker 2023).

> *'The gig economy in which we participate [...] creates a situation for the nervous system, which is beyond our awareness, where we live in a constant state of alertness and arousal that borders on anxiety. I am constantly a little too aroused and a little too high, which makes it very difficult to let go. Resting becomes a task. One more thing to do. One more discipline'.*

How can we pause in a way that saves us from self-optimization?
How can we resist using or abusing rest time for competitive advantage and profitability?
How can this text resist those mechanisms?
How can we protect rest in the field of art?

'The real rest is a passive pleasure.'

But what happened next with Oblomov, Céline?

CK: Even over the next hundred pages of the novel, Oblomov only leaves his divan for short periods of time. What may at first seem like a moment of rest turns out to be a permanent state. This ultimately shapes all relationships – between the characters in the novel, but also between the readers of the novel and its protagonist. As Oblomov remains immersed in his divan, propped by cushions and wrapped in his dressing gown, present time and future plans disappear into the unknown. His body becomes diffuse, enveloped in a garment that lacks discernible contours. Petra Herrmann (as cited in Cheauré 2017: 267) expressed it beautifully when she observed that the name Oblomov with its three O's evokes something heavy and dark like velvet porters, as soft and comfortable as a worn mattress.

MA: I like the way you interpret Oblomov's dressing gown. In psychiatric hospitals around 1900, the nightgowns that patients wore were intentionally revealing so as to keep them in bed: Who would want to leave bed half-dressed and exposed to the eyes of strangers? But there are also photographs from that time that show creative ways that patients used duvets and sheets to dress themselves (see Ankele 2022a).

> *'I had already thoughts about putting a yoga mat in the toilet, but I would then be lying right next to the toilet bowl. And somehow I thought: I haven't sunk that low yet'.*
>
> *'But it could be that I will utilize this option at some point and that will be ok for me after all'.*

AA: Here I think of Oblomov again: this actually very likeable character gradually becomes a pathologized body.

CK: This is very clear in the history of the novel's reception. Oblomov is portrayed as a positive character whose kindness, generosity and honesty, according to the narrator, are written all over his face; there is no sign at all of sadism or tyranny here. In the early reception of the novel, however, Oblomov is as a type: as a member of the Russian landed aristocracy and master of 300 serfs, he signifies the intellectual and social stagnation of his time. These social criticisms are then shifted into the pathological by psychoanalytical and psychiatric readings of the character.

AA: You could tell a story about love but instead interpretation twists the character into a lazy, parasitic, backward-looking figure. And in the end, the guileless Oblomov is declared a psychopath who tyrannizes from the bed.

> *'Lazy is such an overused term. But why do people say it? Because they feel guilty when they're not working'.*

CK: The constant passivity of Oblomov's character, his permanent resting position, is responded to as a tremendous provocation, as if his inaction creates a gap or void that must be filled by interpretation. From the 1920s, Kolnai (1923) and Riemann (1961/1997) offer psychodynamic interpretations of Oblomov as a symbol of depression. In the 1960s and 1970s, Oblomov is programmatically characterized by Heinz Dietrich (1965) as 'a special type of weak-willed psychopath (*Oblomovist*)'.

MA: The term *bed addiction* (see Anonym 1844: 1078) comes to mind. It was coined by psychiatrists in the late nineteenth century to describe a patient's refusal to leave the bed once bed-rest treatment was finished.

> *'The bed is my friend and my protector, but sometimes I am also at odds with the bed. Sometimes the bed gets claws. You have to be careful that you crawl out of bed before that happens. The bed is sometimes also a life bunker'.*

MA: Prescribed bed rest led to irritations on their side. Lying in bed was supposed to be reserved for night-time, while a more upright position was supposed to determine the day. In letters patients often expressed the wish to be 'a useful member of society again' – a usefulness that was (and still is) determined by economic parameters and an upright posture.

> *'My parents and grandparents thought it was antisocial, sacrilegious, almost a mortal sin to lie in bed during the day'.*

CK: And if it is not seen as sinful, then as reflecting a pathology – which does not, however, absolve the patient of moral blame. In this sense, Oblomov has had a short but striking career as a pathological syndrome. From an antisocial type living on his divan at the expense of his serfs, he is gradually reinterpreted as a renitent refuser of labour who refuses to leave his *bed* (!).

> *'There are mainly two rebellious acts in neoliberalism. Liking yourself and exposing yourself not working'.*

CK: The incredible thing is that the reception of this novel still reads like a blueprint for the conversations that you, Angela, had with the women in your bed.

> *'I realize that my need for rest is not accepted. I then feel inferior, flawed and devalued. As if I were a defective product, a deficient specimen'.*

AA: I need to rest in bed because I have a sick nervous system, but I also choose to rest in bed to free myself and my sick sisters. And now I invite you to rest and stay sick with me.

CK, MK, AA: Thank you very much, bed!

References

Acosta, N., F. Sosa and E. Meilicke (2021), 'Black Power Naps', *Zeitschrift für Medienwissenschaft* 24 (13): 88–97. https://doi.org/10.25969/mediarep/15778.

Ankele, M. (2016), 'The patient's view of occupational therapy: The Hamburg-Langenhorn Asylum during the Weimar Period', in W. Ernst (ed.), *Work, Psychiatry and Society, cc. 1750–2000*, 238–61, Manchester: Manchester University Press.

Ankele, M. (2019), 'Horizontal Scenographies. The Sickbed as a Setting of Psychiatric Subjectivation', in L. Friedrich, K. Harrasser and C. Kaiser (eds), *Scenographies of the Subject*, 43–58, Wiesbaden: Springer Verlag.

Ankele, M. (2022a), 'Aspects of Clothing in Mental Institutions around 1900', In Dr. Guislan Museum (ed.), *Mirror Mirror. Fashion and the Psyche*, 73–89, Antwerp: Hannibal Books.

Ankele, M. (2022b), 'From a Patient's View: A Sensual-Perceptual Approach to Bed Rest', in B. Hitzer and R. Boddice (eds), *Feeling Dis/Ease. Experiencing Medicine and Illness in Modern History*, 237–54, London: Bloomsbury, 237–54.

Anonym (1844/39), 'Bettsucht', *Oesterreichische Medicinische Wochenschrift als Ergänzungsblatt der Medicinischen Jahrbücher des k.k. Österreichischen Staates*, 1078.

Cheauré, E. (2017), 'Faulheit. Muße. Kreativität. Überlegungen zur Oblomowerei', in G. Dobler and P. Ph. Riedl (eds), *Muße und Gesellschaft*, 267–88, Tübingen: Mohr Siebeck.

Dietrich, H. (1965), 'Ein besonderer Typ willensschwacher Psychopathen (Oblomowisten)', *Münchener medizinische Wochenschrift* 107: 2225–29.

Green, S., and Baker, L. (2023), 'Quiet Quitting and Cultural Narratives of Resistance'. *Journal of Cultural Studies*, 31(2): 178–95.

Hedva, J. (2016): *Sick Woman Theory. Mask Magazine.* Retrieved from https://www.maskmagazine.com/not-again/struggle/sick-woman-theory

Hersey, T. (2016): 'Founder of "The Nap Ministry"', retrieved from https://thenapministry.com.

Hersey, T. (2022), *Rest is Resistance. A manifesto*, New York: Little, Brown Spark.

Kaiser, C. (2021), 'Oblomow-Syndrom', in R. Gaderer and W. Peeters (eds), *Syndrome. Fiktion und Pathologie*, 203–10, Hannover: Wehrhahn Verlag.

Koetse, M. (2022), *'The Lying Flat Movement. Resisting the Rat Race'*, Goethe-Institut: Magazin STILLSTAND, retrieved from https://www.goethe.de/prj/sti/en/lan/res.html

Kolnai, A. (1923), 'Gontscharows "Oblomow"', *Imago. Zeitschrift für Anwendung der Psychoanalyse auf die Geisteswissenschaften* 9 (1923): 485–94.

Riemann, F. (1961/1997), *Grundformen der Angst. Eine tiefenpsychologische Studie*, Munich, Basel: Reinhardt.

Rosenblum, C. (2021), 'Work is a False Idol', *New York Times*, 22 August.

CHAPTER TWENTY-SIX

Sociality of self-care: Simone Leigh's *The Waiting Room*

Cera Smith

In 2021, over 230,000 healthcare providers in the United States left their professions (Popowitz 2022: 4). Over 145,000 left in 2022 and the number has continued to climb (Popowitz 2023: 4). Globally, 37 per cent of surveyed clinicians are considering switching jobs and 13 per cent are considering leaving healthcare altogether in the next two to three years (Goodchild et al. 2023: 10).

While the stress of the COVID-19 pandemic has pushed clinicians from all backgrounds out, workplace discrimination and continued healthcare inequity add to pandemic factors, pushing many Black physicians to leave (Lemos et al. 2021: 2). Their exodus occurs even as underserved American populations need an additional 180,400 physicians to meet current demand (Skorton 2023: 2). Black patients receive inferior care when Black clinicians leave. But who cares for Black care workers? In this text, I use the terms *care worker* and *caregiver* to refer not only to healthcare providers, but also to the Black public who continuously care for and about Black loved ones in a racist society.

Concern for Black care workers is not restricted to pandemic conditions or hospital settings. Black American artist Simone Leigh's social practice art project *The Waiting Room* (2016) foregrounded this concern.[1] The project – undertaken during Leigh's residency and installed at New York City's New

[1]Despite many Black artists' resistance to the designation 'social practice art', I use the phrase to honour Leigh's strategic labelling of her work as being 'social practice-y' to access institutional funding (Gaines, Leigh and O'Grady 2023: 335).

Museum – addressed the toll that caring for Black wellbeing in a racist society takes. *The Waiting Room*'s installation and series of workshops and treatments called 'care sessions' aimed to facilitate Black healing from the traumas of racist violence and of social disregard for Black suffering.

Centring Black women as its primary audience, *The Waiting Room* recognized that Black women have historically been presumed caretakers and are also among the most likely to receive insufficient care. The project responded to the story of former elderly and youth caretaker Esmin Green, a forty-nine-year-old Black woman who died in a Brooklyn hospital waiting room from medical neglect (Buckley 2008). Green waited twenty-four hours to see a doctor but died on the waiting room floor after lying there unattended to for over thirty minutes. Waiting for racist indifference and subpar treatment to end had devastating consequences then and continues for Black caregivers now.

Leigh defied racism's perpetual delay and denial of care by using her installation to actively treat racialized caregiver fatigue. The artist's airy apothecary combined sterile hospital imagery – clean, white surfaces – with imagery from the root worker's den – jars of herbs, roots, and other medicinal substances – to promptly offer holistic healthcare services to Black people. Unlike typical American waiting rooms, Leigh's reception area featured hard stools rather than rows of chairs. It served as a transitional space where guests entered, viewed the chalkboard listing the day's care sessions, and proceeded to adjoining rooms without having to wait for insurance approval or stop because of overbooked physician schedules.

Jars of herbs lined the walls, but these were not Leigh's primary tools for remedying racialized stress. Care sessions – including guided meditations, Afrocentering, massage, acupuncture, herbalism, music, conversations about aging and talks on toxicity and disobedience – produced the real healing. Leigh's friends and health practitioners facilitated sessions on a first-come-first-served basis. Uncluttered session rooms created a peaceful environment with subdued lighting. White sandbags stacked like pillows conveyed protected rest.

Despite being its creator, Leigh doubted *The Waiting Room*'s ability to meaningfully improve racialized living conditions. When asked if an unknown substance in her apothecary – what Leigh called 'Black-Lives-Matter powder' – protects her from police brutality, the artist responded: 'That's the problem. It would if I had faith that it would work, but I don't' (Trouillot 2016). Leigh's simultaneous disbelief in and conviction about the medicine's efficacy prompts me to ask: Why would she run the installation and care sessions if she doubted their ability to help, especially after piloting similar sessions in her 2014 *Free People's Medical Clinic*?[2] Should *The*

[2]Held at Stuyvesant Mansion, the historic home of Dr Josephine English (the first Black woman with an Obstetrics and Gynecology practice in New York), Leigh's social art project *Free People's Medical Clinic* featured workshops, performances and Q&A sessions that provided health services to Brooklyn's Black communities.

Waiting Room be viewed as an ineffective repetition and ultimately, as she called it, 'one of [her] failed projects' (Tomkins 2022)?

Measuring *The Waiting Room*'s success by its (in)ability to vanquish racism or permanently fix Black caregiver burnout misses, however, its beneficial promotion of self-care as a critically social practice. Leigh's project removed Black care workers from settings that cause hypervigilance and invited them to prioritize their own healing so that they could reenter the collective fight for Black wellbeing and racial justice. Unlike Leigh's *Free People's Medical Clinic*, which was held in the community space Stuyvesant Mansion, *The Waiting Room* utilized the art museum's rarified status to prompt curiosity, sustained attention, and reflection on the significance of participants' well-being. They had to see their own lives as the art worth protecting.

While some critics praise Leigh for configuring community healthcare, she clarified that her goal was not to 'set up a mock NGO pretending to rescue Black people from some abject situation' – a perverse 'post-colonial fantasy' – but rather to 'expose [...] a gold mine of knowledge that we have ignored, or even that we don't know exists' (Simmons 2016). Here, Leigh identifies highlighting Black health knowledge as her goal, but hindsight reveals that the installation may have served other purposes, too. Instead of focusing outward, I hypothesize that Leigh may have used the residency to focus inward, giving herself some relief from the weight of bearing witness to anti-Blackness in her art. In a society that glorifies Black women's sacrificial care for others, Leigh foregrounded her own healing needs and invited other Black care workers to do the same. As she testified later, '[I] make work about myself for myself, for my own community' (Gaines, Leigh and O'Grady 2023: 342). While Leigh's statement connects her to her community, it also suggests that her '[s]elf-thought' was the foremost motivator for her social practice art (Gaines, Leigh and O'Grady 2023: 336).

Counterintuitively, the medicine Leigh needed was community. Exhausted by Black death, Leigh used her residency to surround herself with Black life. For example, she organized a party for herself and Black women to find relief, convening a group called Black Women Artists for Black Lives Matter at the museum. Over 100 attendees prioritized their own wellness by joining workshops, performances, and exchanges like those in *The Waiting Room*. The gathering was a joyful demonstration of individual self-care as a practice of communal defence for Black lives.

Leigh's temporary solution to racial weariness exemplifies the collective benefit of Black people prioritizing their own health. For many Black caregivers, especially in the wake of pervasive racial violence and the COVID-19 pandemic, self-care may mean leaving the healthcare industry or other caregiving roles. Importantly, *The Waiting Room* reframes this move not as selfish avoidance, but as an energizing pathway that reenables Black caregivers to support Black people inside formal healthcare institutions and beyond.

References

Buckley, C. (2008), 'A Life Celebrated, and a City Criticized', *The New York Times*, 7 July. Available online: https://www.nytimes.com/2008/07/07/nyregion/07funeral.html (accessed 11 November 2024).

Gaines, M., S. Leigh and L. O'Grady (2023), 'Malik Gaines, Simone Leigh, and Lorraine O'Grady Conversation', in E. Respini (ed.), *Simone Leigh*, 334–51, Boston: Institute of Contemporary Art/Boston.

Goodchild, L., A. Mulligan, C. West, M. A. Calero, N. Mansell and T. Mueller (2023), 'Clinician of the Future 2023', Elsevier Health, available online: https://www.elsevier.com/insights/clinician-of-the-future#2-2023-report (accessed 11 November 2024).

Lemos, D., L. Carlasare, N. Okeke, Z. Qusair and F. DeMaio (2021), 'Summary Report: Experiences of Racially and Ethnically Minoritized and Marginalized Physicians in the U.S. during the COVID-19 Pandemic', American Medical Association, available online: https://www.ama-assn.org/delivering-care/public-health/experiences-minoritized-marginalized-physicians-us-during-covid-19 (accessed 11 November 2024).

Popowitz, E. (2022), 'Addressing the Healthcare Staffing Shortage', Definitive Healthcare, October, available online: https://www.definitivehc.com/sites/default/files/resources/pdfs/Addressing-the-healthcare-staffing-shortage.pdf (accessed 11 November 2024).

Popowitz, E. (2023), 'Addressing the Healthcare Staffing Shortage', Definitive Healthcare. September, available online: https://www.definitivehc.com/sites/default/files/resources/pdfs/addressing-the-healthcare-staffing-shortage-2023-report.pdf (accessed 11 November 2024).

Simmons, W. J. (2016), 'Artists at Work: Simone Leigh', *Interview Magazine*, 26 July, available online: https://www.interviewmagazine.com/art/artists-at-work-simone-leigh (accessed 11 November 2024).

Skorton, D. J. (2023), 'How Can We Improve Health Workforce Diversity and Address Shortages? A Conversation with Historically Black College and University Leaders and Students', *Committee on Health, Education, Labor and Pensions (HELP) U.S. Senate*, Morehouse School of Medicine: Association of American Medical Colleges, 12 May. Available online: https://www.help.senate.gov/imo/media/doc/Skorton%20Testimony.pdf (accessed 11 November 2024).

Tomkins, C. (2022), 'The Monumental Success of Simone Leigh', *The New Yorker*, 21 March. Available online: https://www.newyorker.com/magazine/2022/03/28/the-monumental-success-of-simone-leigh (accessed 11 November 2024).

Trouillot, T. (2016), 'Simone Leigh's *The Waiting Room*', *BOMB Magazine*, 25 July, available online: https://bombmagazine.org/articles/2016/07/25/simone-leigh-s-em-the-waiting-room-em/ (accessed 11 November 2024).

CHAPTER TWENTY-SEVEN

Kintsugi and the art of self-repair

Suzannah Biernoff

In January 2018, the New York–based Instagrammer Isabella Santa Maria posted a photo of herself with the caption 'Kintsugi – the Japanese art of mending broken pottery with gold lacquer'. A golden seam curves down the right side of her face, stretching from just below her lower eyelid to her chin. A second, fainter, line runs from tear duct to lip. Santa Maria has returned to the theme of *kintsugi* in subsequent Instagram posts, and in a 2019 video interview where you can watch her applying gold pigment to her scar (she calls it 'putting the *kintsugi* on') while she talks about learning to see beauty in her imperfections. We bear the traces of our history, she says, our bodies a living chronicle that is inscribed and re-inscribed with meaning: the trauma of a childhood accident, the deep emotional wounds of stigma, and now new, more sustaining associations of growth and transformation. 'Perhaps we are just taking on a new form, we are evolving, we are blossoming' she reflects in the interview (*BBC World Service* 2019).

The object I have chosen for my story is perhaps not an obvious one for a volume on art and the critical medical humanities. It is a simple stoneware tea bowl with a sandy coloured ash glaze, made in central Japan in the Muromachi period. The label on the display case in the Victoria and Albert Museum gives the date range 1400–1500. It has been badly broken and, at some point, repaired in the traditional manner with lacquer and gold. Seto ware tea bowls like this were often fired in stacks, the online catalogue explains, and part of the rim of the bowl beneath is fused to the underside (V&A 2009). Maybe it was excavated from a kiln waste heap and restored.

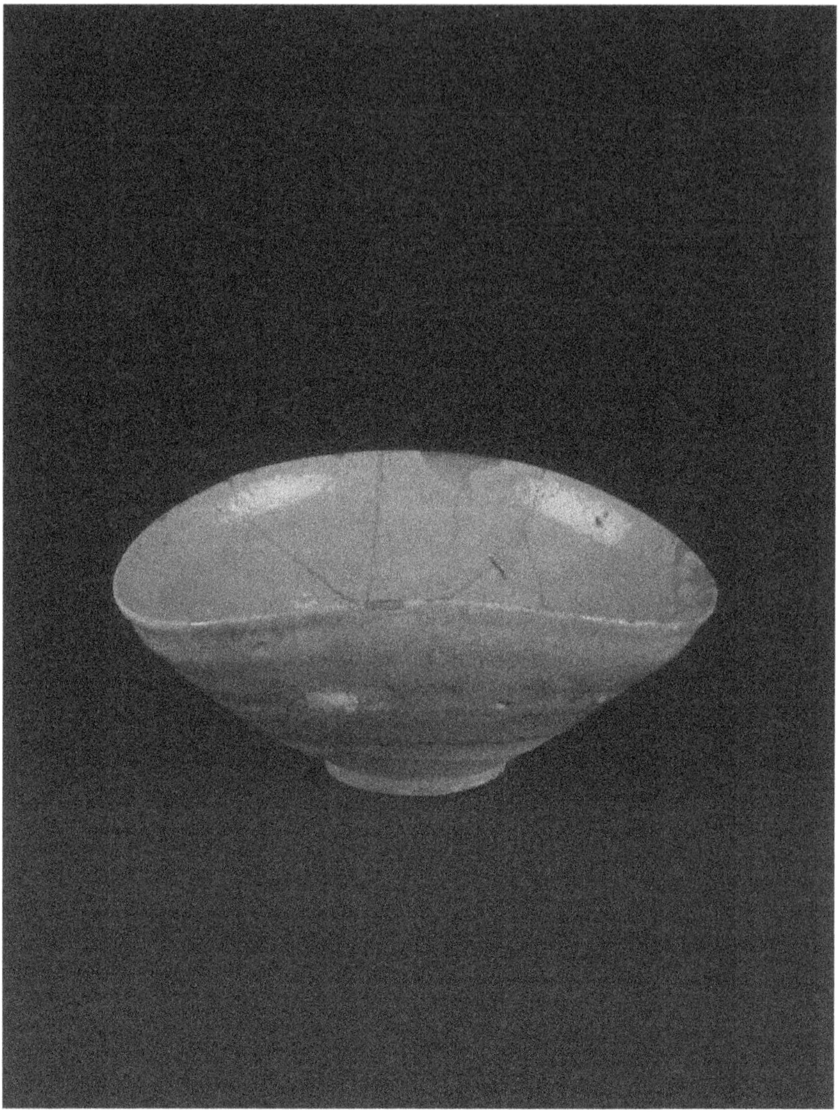

FIGURE 27.1 Tea bowl, stoneware with yellowish green ash glaze; Japan, Seto/Mino, Muromachi period, 1400–1500. © Victoria and Albert Museum, London. https://collections.vam.ac.uk/item/O437411/tea-bowl-unknown/

In its most recent incarnation as museum artefact, it will only be touched by a conservator or curator, but I imagine cupping it in two hands. It is surprisingly large, with gently curving sides; it would be easy to spill my tea in a moment of distraction. I imagine its warmth and asymmetry as I raise it to my mouth. The finer cracks are infilled with gold, like miniature flows of molten lava, the metal retaining a memory of its liquid state. In several places the rim has been repaired where fragments are missing. I can feel it on my lips: the smooth transition from ceramic to gold. It is elemental.

What can we do with an object like this? Santa Maria provides one answer: the repair of this tea bowl is an object lesson in self-care; it teaches us that signs of past damage are not ugly or shameful, that there is aesthetic value in asymmetry, irregularity and change. She implies that the self is like this bowl; we are fragile things, we can crack and break in a multitude of ways, through accident, neglect, deliberate harm, or natural disaster – Japan's history of earthquakes is one possible explanation for the development of *kintsugi* as a practice.

For the Japanese American philosopher Yuriko Saito, the contemporary interest in *kintsugi* and the related Japanese principle of *wabi-sabi* – finding beauty in imperfection and impermanence – are part of a global concern to develop a more caring and sustainable relationship with objects and the material world. As a cultural practice with roots in Zen Buddhism, *kintsugi* embodies an attitude of respect for the other (both human and non-human), and a conviction that the damaged object has 'its own integrity' or Buddha nature (Saito 2022: 155). For me, crouching in front of the display case for a better view, the tea bowl is a tiny window onto an unfamiliar world: a different way of seeing imperfection; perhaps even an antidote to late capitalism's 'growing epidemic of socially prescribed perfectionism' (Flett et al 2022).

By the time Santa Maria's story was picked up by the media in 2019, *kintsugi* had found its way into the self-help literature with titles like Candice Kumai's *Kintsugi Wellness: The Japanese Art of Nourishing Mind, Body, and Spirit* (2018) and Céline Santini's *Kintsugi: Finding Strength in Imperfection* (2019). Bonnie Kemske's *Kintsugi: The Poetic Mend*, published a few years later in 2021, is about ceramics, but the final chapter, 'A Metaphoric World', makes a more explicit set of claims about the value of *kintsugi* at a time (during the COVID-19 pandemic) when so much seemed broken or unbearably fragile. *Kintsugi* is beautiful and valuable in itself, Kemske writes, but its real power 'lies in the metaphoric overlay that we, as the flawed humans we are, apply to it' (137).

These ideas have started to inform medical ethics, patient care, and arts in health initiatives. In a recent discussion piece, Dominic Wilkinson suggests that *wabi* aesthetics (including the practice of *kintsugi*) has the potential to change the way healthcare professionals and patients think about physical imperfection, disability, disease, and death. His article begins with a description of a stoneware tea bowl not unlike the one in the V&A; he notes its asymmetry, the tiny indentations in its surface, and evidence of past damage and repair. Rather than 'defects', these signs of use and age are what make it unique and precious, like the 'ageing face or hand of a grandparent'

(2022: 937). Instead of seeing impairment, illness, and injury as unfortunate or treatable deviations from an ideal of perfect health, we could embrace 'the notion that these are natural and inevitable, and can at least sometimes bring special value and beauty' (Wilkinson 2022: 937).

In these sources, and in several recent exhibitions, we see *kintsugi* being instrumentalized as a metaphor. *Eternally Yours*, an exhibition in London in 2022, showcased historical and contemporary practices of visible mending and creative reuse, including pottery salvaged in the aftermath of Japan's devasting 2011 earthquake and repaired by Aono Fumiaki. As I write this, the Medical Museion in Copenhagen has on display a collection of objects showing the ingenious ways in which the human body has been repaired, and repairs itself: carved prosthetic hands and intricate metal arteries, bones that have been reset, hearing aids and dentures, even a hand-sewn aorta. The exhibition and accompanying learning activities challenge 'the common understanding of aging as a process marked by decay and decline' (*Kintsugi: Golden Body Repairs* 2023).

Like all metaphors (from the Greek *metaphero*, 'to transfer or carry over'), the examples I have given here borrow some meanings and leave others behind. There are always other stories we could tell about the conditions and impacts of cultural transfer and the nuances of meaning that get lost in translation. Our tea bowl might invite a deeper enquiry into the aesthetics of Zen Buddhism, a religious tradition concerned with transcending the self – not with self-realization or self-repair. Or we might wonder why *kintsugi* is so popular in the West. How has imperfection, as an aesthetic value, become entangled with the neoliberal rhetoric of self-help and resilience? The contemporary *kintsugi* phenomenon is ostensibly about embracing a non-Western and pre-capitalist perspective on the world. Buetow and Wallis (2019) make this explicit when they refer, in an article published in *Medical Humanities*, to 'Lessons from the East'. But as a metaphor, *kintsugi* is easily co-opted into modern, Western therapeutic narratives (Illouz 2007: 43–63). There are other stories too, if we search for them. The V&A catalogue entry includes the note: 'purchased from the Japanese Commissioners for the Philadelphia Exposition of 1876'. The Western fascination with Japanese culture is not new.

John Berger uses the term *confabulation* to denote the inarticulacy that prefaces language and representation: a generative opacity where bodily experience is translated, always imperfectly, into words or images. It captures, as well, the imaginative slippages and elisions, and the inevitable fabrications, that accompany any act of translation – and every act of writing. If a tea bowl can be an object lesson in the beauty of imperfection, or the ethics of care, it is because objects, like words and images, can be proxies for the human body and self, and sometimes they can seem to speak with more fluency. Or maybe the work of translation is simply less effortful, between bodies of clay and bodies of flesh, the distance closer than that between flesh and word.

References

BBC World Service (2019), 'Heart and Soul – The Instagrammer Inspired by Kintsugi', 21 March. Available online: https://www.bbc.co.uk/programmes/p073nh01 (accessed 1 May 2024).

Buetow, S., and K. Wallis (2019), 'The Beauty in Perfect Imperfection', *Journal of Medical Humanities* 40 (3): 389–94.

Eternally Yours: An Exhibition about Care, Repair and Healing (2022), Terrace Rooms, Somerset House, London, 16 June to 25 September, https://www.somersethouse.org.uk/whats-on/eternally-yours (accessed 1 May 2024).

Flett, G. L., P. L. Hewitt, T. Nepon, S. B. Sherry and M. Smith (2022), 'The destructiveness and public health significance of socially prescribed perfectionism: A review, analysis, and conceptual extension', *Clinical Psychology Review* 93: 102130.

Illouz, E. (2007), *Cold Intimacies: The Making of Emotional Capitalism*, Cambridge: Polity.

Kemske, B. (2021), *Kintsugi: The Poetic Mend*, London: Herbert.

Kintsugi: *Golden Body Repairs* (2023), Medical Museion, Copenhagen, https://www.museion.ku.dk/en/kintsugi_/ (accessed 1 May 2024).

Saito, Y. (2022), *Aesthetics of Care: Practice in Everyday Life*, London: Bloomsbury.

Santa Maria, I. (2018), 'Kintsugi—the Japanese art of mending broken pottery with gold lacquer' [Instagram], 12 January, available online: https://www.instagram.com/p/Bd1YSivBzEl/?hl=en (accessed 1 May 2024).

V&A (2009), Tea Bowl, object record, 25 June, available online: https://collections.vam.ac.uk/item/O437411/tea-bowl-unknown/ (accessed 1 May 2024).

Wilkinson, D. (2022), 'Wabi-Sabi: A Virtue of Imperfection', *Journal of Medical Ethics*, 48 (11): 937–38.

CHAPTER TWENTY-EIGHT

Being Horizontal: a visual essay

Nora Heidorn

The standard enlightenment representation of the human body is of a singular, upright, able-bodied man, gazing forward. *Being Horizontal* is an ongoing curatorial project concerned with imagery of reclined and inclined bodies that contest this ideal. The feminist philosopher Adriana Cavarero, whose book *Inclinations: A Critique of Rectitude* (2016) has informed my thinking, theorizes inclination as a model of the subject that is mutually dependent with others and situated in its world: it leans out of the vertical axis of the 'I' towards other creatures and things. This model contrasts with the masculinist ideal of *homo erectus*, who is self-sufficient, rational, righteous, sexually straight and literally upright.

We encounter reclined bodies in different situations in art and culture: persons sleeping, resting, or making love; the unwell, the injured, the deceased. Common tropes include the reclined nude, the fallen soldier, the psychoanalytic patient and the birthing woman. Representations of horizontal figures tell stories about what it means to occupy a human body that is gendered, raced, classed, medicalized; a body which requires, lacks, or receives care; that depends on others, that is supported by objects, that is examined and watched. At the same time, reclining persons elicit particular types of gaze: medicalizing, sexualizing, caring, objectifying, worried, desiring, compassionate…

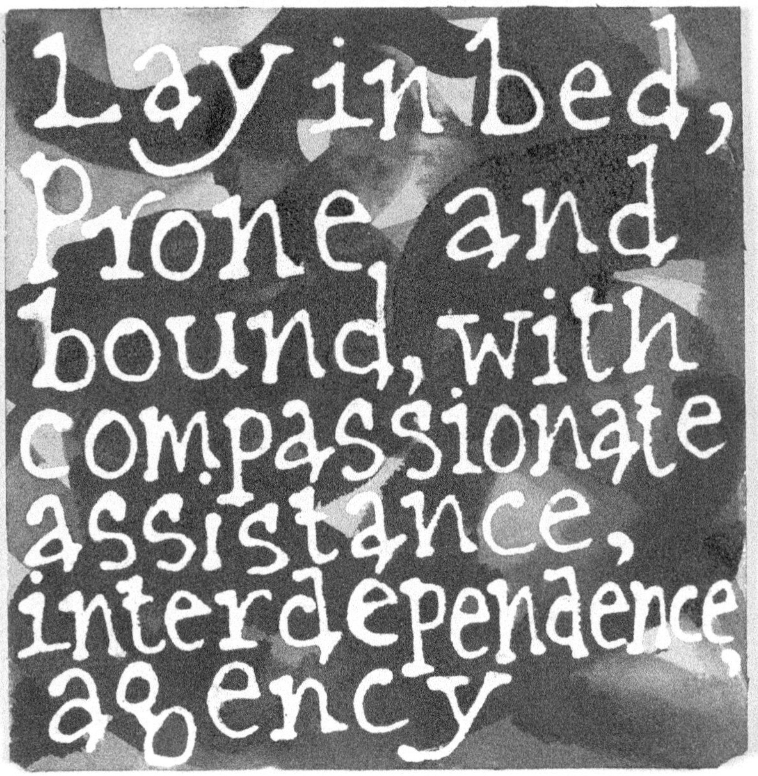
Lay in bed,
Prone and
bound, with
compassionate
assistance,
interdependence,
agency

28.1

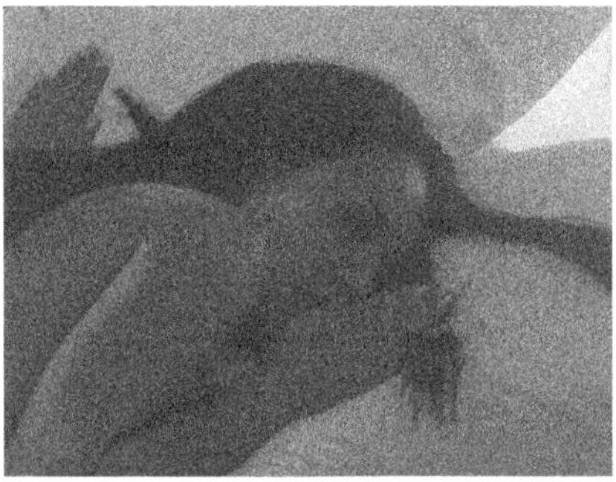

28.2

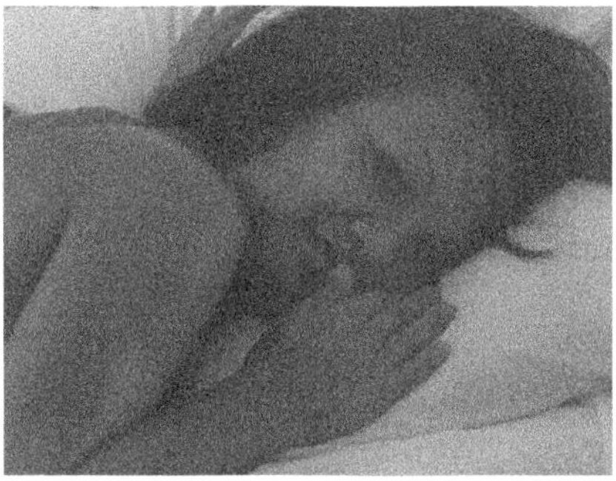

28.3

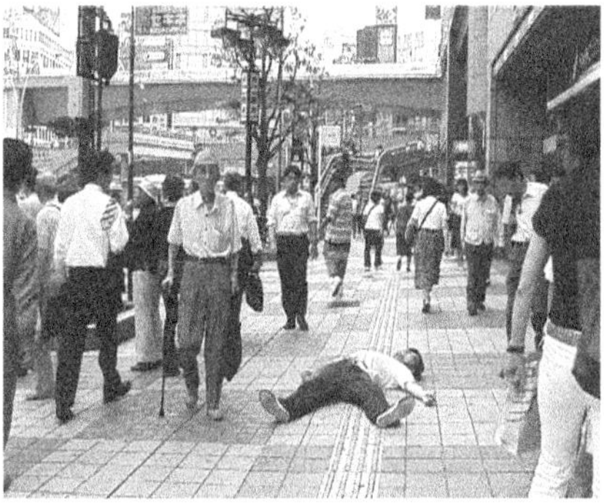

28.4

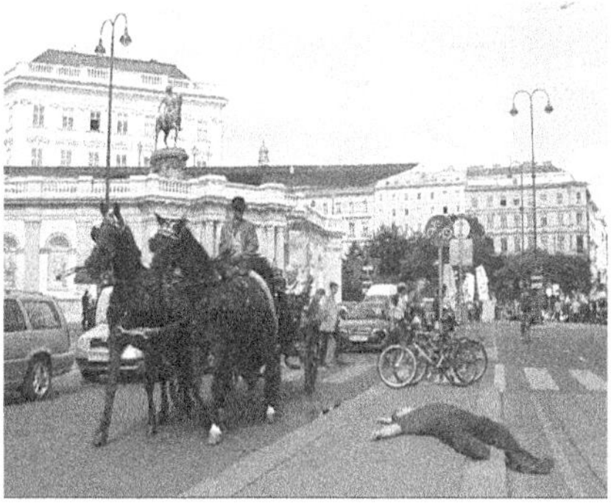

28.5

From her sickbed at home, Felicity Callard observes that 'what we perceive, and how we think, depends on where we are and how our body is positioned. [A] horizontal body ... is in a cognitively and affectively different place from that inhabited by vertical others' (2020: 728). In this volume, in relation to Angela Alves's performance and sound installation *REST* (2019), Alves, Monika Ankele and Céline Kaiser explore the sociocultural contexts and clinical histories of lying in bed, noting the 'radical readjustment of the whole body-mind system' provoked by horizontality. Tala Khanmalek and Heidi Andrea Restrepo Rhodes read the reclined subject as a 'symbol of queer, disabled failure, but one which intimately knows the fleshly secrets that abound in recumbent life' (2020: 49–51); for them, 'rest, like poetry, is not escape or luxury or relinquishing political life or accountability to the world' (52).

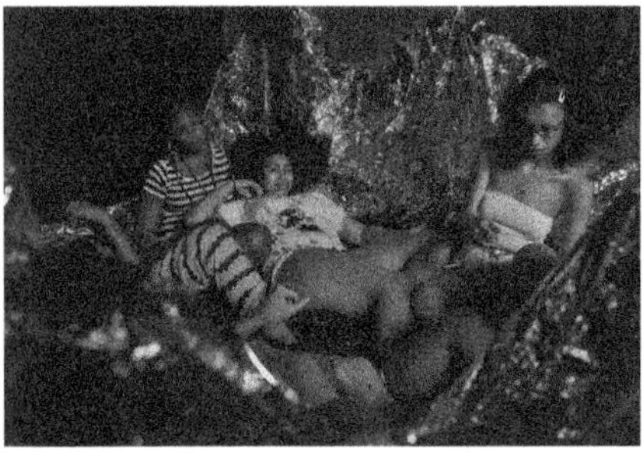

28.6

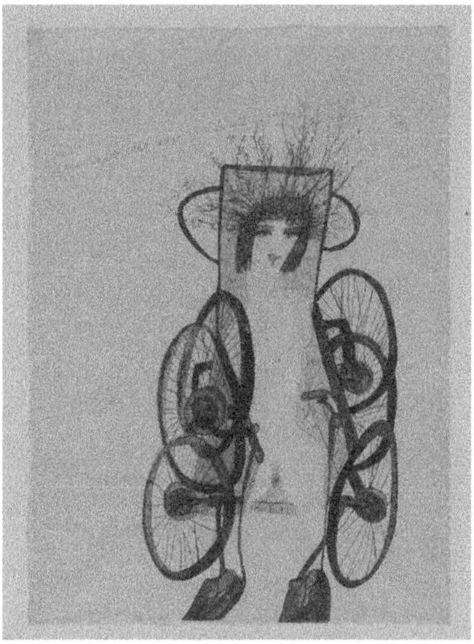

28.7

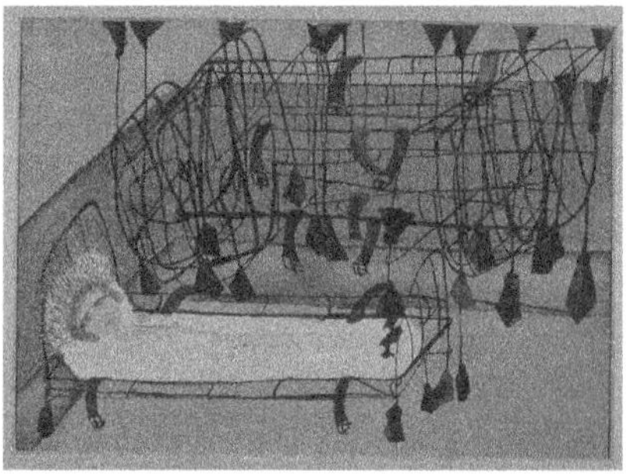

28.8

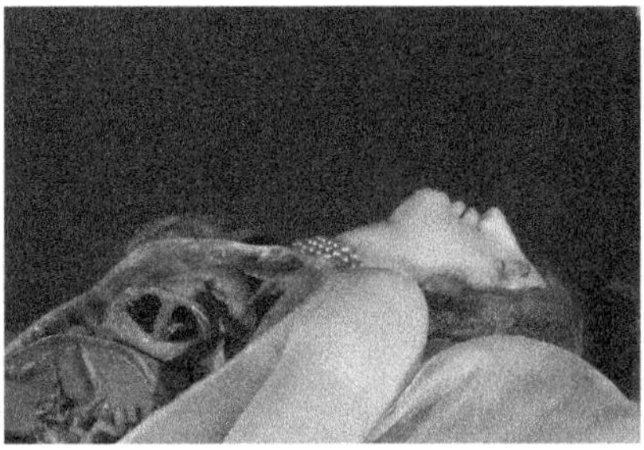

28.9

In addition to the affects and knowledges which horizontality produces in the reclining subject, what does their representation produce in their witnesses? What are the politics, ethics and affects of looking at prone bodies? How do horizontal bodies address and implicate the observer differently to upright figures? Carol Rama's *Appassionate* watercolours were a starting point for *Being Horizontal*. Her institutionalized and disabled subjects are 'sick women' as invoked by Johanna Hedva in their manifesto that politicizes the sick woman as a multigendered and intersectionally defined identity (2022). The *Appassionate* look back at us from wheelchairs and hospital beds, flicking their tongues; they have a penchant for red pumps. They are at once sick and desiring, defying the passivity and un-sexing associated with the institutionalized patient. By being with the images that make up my small archive of *Being Horizontal*, I realized that many of them challenge the correlating binaries of power/powerlessness and uprightness/horizontality.

In *Metre*, a poem I commissioned from Julie Morrissy for the exhibition *Being Horizontal* I curated at Project Arts Centre in Dublin in 2023, Morrissy considers recline in relation to friendship and trust:

we do not lie down with everyone   the
flatness requires an invitation   or
understanding   it is like touch   when we
peel off layers and collapse

(2023)

Looking at images of horizontal bodies, I recognize the intimacy Morrissy describes, or rather, the discomfort produced when there is no intimacy with the reclined other: when a person cannot be upright, or lies prone against their will, or is compelled by economic factors or lack of agency to assume this position for the visual consumption and pleasure of others.

When I curated *Being Horizontal* as an online event (in 2022) for the series that shaped this book, I invited the artist Harold Offeh to perform his work *Lounging* (2017–20) to a live audience on Zoom through his webcam. Imitating the Black singer Teddy Pendergrass' album cover portrait, Offeh struck a pose lying on his side with his head resting on his propped-up elbow. For three or four minutes, we watched Offeh breathe and blink his eyelids, looking back at us watching him strain to remain still in the supposedly leisurely pose. As part of the virtual audience, I found my feelings shift from curiosity to embarrassment, tenderness, and amusement. The intentional deployment of horizontality by Offeh offered an affective, political, and

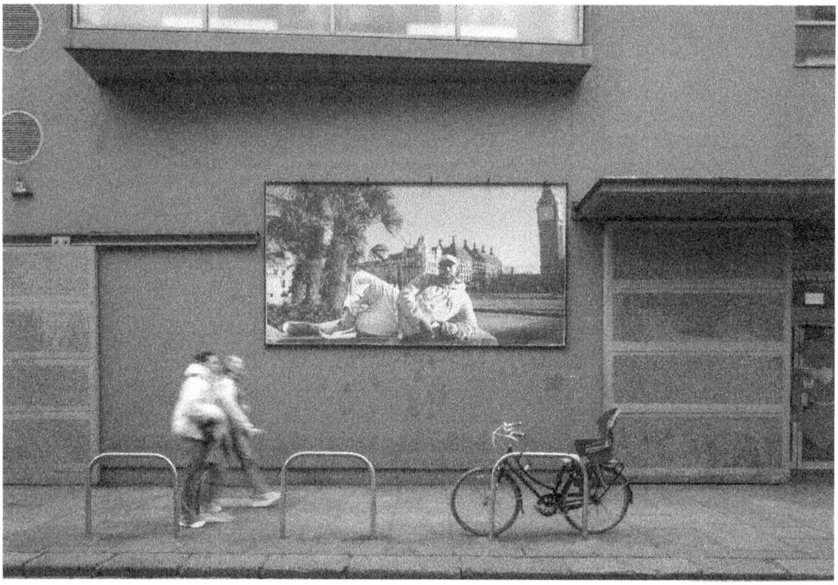

28.10

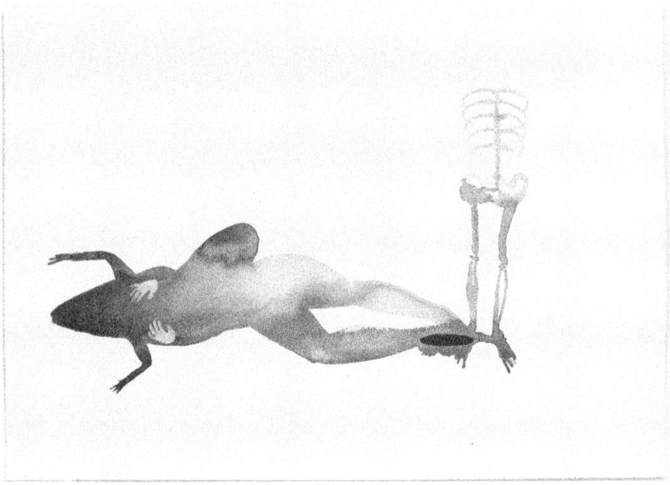

28.11

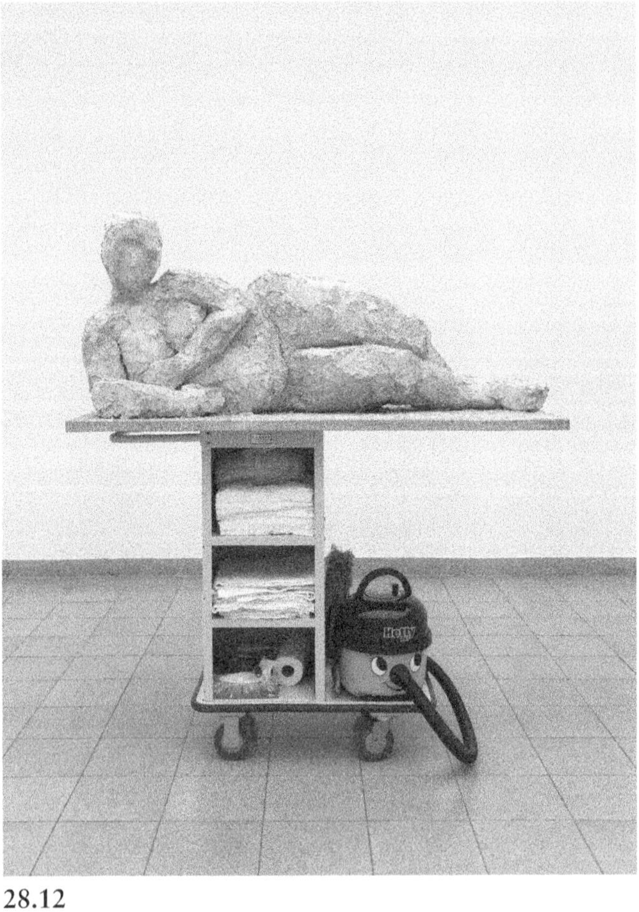

28.12

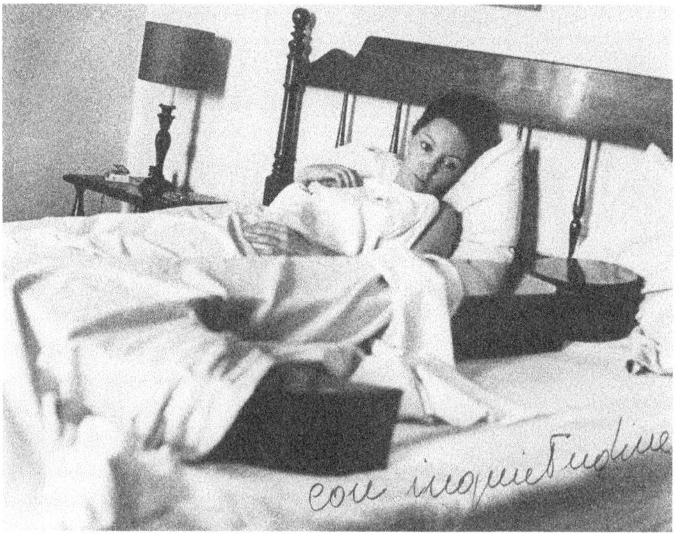

28.13

intellectual challenge to those watching, as it prompted us to reconsider its associations with a loss of agency or power.

Collapsing in public space together with others, and remaining communally prone on the ground, is a protest strategy. Collective horizontality has been employed to create attention and enact resistance: by ACT UP, against the indifference of politicians toward queer people infected with HIV; by cyclists protesting unacceptable death rates in dangerous city traffic; and by Extinction Rebellion activists staging funeral processions for destroyed species and ecosystems. The media images generated by these

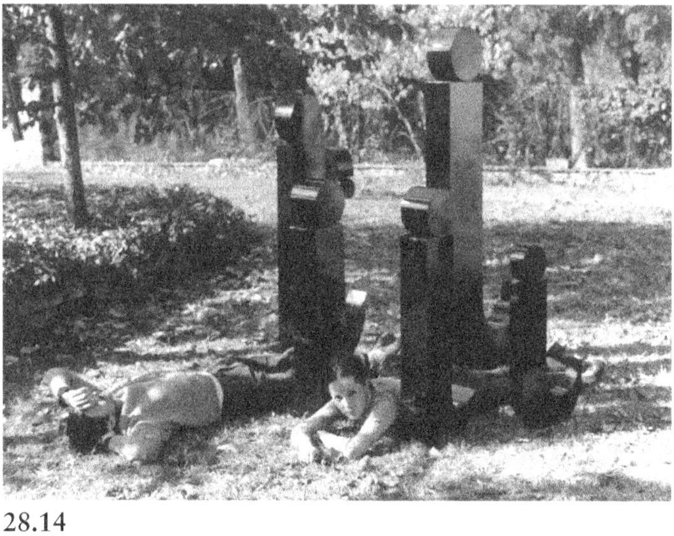

28.14

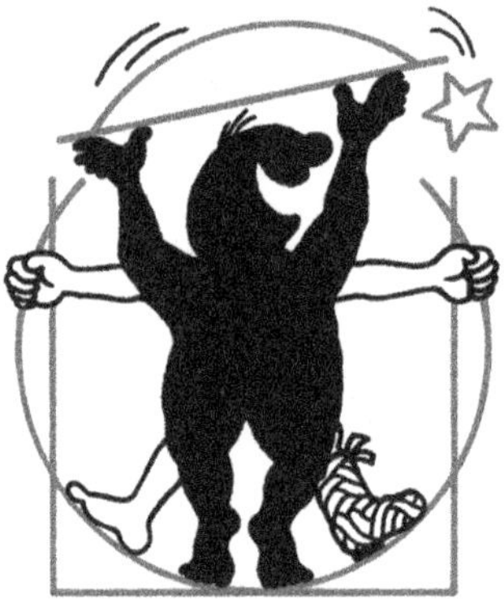

28.15

protests address us emotionally and appeal to our most basic responsibility to care for one another and our world (D'Souza 2024: 24, 48). We might begin to address this responsibility to mutual care by paying serious attention to the affects, knowledges and politics generated by horizontal bodies and their representations.

Note: I would like to thank the editors of this book; Sara Greavu from Project Arts Centre (Dublin); and Giulia Crispiani from NERO (Rome), for supporting and intellectually engaging with this ongoing project. My research was funded by a PhD studentship from the London Arts and Humanities Partnership.

Figures

28.1 Jade de Montserrat, *Lay in bed, prone and bound, with compassionate assistance, interdependence, agency,* 2021. Watercolour and ink on paper, 20 × 20 cm. Image courtesy of Manchester Art Gallery.

28.2 and 28.3 Nashashibi/Skaer, *Why Are You Angry?* (video still), 2017. Courtesy of the artists and Peter Freeman Gallery.

28.4 Kinkaleri, *WEST* (*Tokio*), 2007. Video still. Courtesy of the artists.

28.5 Kinkaleri, *WEST* (*Wien*), 2004. Video still. Courtesy of the artists.

28.6 *Polycrastination Station of Black Power Naps, the Black Bean Bed,* 2018, at Matadero Madrid. Courtesy of Navild Acosta and Dr. Shadow F. Sosa. Photograph by Bego Solis.

28.7 Carol Rama, *1930–1931 brevetto n. 7H1261R* (*Appassionata*), 1940. Acquerello, tempera e matita colorata su carta, 41.5 cm (h) × 30.5 cm (b). Inv. FD/210, Torino, GAM – Galleria Civica d'Arte Moderna e Contemporanea, Fondazione Guido ed Ettore De Formaris. Courtesy of the Fondazione Torino Musei. Photo: Studio Fotografico Gonella, 1986.

28.8 Carol Rama, *Appassionata*, 1940. Acquerello, tempera e matita colorata su carta, 23 cm (h) × 33 cm (b), inv. FD/211, Torino, GAM – Galleria Civica d'Arte Moderna e Contemporanea, Fondazione Guido ed Ettore De Formaris. Courtesy of the Fondazione Torino Musei. Photo: Studio Fotografico Gonella, 1986.

28.9 Clemente Susini, *Venerina or the Female Recumbent Body with Removable Anatomical Parts*. Courtesy of Alma Mater Studiorum, University of Bologna, Sistema Museale do Ateneo, Museo di Palazzo Poggi. Photo: Fulvio Simoni.

28.10 Harold Offeh, *Lounging (Westminster)*, 2023, billboard. Commissioned for the exhibition *Being Horizontal* curated by Nora Heidorn, February–March 2023. Courtesy of Project Arts Centre, Dublin. Photography by Ste Murray.

28.11 Caroline Boileau, *Double et doublée* de la série *Hors d'elle*, 2019. Watercolour on paper, 35.6 cm × 50.8 cm. Courtesy of the artist. Photo: Paul Litherland.

28.12 Nicole Wermers, *Reclining Female* #2, 2022. On display in Nicole Wermers, *Reclining Fanmail*, curated by Melanie Ohnemus, Kunsthaus Glarus, 2022. Photo: Gunnar Meier.

28.13 Ketty La Rocca, *Con inquietudine*, 1971, gelatin silver print and felt-tip pen, 12.5 cm × 17.8 cm. Courtesy Archivio Ketty La Rocca | Michelangelo Vasta.

28.14 Ketty La Rocca, *Performance with J (3)*, 1969–70, gelatin silver print, 13 cm × 18 cm. Courtesy Archivio Ketty La Rocca | Michelangelo Vasta.

28.15 Logo of the Gesundheitstag [Health Day], an annual political and activist gathering about the topic of (alternative) health in Germany in the 1980s, designed by Roland Matticzk/Sehstern.

References

Being Horizontal / Sínte (2023) *Project Arts Centre*. Available at: https://projectartscentre.ie/event/being-horizontal-sinte/ (accessed 24 April 2023).

Being Horizontal: Vulnerability, Interdependence and Resistance (February 2022) (2022) *Confabulations: Art Practice, Art History, Critical Medical Humanities*. Available at: https://confabulationsdotorg.wordpress.com/current-programme/being-horizontal-vulnerability-interdependence-and-resistance/ (accessed 27 April 2023).

Callard, F. (2020), 'Epidemic Time: Thinking from the Sickbed', *Bulletin of the History of Medicine*, 94 (4): 727–43.

Cavarero, A. (2016), *Inclinations: a critique of rectitude*, Stanford: Stanford University Press.

D'Souza, A. (2024), *Imperfect Solidarities*, Berlin: Floating Opera Press.

Hedva, J. (2022), 'Sick Woman Theory', *Tropical Cream*, 12 March, available at: https://topicalcream.org/features/sick-woman-theory/ (accessed 9 April 2024).

Heidorn, N. and G. Crispiani (2022), *Laying Horizontal*, *NERO Editions*, available at: https://www.neroeditions.com/laying-horizontal/ (accessed 6 October 2023).

Khanmalek, T. and H. A. R. Rhodes (2020), 'A Decolonial Feminist Epistemology of the Bed: A Compendium Incomplete of Sick and Disabled Queer Brown Femme Bodies of Knowledge', *Frontiers: A Journal of Women Studies*, 41 (1): 35–58.

Morrissy, J. (2023), *Metre* [Poem printed on paper strip, 100 × 3 cm].

CHAPTER TWENTY-NINE

Lifeblood – Edvard Munch: towards a curatorial medical humanities

Allison Morehead

The Norwegian artist Edvard Munch (1863–1944), author of *The Scream* (1893), aimed to create universally intelligible works on themes such as illness and death, sex and puberty, melancholy and despair. He approached these subjects within the specific context of modernity, including medical modernity, and often through the lived experiences, including medical experiences, of himself and his family and friends. As the son and brother of doctors, friend and favoured artist of numerous medical practitioners, Munch was deeply embedded in medical communities from an early age, frequently accompanying his father on house calls and on lengthy stays at military installations where the elder Munch worked. During his long career, medical professionals provided Munch with privileged access to medical institutions and treatment, and to the vulnerable people that he often depicted in his works.

The exhibition *Lifeblood – Edvard Munch*, at the Munch Museum in Oslo in 2025, transforms these observations into a curatorial project (see Morehead 2024). The title refers to the artist's claim that his art was one's 'lifeblood' as well as a 'healthy reaction' to illness, in and of themselves a form of life, healing and care. Just as importantly, the exhibition hypothesizes that Munch's proximity to biomedicine and his medical experiences afford his work a unique and at times critical view of the medicalization of modern life. The term *medicalization* is intended not as de facto critique but to describe how 'the practices of medicine have modified the very life form that is the contemporary human being' (Rose 2007: 700).

Take Munch's painting *On the Operating Table* (1902–3; Figure 29.1), which allegorizes a significant medical experience from 1902, when the artist had a bullet surgically removed from his hand. The operation took place at Rikshospitalet, Norway's state teaching hospital, hence the gallery of spectators observing the clinical scene. Although rooted in the artist's experience, the painting is filled with improbabilities, from the naked surgical subject to that body's indiscernible genitals; from the nearly faceless doctors and nurse to the similarly anonymized students watching the operation; from the donut of red paint at the level of the nurse's abdomen to the red paint that floats on the surface of the work in a suggestive uterine-like shape. These expressive liberties raise crucial and troubling questions about medical expertise, agency, the spectacularized and medicalized body, the complex nature of care, and the gendering and ungendering of medical practice and patienthood.

To support visitors in accessing historical medical contexts, the exhibition juxtaposes works such as *On the Operating Table* with carefully selected and arranged objects from the history of medicine, many owned by Munch or used in institutions he knew: an X-ray of the artist's hand, surgical tools,

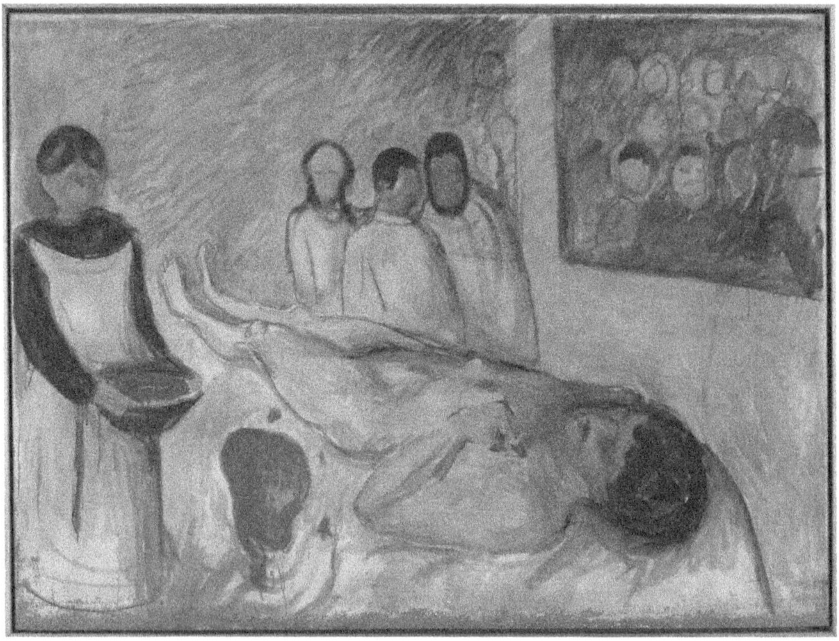

FIGURE 29.1 Edvard Munch, *On the Operating Table*, 1902–3. Oil on canvas, 109 cm × 149.5 cm. Munch Museum, Oslo. Photo © Munchmuseet / Juri Kobayashi.

a chloroform mask, and a uniform of the deaconess nurses who staffed Rikshospitalet. Assembled in the space of a public exhibition, these things – supported by text, seating, lighting, and audio – mediate each other, offering prompts and provocations for visitors to consider how modern surgery, facilitated by new diagnostic and imaging technologies, an anaesthesia and antisepsis, might have radically altered – and continue to affect – subjectivities and intersubjectivities. This curation draws inspiration from the 'thing methods' project at Norsk Teknisk Museum (Huseby and Treimo 2018).

Curators, conservators, and other staff members of museums take extraordinary and often controversial measures to care for, display, and mediate their collections. Curatorial work is fundamentally care-work; the words derive from the same Latin root. And it is care-work that must acknowledge the profound entanglements among visitors, things, and space, as well as a host of practical and ethical challenges related to vulnerable bodies and vulnerable things, including accessibility, security, and aesthetics. *Lifeblood* as an experiment in *curatorial medical humanities*, centring the complexities and possibilities of curatorial work as care-work, with entangled relationalities in mind among people, among things, among people and things. Like the critical medical humanities, it avoids assuming care as a fundamental good, but rather probes the curatorial, as a 'concrete work of maintenance, with ethical and affective implications' (Puig de la Bellacasa 2017: 5). It risks the fraught potentials of care-work to assemble things and people together in the hopes that some relationalities might be reconfigured and new ones might emerge.

References

Huseby, H. B. and H. Treimo, eds (2018), *Tingenes metode: Museene som tingsteder*, Oslo: Norsk Teknisk Museum.

Morehead, A. (2024), 'Edvard Munch and the Medicalization of Modern Life: Towards a Curatorial Medical Humanities', *Journal of Medical Humanities* (published 4 September 2024). https://link.springer.com/article/10.1007/s10912-024-09893-7

Puig de la Bellacasa, M. (2017), *Matters of care: Speculative ethics in more than human worlds*, Minneapolis: University of Minnesota Press.

Rose, N. (2007), 'Beyond Medicalisation', *The Lancet* 369: 700–702.

AFTERWORD

Tanya Sheehan

Productive tensions: I would use this phrase to describe the three days in June 2024, when many of the contributors to this book came together in conversation in London. A call to explore the intersections of visual art and the critical medical humanities had occasioned the convening of artists, curators, and academics. As a member of this last category, I had joined the workshop with the notion that the research presentations and intellectual exchanges might result in a manifesto of the kind recently generated by art historians Fiona Johnstone and Suzannah Biernoff (Johnstone 2018; Biernoff and Johnstone 2024). Instead, the gathering stimulated a diverse and complex collection of ideas which mapped the tensions between disciplines and interdisciplinarity, individuality and collaboration, historical and contemporary, making and analysis. Emerging from differences in perspectives and practices was a collective resistance to arriving at a 'magical endpoint' where conflicts would melt away to reveal a singular critical path forward. By the workshop's end, I knew that this book needed to preserve the tensions which surfaced *between* and *within* these worlds of 'art' and the 'critical medical humanities', while not losing sight of the shared matters of concern that bring them together.

Poring over the thousands of transcribed words derived from those conversations in London, I return again and again to the questions within that archive circling the subjects of human agency and experience, perhaps because they have motivated my own writings on the visual culture of medicine. *Who is allowed to speak? Who cares? Where does an experience begin and end? Who is a reliable witness?* and *Who owns images?* are all essentially political matters, insofar as they concern power structures that variously define, constrain, authorize and disallow. Related to this probing of boundaries is the workshop's interrogation of the value and constraints of disciplinary perspectives, like *What is history good for?*, *Who has given us the terms we identify ourselves by?*, and *How do we do otherwise?* Repeated among my notes is the particular phrase 'disciplined by disciplines', which points to the ways in which fields of knowledge operate as systems of rules that define how their members are supposed to think and act. According to the logic of those systems, to engage in scholarship otherwise constitutes field *breaking*, which can carry both negative and positive connotations; in academic circles, 'bad' scholarship is condemned, field-making rewarded.

That concerns with discipline(s) would surface in the production of this volume is no surprise, given that an experiment in interdisciplinarity sits at its core. The motivation for *Art and the Critical Medical Humanities*, after all, is not merely to collect together little histories of art as they relate to medicalized bodies, technologies, and cultures. That work has been done, by many scholars, for many decades. Rather, it is to ask with genuine curiosity: What happens when 'art', understood as the purview of both artistic practice and art history, interacts with the field of critical medical humanities, which itself has been forged through collaborative and interdisciplinary enquiry into human health and its contexts? In a single, ambitious gesture, the book engages long-standing debates about how the work of criticism and making, humanistic enquiry and medical discourse can be integrated, precisely to challenge entrenched notions of fixed or inflexible boundaries between fields and to insist instead on their entanglement.

Readers who approach this volume from a position outside the art world, such as that of healthcare or the medical humanities, may be surprised to learn of the tensions that often exist between the making and the analysis of art. *Art* – the thing to which the book's title connects the critical medical humanities – is hardly coherent or uncontested within contemporary practice, which sets up additional challenges and opportunities with respect to disciplinary interrelations. While approximately half of the volume's contributors identify as historians of art (including its three editors) and its primary mode of communication is academic prose, the project as a whole embraces creative ideation, intellectual playfulness, boundary pushing, iterating – in sum, artistic thinking.

That this volume seeks to explore possibilities, rather than definitively solve problems, is consistent with its embrace of artistic thinking. Consider its title: the conjunction 'and' leaves intentionally open the nature of the relationship between the entities it brings together. Artists and art historians might find it tempting to call for an arts-led or arts-centred critical medical humanities, but would that not effectively replace one hierarchy with another? To create space for shared sets of practices, questions, and provocations to emerge, and to hold them in relation without assigning priority or dominance: that is this book's critical challenge.

References

Biernoff, S. and F. Johnstone (2024), 'What Can Art History Offer Medical Humanities?', *Medical Humanities*, 50: 529–38.

Johnstone, F. (2018), 'A Manifesto for a Visual Medical Humanities', *BMJ Medical Humanities* (blog). https://blogs.bmj.com/medical-humanities/2018/07/31/manifesto-for-a-visual-medical-humanities

INDEX